Encyclopedia of Electromyography: Principles, Methods and Techniques

Volume I

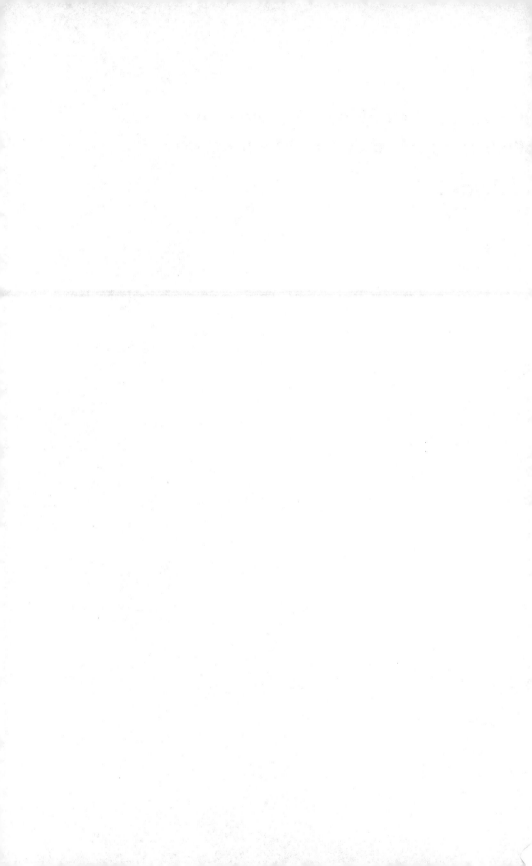

Encyclopedia of Electromyography: Principles, Methods and Techniques

Volume I

Edited by **Michael Backman**

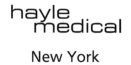

hayle medical

New York

Published by Hayle Medical,
30 West, 37th Street, Suite 612,
New York, NY 10018, USA
www.haylemedical.com

**Encyclopedia of Electromyography: Principles,
Methods and Techniques
Volume I**
Edited by Michael Backman

International Standard Book Number: 978-1-63241-159-4 (Hardback)

Contents

Preface

This book on Electromyography focuses on key principles of using and examining EMG and encompasses a broad range of subjects including Principles and Methods, Signal Processing, and Diagnostics. The authors have varied in their approach to their subjects, from reviews on different aspects of the field to experimental studies with exciting new findings. The experts have analyzed literature related to applied surface electromyography parameters for evaluating muscle function and fatigue to the constraints of different analysis and processing techniques. It also describes emerging applications where electromyography is employed as a means to regulate electromechanical systems, water surface electromyography, scanning electromyography, EMG measures in orthodontic appliances and in ophthalmological field. These original approaches to the usage of EMG measurement will be of great interest to readers.

The researches compiled throughout the book are authentic and of high quality, combining several disciplines and from very diverse regions from around the world. Drawing on the contributions of many researchers from diverse countries, the book's objective is to provide the readers with the latest achievements in the area of research. This book will surely be a source of knowledge to all interested and researching the field.

In the end, I would like to express my deep sense of gratitude to all the authors for meeting the set deadlines in completing and submitting their research chapters. I would also like to thank the publisher for the support offered to us throughout the course of the book. Finally, I extend my sincere thanks to my family for being a constant source of inspiration and encouragement.

Editor

Part 1

Principles & Methods

A Critical Review and Proposed Improvement in the Assessment of Muscle Interactions Using Surface EMG

James W. Fee, Jr. and Freeman Miller
Alfred I. DuPont Hospital for Children
USA

1. Introduction

The purpose of this chapter is to propose a mathematical relationship between EMG excitation recorded from muscles in opposition to, or in coordination with each other. The concept of correlating co-activation between muscles with EMG parameters is not new. Cowan et al. (1998) investigated the use of the Pearson Product-Moment correlation coefficient to quantify muscle co-activation using electromyography. They concluded that this method shows promise for describing side differences in diplegics and for assessing the effects of physical therapy and other interventions. Careful reading of this work shows that only "select" intervals of the EMG data were compared. These intervals were selected on the basis of "burst activity" of one muscle. This selection is done by hand and for large quantities of data, typical of a gait laboratory, would be labor intensive. In our laboratory the authors have found the Pearson Product-Moment unable to distinguish between two noisy signals from inactive muscles and two that are fully active. Using insights from the literature review, presented below, this chapter will propose an alternative, continuous function for describing muscle interaction over any and all portions of a gait cycle.

2. Background

The history of the development of EMG's as an assessment tool follows closely the development of mathematics over the last century and a half. In an extensive review, Reaz et al.(2006) traces this history from Francesco Redi's documentation of electrical activity in a muscle in 1666, to its present use as a controlling mechanism for modern human computer interaction. Most of the mathematical analysis applied to EMG signals concerns itself with the relationship between various parameters of the signal and the forces generated in the muscle.

In its simplest form, an isometric contraction results in electrical activity in the muscle. De Luca (1997) states that while a simple equation describing this relationship would be extremely useful, such a simple relationship does not exist. In spite of this, numerous researchers have applied a countless variety of methods to the extraction of force from EMG signals.

Christensen et. al. (1986) compared the number of zero crossings with force production and found a linear relationship up to 50% of a maximum voluntary contraction. At low levels of maximum contraction the number of spikes was found to increase with increasing force

(Haas, 1926). At higher force levels, the mean rectified value of the signal was found to exhibit linearity with force (Fuglsang-Frederiksen, 1981). Other investigators turned to the frequency domain and demonstrated an inverse relationship between force and frequency (Ronager et al, 1989). At the same time it has been shown that mean power frequency increases with increasing force (Li & Sakamoto, 1996). A study in 1999 showed that the median frequency increases with force up to a point equal to 50% of the maximum contraction (Bernardi M, et al. 1999). In a review article on surface EMG and muscle force, Disselhorst-Klug, et al. (2009) conclude that muscle force can be estimated from EMG signals in geometrically well-defined situations during isometric contractions.

When limb motion and coordination are involved the relationship between (dynamic) EMG and force takes on greater dimensions of complexity. There are three basic types of data utilization involved in the study of dynamic EMG. Most common is the interest in the presence or absence of the particular muscle's activity during a portion of some movement, for example a gait cycle. A second interest is in the envelope shape of the EMG waveform over an entire movement. Lastly, there is the interest in relating the force generated by a muscle to itself (at some other part of the movement) or to some other muscle (Rechtien, et al. 1999). In order for the EMG representation of forces to be related to one another, each must be normalized to some standard value.

Burden (2002) gives an extensive review of research, performed over the last two and a half decades, on normalization methods. The author identifies eight methods of normalization. Of these eight, two are of the most interest: first, a method whereby an EMG signal is divided by the maximum of itself (Peak Task, PT), and a second (Mean Task, MT) whereby an EMG signal is divided by the mean of itself. The author reports that, with respect to other more complex methods, both the PT and the MT methods reduced inter-individual variability, and improves the sensitivity of surface electromyography as a diagnostic gait analysis tool. The use of these methods also increases the effect size and hence the power of statistical comparisons between groups in relation to the output from other methods. The drawbacks of these methods are, first in the case of PT, the selected maxima could easily be an artifact in the recording of the signal. In the second method, normalizing to the mean of the signal could easily result in the existence of normalized EMG points in excess of 100%. If these points are attenuated to 1.00 as is often the case, the normalized task EMGs may not reveal the proportion of an individual's muscle activation capacity required to perform a specific task.

To compare EMG patterns between muscles groups, it is necessary to use a time-normalization technique so that a point-by-point comparison of EMG activity is possible. Carollo JJ & Matthews (2002) suggest that this can be done by breaking the EMG pattern up into individual stride cycles, which are considered the period between successive heel-strikes in the same leg. The individual EMG stride patterns are then time normalized, expressed as a percentage of total cycle. In a review paper on muscle coordination, (Hug, 2011) finds fault with this method because of the variability of the point of toe-off (between 58 and 63% of the gait cycle). To correct this, Sadeghi et al. (2000) and Decker et al. (2007) use "curve registration" or "Procrustes analysis" methods, respectively. Curve registration relies on finding the peak points in the joint power curves and aligning gait cycles accordingly. The Procrustes method describes curve shape and shape change in a mathematical and statistical framework, independent of time and size factors. Thus the method normalizes both time and stride magnitude at the same time.

Hodges & Bui (1996) state that, in order to allow comparisons between muscles, experimental conditions and subjects or subject groups, accuracy of onset determination is crucial. Onset is most often recognized as the point where the EMG values cross and remain above a pre-chosen threshold value. The choice of this threshold value varies among researchers. Some place it at two standard deviations above the noise level (Micera et al. 1998). Lidierth (1986) added to this method by specifying that the threshold value be exceeded, and remain so, for a specific time constant. Others use a percentage of the peak EMG, and report that this percentage varies from 15 to 25% of the maximum signal (Staude, 2001). More sophisticated methods evaluate statistical properties of the measured EMG signal before and after a possible change in excitation level (Staude & Wolf, 1999).

De Luca (1997) suggests that, at least in the case of the threshold method, off time be found as the opposite of on time, that is when the amplitude falls below the same percentage of maximal contraction. He further suggests that when comparing on and off times of two muscles, that a 10ms window of error is the best that can be expected.

Having extracted a measure of force from the EMG signal by whatever means, and knowing when a muscle is active or inactive, attention turns toward the comparison of activity in two or more groups of muscles. The most elementary technique for the examination of two coordinating muscles groups is the visual inspection of the raw EMG signal together with appropriate graphics of the joint angles. Conclusions drawn from such observations are subjective at best, thus a more quantitative method is needed (Kleissen et al. 1998).

De Luca (1997) defines two parameters that are commonly used to represent the EMG signal: the average rectified value and the root mean square value:

$$RMS = 1 / n \sum x^2 (i)$$

Here x is a sample point with the sum taken over sample size n.

For comparison purposes Fukuda et al.(2010) state that the RMS value is prefered because it is a parameter that better reflects the levels of muscle activity at rest and during contraction, and for this reason, it is one of the most widely used in scientific studies. A slightly more complex method of analysis was reviewed by Fuglsang-Frederiksen (2000). When comparing the activation of different muscles, he found that the turns/amplitude analysis method was more useful than other methods. Turns analysis consists of counting the number of positive and negative potential changes exceeding 100ʋv ("turns") and their amplitudes. The turns ratio is computed by dividing the mean amplitude (of the turns) by the number of turns. The method was used by Garcia et al.(1980) as a quantitative assessment of the degree of involvement of antagonist muscles.

In a variation on the turns counting method, Jeleń & Sławińska (1996) compared the activation of two muscles using a spike counting method. This method counts the number of times the EMG signal crosses a "noise level" threshold. These authors showed that this count is in good agreement with muscle activity.

Area under the EMG curve has been used successfully to compare co-contraction. In a unique normalization scheme, reported by Poon & Hui-Chan (2009), EMG co-contraction ratios were calculated as ratios of the antagonist EMG area to the total agonist-plus-antagonist EMG areas. The authors claim this technique allowed the comparison of data obtained on different days for within- or between-subjects.

Work presented in the next section will demonstrate that the method to be outlined in this chapter is quite similar to Poon's (Poon & Hui-Chan, 2009). However a simple mathematical construct reveals that the author's ratio is not unique:

$$A / (A + a) = B / (B + b)$$

Let: $B = 2 * A$ and $b = 2 * a$

If "A" in the above equation is antagonist EMG area and "a" is agonist area, it is possible to conceive of another muscle group such that antagonist area "B" is twice that of "A" and agonist muscle "b" is twice the area of "a". The calculation for both muscles groups will produce the same co-contraction ratio, however a clinician, observing the muscle group's behavior, would find the two levels of co-contraction to be quite different. The authors of this chapter will assert that it is not possible to represent the co-activation of two muscles by a single parameter. One must consider the activation of both relative to the normalized value and the ratio of each to the other.

The next level of sophistication in the analysis of EMG data is the examination of the frequency content of the signal. Several parameters are obtained from the power spectrum (the Fourier transformation of the EMG signal). The mean frequency is defined as the mathematical mean of the spectrum curve, the total power is the integral under the spectrum curve, and the median frequency is defined as the parameter that divides the total power area into two equal parts. Finally the peak power is the maximum value of the total power spectrum curve.

The most commonly used parameter in the frequency domain is the median frequency. Hermens et al.(1992) report that this parameter deviates from its normal value in a number of neuromuscular disorders, therefore the parameter is often used in clinical settings. In a comparative study this parameter, like the turns ratio and the spike count, would be calculated for each muscle group and then compared using a statistic such as the ANOVA or a paired t-test (Lam, 2005). A slight variation on this is the mean power frequency which is found by dividing the summed product of the frequency and power by the summed power. Feltham et al. (2010) used this parameter to demonstrate differences in co-contraction levels between the right and left sides in children with spastic hemiparetic cerebral palsy and both arms of typically developing children. In the case of the other two variables peak power has been shown to be related to muscle fiber conduction velocity and total power to muscle force (Li & Sakamoto, 1996; Farina et al. 2004).

Among the newest methods of EMG analysis are those involving wavelet analysis, which examines both the frequency and time domain combined. A wavelet transform is a Fourier transform performed on a particular section of an EMG signal. Further, the time width (or window) of the "section" can be dependent on the frequency content of that section. That is, the window is narrowed for high frequencies and widened for low frequencies. Karlsson et al.(2009) define this as a mathematical microscope in which different parts of the signal can be observed by adjusting the focus. When testing children with cerebral palsy, Prosser et al.(2010) point out that wavelet analysis eliminates the need for amplitude normalizations. This is beneficial because many of these subjects cannot make a maximal contraction.

In a paper presented at the IEEE conference on Engineering in Medicine and Biology Dantas, et al.(2010) compared Fourier analysis with wavelet transform analysis. They point out that Fourier analysis assumes signal stationarity, which is unlikely during dynamic contractions. Wavelet based methods of signal analysis do not assume stationarity and may be more appropriate for joint time-frequency domain analysis.

The nature of the Fourier analysis is that it transforms the signal into a series of sine-cosine functions and is therefore especially well adapted for analyzing periodic signals. Herein lies its major drawback, EMG signals are not only non-stationary, but non-periodic, "fractal" and seemingly chaotic. Borg (2000) points out, that instead of decomposing and reconstructing a signal in terms of the sines and cosines functions, wavelet analysis allows the use of an array of waveforms such as: saw tooth functions, rectangle waves (Walsh functions), or finite time pulses. In a paper published last year, Bentelas (2010) demonstrated how the Continuous Wavelet Transform (CWT) is mathematically similar to surface EMG signals with noise and is therefore the favorite candidate for analyzing these signals.

The wavelet transform method has been applied with increasing success. In a paper on the ergonomics of driving, Moshou et al. (2000) clearly demonstrate the ability to remove noise from the EMG signal. As a result, small coordinated muscle activity of the shoulder can be observed, that would otherwise have been hidden in the noise. The use of this method to investigate dynamic muscle dysfunction in children with cerebral palsy has lead to clear distinctions between this population and the normally developing group (Wakeling et al. 2007). Lauer et al. (2007) expanded on this and were able to show differences in levels of co-contraction between the less and more involved side.

3. Methodology

With the above review in mind, the authors propose a method of comparing two EMG signals. While most of the illustrations presented will be of raw or stylized raw EMG data, the method will be demonstrated to work equally as well on filtered, enveloped data. The method begins with a full wave rectification of surface EMGs recorded as gait data. The gait data presented here will be from multiple walks; each walk will have been cut into cycles beginning and ending either at toe-off or heel-strike and then pieced together end to end (i.e. toe-off to toe-off or heel-strike to heel-strike). For simplified illustrative purposes only one cycle will be presented, however all mean values will have been calculated over the entire ensemble.

The method of normalization is a combination of both the "Peak Task" and "Mean Task" methods of (Burden, 2002). Figure 1, below, is an illustration of the method. For illustrative purposes a stylized EMG signal is presented. The signal consists of two sine waves, of different

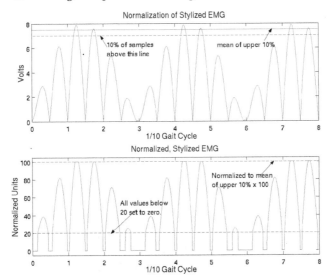

Fig. 1. Normalization method stylized EMG data constructed from several sin waves is used to demonstrate a method of normalization.

amplitude and frequency summed together. The timing of half a "wave" will be considered one tenth of a gait cycle. For the normalization process, a set of points are found such that they are the upper 1/10 of all samples in the particular gait cycles of interest. The mean of these samples (in the illustrative case 80 points are found to have a mean of 7.8 volts) is taken as the normalizing value. All points in the ensemble are then divided by this mean. The result of this division will be a signal with several points that have a value higher than unity. These will be considered artifacts and set to the value one. The signal is then multiplied by 100. After this multiplication, all values below 20 are considered to be noise and are set to zero.

The comparison of two muscle excitations requires the defining of two parameters. The first of these parameters will be called the "Excitation Index". If it can be imagined for a moment that, for a tenth of a gait cycle, the EMG were at maximum potential, the signal over that time period would be a full ten volts. The normalized value would be 100 over the entire time period (tp). The integration of this full excitation would equal the area of a rectangle (100 x tp). When two signals are involved, both maximally on for the same time period (tp), the total possible area under both signals is (200 x tp). This will be considered the "standard" Excitation. The excitation index will be defined as the sum of the integration of the two EMG signals over a tenth of a gait cycle divided by that tenth's "standard". It should be noted here, that tp is not a constant and is likely to vary over each gait cycle, as a result a "Standard Excitation" must be calculated for each tenth cycle.

The second parameter to be defined will be called the co-activation ratio. This ratio will be defined simply as the smaller of the two integrated EMG signals divided by the larger. The result will always be a number between zero and one. An illustration of the calculation of the two parameters is presented in figure 2. In this case the second EMG signal is

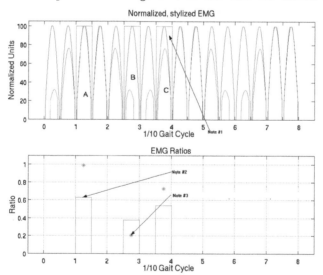

Note:
#1 Area under the rectangle equals the total area of a 1/10 gait cycle. Twice this area is the maximum integral of the combined EMG signals (The Standard Excitation (SE)).
#2 Bar Height = The ratio of the sum of the integral of both EMG signals / SE.
#3 Point Value = Ratio of the two "stylized" EMG signals in "B" above.

Fig. 2. Stylized assessment method

represented as a full wave rectified sine wave whose frequency was set to the combined frequency of the first. In the case of the A'th tenth cycle both EMG signals are almost the same, however the area of a sin wave is not equal to a square wave. The height of the bars of the graph in the lower half of the figure represents this difference in area. In the case of "A" the area under the two stylized EMG signals is 0.6 of 60% of the "Standard Excitation". The red dot represents the ratio of the two signals, slightly less than one because the two areas are almost equal. The B'th and C'th tenths can be similarly interpreted. The assessment system can be applied to the co-activation of two antagonistic muscles (better known as co-contraction) as shown in figure 3. This figure delineates the differences between co-contraction in a normally developing limb and one with hemiplegia. Clearly, in this gait cycle, there is almost no co-contraction evidenced in the normally developing subject. This is not the case in the subject with hemiplegia. A quick review of the profiles reveals that, while the highest co-contraction occurs in the eight tenth of the gait cycle, the total excitation of both muscles is less than 10% of maximum. From the mean values it can be seen that, while the excitation index is just below 9%, the co-activation ratio is just below 17% (the rounded off value). With these values presented, it is left to the clinician to decide if this co-activation is significant.

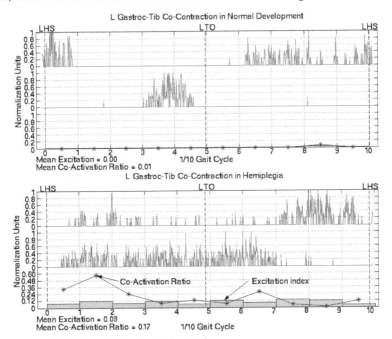

Note: Means are calculated over 14 cycles (140 points).

Fig. 3. Assessment of a Co-Contracting Muscle- This figure illustrates a clear difference between hemiplegia and normally developing gait cycles on a 1/10 cycle by cycle basis.

Turning to the original motivation for this work, Figure 4 demonstrates the use of the assessment method to explore excitation in contralateral muscles. Our hypothesis states that if "mirrored excitation" exists, it is most likely to be seen at mid-stance/mid-swing, where the muscles of the "swinging" limb should be inactive and the supporting limb's muscles should be most active. While it is not the intent of this chapter to prove or disprove our working hypothesis, some results will be presented in order to demonstrate the efficacy and efficiency of the method of assessment outlined and advocated.

With regard to mirrored excitation, it is expected, that the excited muscle will be mirrored onto the inactive muscle. In the example below, for the normally developing subject, it can be seen that the co-activation ratio for this gait cycle is highest at mid-stance of both limbs. This is actually an atypical gait cycle, chosen so the numbers would be large enough to be seen on the graph. The mean values were in fact 0.07 on the left and 0.04 on the right. An examination of the means of these values over the 10 cycles, in the subject with hemiplegia, reveals a mean excitation index on the left of 0.14 (slightly higher than the value of the complete gait cycle) and a mean ratio of 0.44 (almost twice the value for the complete cycle). While the values at mid-stance on the right are 0.08 and 0.62 respectively. From this, one would conclude that there is an influence at left mid-stance, but without the greater excitation index at right mid-stance, information from other muscles would be needed to draw any conclusions.

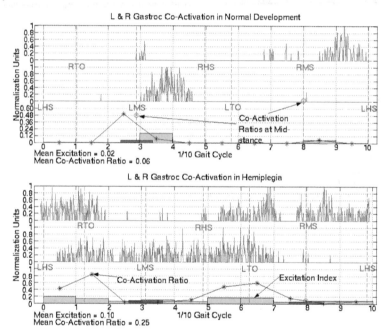

Note: Mid-stance (L & R MS) values are calculated from data taken between 1/20th cycle on either side of the mid-stance point.

Fig. 4. Left and right side co-activation.

The previous two graphics presented EMG data in raw, rectified, normalized form, with the assessment analysis being performed on this raw data. This is simply the authors' preference and should not be interpreted as the only way the analysis can be done. The next graphic, Figure 5, presents a comparison of the analysis performed on both raw and filtered data. To be noted here is the fact that both profiles, that of the excitation index and the co-activation ratio appear very much alike. The mean excitation index is slightly less (0.06 vs. 0.10) while the mean co-activation ratio is slightly greater (0.37 vs. 0.25). Each of these differences makes sense when considering what filtering does. By lowering the peak values of the EMG data, the excitation index has a smaller numerator and thus a smaller value for each 1/10 cycle. At the same time that peaks are made lower the data is spread over a larger region of time, this causes the regions with the higher peaks to take up greater area. Since the co-activation ratio is calculated by dividing the smaller number by the larger, an increase in the smaller number (in this case) is reflected by a larger ratio.

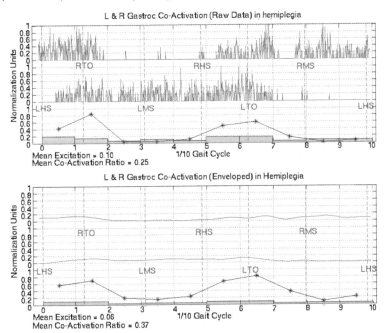

Fig. 5. Raw and filtered EMG and their resulting parameters.

The presentation of this data in a meaningful way so that different muscle groups among different subjects can be compared, is not a trivial matter. A method for plotting twenty points per muscle per gait cycle for several muscles of interest must not overwhelm the reader with data while at the same time allow a readily recognizable comparison of pertinent information. In the case of the authors, the interest is in comparing contralateral co-activation with co-contraction in both limbs. At the least this involves three muscle groups, adding to this is the desire to compare these muscle groups at particular points in each gait cycle (mid-stance) thus adding an additional two comparison groups to the representation task.

The method to be suggested here will utilize two distinct graphing methods; in the first, line graphs will present the excitation index and co-activation ratios in their pure calculated form. In the second, bar charts will compare normalized values of the excitation indices. It is felt that both are of value and both have a valid place. The bar charts provide an immediate means of comparing muscle groups within the same subject. Line graphs provide a means of comparing data across subject.

To construct the graphs, the authors calculate a mean value of each parameter over the ensemble of gait cycles recorded for each subject. From each ensemble of muscle groups to be compared, the maximum muscle excitation index is chosen and all other excitation indices are normalized on this value. Each normalized value now represents the comparative excitation of each muscle group. Since the co-activation ratio represents the comparison of activation between the two muscles of a given group, multiplying the normalized excitation index by this ratio, preserves its comparative property between the groups. The process lends itself well to a graphical representation by means of a stacked column graph. Figure 6 presents a comparison of Gastrocnemius-Anterior Tibialis interaction in seven subjects with hemiplegic cerebral palsy. The data presented represent a number of interesting interactions between the groups. In the third, fourth and sixth subject, co-contraction is the dominant muscle activity. In the other 4, the dominant activity is the co-activation between the right and left sides. In two of the subjects (#1 and #7) this dominance is seen across the entire gait cycle, in the remaining two the dominance occurs only at the points of mid-stance. While the method of presenting the normalization of means clearly has its value in the intragroup comparison for a single subject, it can give misleading results when comparisons are made across subjects. To address the issue, data is presented as it was before normalization. These two added sets of data insures that a very strong excitation, when normalized to unity, is not seen as comparable to a weak excitation that might happen to the maximum value for another subject.

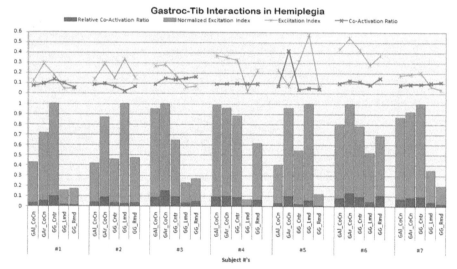

Legend: GAl = Gastroc-Tib left, GAr = Gastroc-Tib right, CoCn = Co-contraction,
Cntr = contralateral co-activation (measured over the complete cycle), GG = Gastroc-Gastroc, Rmd = Right Mid-Stance, Lmd = Left Mid-Stance
Bar charts are normalized data, line graphs are actual values.

Fig. 6. Excitation indices and co-activation ratios for seven subjects

In the example presented in Figure 6, maximum excitation is almost the same for subjects 1, 2, 3, 4, and 7. Comparison of these subjects would be fairly reasonable. Comparison of these with subjects 5 and 6 becomes more problematic because their maximum excitations are clearly more intense.

As a final step Figure 7, below, provides a comparison to data from three normally developing subjects for the same muscle groups. This graph demonstrates the value of both

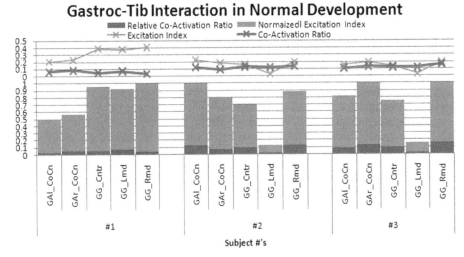

Legend: GAl = Gastroc-Tib left, GAr = Gastroc-Tib right, CoCn = Co-contraction,
Cntr = contralateral co-activation (measured over the complete cycle), GG = Gastroc-Gastroc,
Rmd = Right Mid-Stance, Lmd = Left Mid-Stance
Bar charts are normalized data, line graphs are actual values.

Fig. 7. Normalized mean excitation indices for three normally developing subjects

the bar and line graphics. While the bar graphs suggest that it may not be unusual for co-activation across the body to exist at mid-stance, the line graphs make it clear that it is not a dominant form of excitation. The most obvious difference between the normally developing subjects and those with hemiplegia are the obviously consistent indices and ratios seen in the normal developing subjects. All interaction in this data seem to be at about the same level. The slight elevation in excitation index of contralateral muscle groups of subject #1 may not be indicative of all normal subjects, a larger subject population would be necessary to identify true trends in normal developing subjects.

While the normalization method presented above may provide a good tool for visualization, the set of values calculated from tenths of a gait cycle should easily form the basis of a statistical analysis using a paired t-test or a two-way ANOVA.

4. Conclusion

It has been the purpose of this chapter to present a method whereby the co-activation of two muscles can be compared and presented to the clinician in a meaningful way. It has been shown, with the use of both stylized EMG data, and real data from ongoing experimentation, that the method presented provides two unique numbers which completely define the state of excitation of a muscle group. It has been demonstrated further that this method overcomes the pitfalls of previous attempts. Among its attributes are the method's ability to deal with both active and inactive muscle activity and to easily fit into many standard gait analysis reports.

The method begins with a normalization that combines two previously described methods. This combination of normalization on peak values and mean values of the data set itself eliminates drawbacks of both methods. Additionally it eliminates the need for a maximal contraction which many of those in the cerebral palsy population cannot perform.

The assessment method provides two numbers, the first, the Excitation Index, measures the activation of both muscles of interest in combination. The second number, the Co-activation Ratio, provides a measure of each muscle's excitation relative to the other. In combination, the two measures completely define the comparative excitation of any two muscles of interest.

The chapter presents several graphical methods of presenting the assessment method so that it can be used to compare a single set of muscles in a gait analysis, or to compare multiple groups of muscles across a sample population.

Although the data analyzed have largely been raw, unfiltered EMG data, the method can be applied equally as well to filtered "enveloped" data. In the case of one such analysis presented, while the mean values were somewhat different for filtered data, the overall profiles of both the excitation indices and the co-activation ratios remain consistent over the gait cycle presented.

Finally the chapter has demonstrated that the method can be applied to ongoing research in the author's laboratory. The authors believe that this demonstrates the value of the method in a real application.

5. References

Bentales Y (2010) An Algorithm of Wavelets for the Pretreatment of EMG Biomedical Signals. Contemporary Engineering Sciences, Vol. 3, No. 6, (2010) pp. 285 - 294, ISSN 1313-6569.

Bernardi M, Felici F, Marchetti M, Montellanico F, Piacentini MF, & Solomonow M. (1999) Force generation performance and motor unit recruitment strategy in muscles of contralateral limbs. *J Electromyogr Kinesiol* Vol. 9, (1999) pp. 121–30, ISSN: 1050-6411.

Borg F. (2000) EMG and Wavelet Analysis – Part I. Technical Report HUR – FB 07/16/00. 1. HUR Ltd.

Burden A. (2002) How should we normalize electromyograms obtained from healthy participants? What we have learned from over 25 years of research. *Journal of Electromyogr Kinesiol.* Vol. 20, (2010) pp. 1023–1035, ISSN: 1050-6411.

Carollo JJ & Matthews D. (2002) Strategies for clinical motion analysis based on functional decomposition of the gait cycle, *Phys. Med. Rehabil. Clin. N. Am.*, Vol. 13 (2002) pp. 949–977, ISSN:1047-9651.

Christensen H & Fuglsang-Frederiksen A. (1986) Power spectrum and turns analysis of EMG at different voluntary efforts in normal subjects. *Electroencephalogr Clin Neurophysiol* Vol. 64, No. 8, (Aug., 1986), pp. 528–35, ISSN: 0018-9294.

Cowan MM, Stilling DS, Naumann S & Colborne GR. (1998) Quantification of antagonist muscle coactivation in children with spastic diplegia. *Clin. Anat.* Vol. 11 No. 5. (May, 1998), pp. 314-9, ISSN: 0897-3806.

Dantas JL, Camata TV, Brunetto MA, Moraes AC, AbrÃ£o T, & Altimari LR. (2010) Fourier and wavelet spectral analysis of EMG signals in isometric and dynamic maximal effort exercise. Proceedings of the IEEE Eng Med Biol Soc. 2010:5979-82, (2010), ISBN: 978-1-4244-4123-5

Decker L, Berge C, Renous S, & Penin X. (2007) An alternative approach to normalization and evaluation for gait patterns: Procrustes analysis applied to the cyclograms of sprinters and middle-distance runners. *J Biomech*, Vol. 40, No. 9 (Sept., 2007) pp. 2078-87, ISSN: 0021-9290.

De Luca CJ. (1997) The use of surface electromyography in biomechanics. *Journal of Applied Biomechanics*, Vol. 13, No. 2, (May, 2006), pp. 135-163, ISSN: 1065-8483.

Disselhorst-Klug C, Schmitz-Rode T, & Rau G. (2009) Surface electromyography and muscle force: limits in sEMG-force relationship and new approaches for applications. *Clin Biomech (Bristol, Avon)*, Vol. 24, No. 3 (Mar., 2009) pp. 225-35, ISSN: 0268-0033.

Farina D, Merletti R, & Enoka RM (2004) The extraction of neural strategies from the surface EMG. J Appl Physiol Vol. 96 (2004) pp. 1486-1495, ISSN: 8750-7587

Feltham MG, Ledebt A, Deconinck FJ, & Savelsbergh GJ (2010) Assessment of neuromuscular activation of the upper limbs in children with spastic hemiparetic cerebral palsy during a dynamical task. *J Electromyogr Kinesiol.* 2010 Jun; Vol. 20, No. 3 (Jun, 2010) pp. 448-56, ISSN: 1050-6411.

Fuglsang-Frederiksen A (2000) The utility of interference pattern analysis. *Muscle Nerve*, Vol. 23, No. 1 (Jan, 2000) pp. 18-36, ISSN: 0148-639X.

Fuglsang-Frederiksen A. (1981) Electrical activity and force during voluntary contraction of normal and diseased muscle. *Acta Neurol Scand,* Vol. 63(Suppl. 83), (1981) pp. 1–60, ISSN: 0065-1427.

Fukuda TY, Echeimberg JO, Pompeu JE, Lucareli PRG, Garbelotti S, Gimenes RO, & Apolinário A (2010) Root Mean Square Value of the Electromyographic Signal in the Isometric Torque of the Quadriceps, Hamstrings and Brachial Biceps Muscles in Female Subjects, *J. Applied Research*, Vol. 10, No. 1 (2010) pp. 32-39, ISSN: 1537-064X.

Garcia HA, Milner-Brown HS, & Fisher MA (1980) "Turns" analysis in the physiological evaluation of neuromuscular disorders. *J Neurol Neurosurg Psychiatry* Vol. 43 (1980) pp. 1091-1097, ISSN: 0022-3050.

Haas E. (1926) Uber die Art der Tatigkeit unserer Muskeln beim Haltenverschieden schwerer Gewichte. Pflugers Archiv fur die gesamte, *Physiologie*, Vol. 212, (1926) pp. 651–6, ISSN as 0031-6768

Hermens HJ, Bruggena TAM, Batena CTM, Rutten WLC & Boom HBK (1992) The median frequency of the surface EMG power spectrum in relation to motor unit firing and action potential properties, *Electromyogr Kinesiol.* Vol. 2, No. 1, (1992) pp 15-25, ISSN: 1050-6411.

Hodges PW & Bui BH (1996) A comparison of computer-based methods for determination of onset of muscle contraction using electromyography. *Electroenceph. Clin. Neurophysiol.* Vol. 101 (1996) pp. 511–519, ISSN: 1388-2457.

Hug F (2011) Can muscle coordination be precisely studied by surface electromyography? J *Electromyogr Kinesiol.* Vol. 21, No. 1 (Feb, 2011) pp. 1-12, ISSN: 1050-6411.

Jeleń P & Sławińska U (1996) Estimation of the distribution of the EMG signal amplitude, *Acta Neurobiol Exp* (Wars). Vol. 56, No. 1 (1996) pp. 189-96, *ISSN*: 0065-1400.

Karlsson JS, Roeleveld K, Granlund C, Holtermann A & Ostlund N (2009) Signal processing of the surface electromyogram to gain insight into neuromuscular physiology. *Philos Transact A Math Phys Eng Sci.* Vol. 28, No. 367 (Jan, 2009) pp. 337-56, ISSN = 1364-503X.

Kleissen RF, Buurke JH, Harlaar J & Zilvold G (1998) Electromyography in the biomechanical analysis of human movement and its clinical application, *J. Gait Posture*, Vol. 1, No. 8(2) (Oct., 1998) pp. 143-158, ISSN: 0966-6362.

Lam WK, Leong JC, Li YH, Hu Y, & Lu WW (2005) Biomechanical and electromyographic evaluation of ankle foot orthosis and dynamic ankle foot orthosis in spastic cerebral palsy. *Gait Posture.* 2005 Nov; Vol. 22, No. 3 (Mar, 2005) pp. 189-97, ISSN: 0966-6362.

Lauer RT, Stackhouse CA, Shewokis PA, Smith BT, Tucker CA, & McCarthy J (2007) A time-frequency based electromyographic analysis technique for use in cerebral palsy. Gait Posture, Vol. 26, No. 3 (Sep, 2007) pp. 420-7, ISSN: 0966-6362.

Li W & Sakamoto K (1996) The influence of location of electrode on muscle fiber conduction velocity and EMG power spectrum during voluntary isometric contraction measured with surface array electrodes. Appl Human Sci. Vol. 15, No. 1 (Jan, 1996) pp. 25-32, ISSN: 1341-3473.

Lidierth M (1986) A computer based method for automated measurement of the periods of muscular activity from an EMG and its application to locomotor EMGs, *Electroenceph. Clin. Neurophysiol.,* vol. 64, (1986) pp. 378–380, ISSN: 0018-9294.

Micera S, Sabatini AM, & Dario P (1998) An algorithm for detecting the onset of muscle contraction by EMG signal processing, *Med. Eng. Phys.* Vol. 20 (1998) pp. 211–215, ISSN: 1350-4533.

Moshou, D, Hostens I, Papaioannou G, & Ramon H (2000) Wavelets and self-organising maps in electromyogram (EMG) analysis, in *Proceedings of the European Symposium on Intelligent Techniques (ESIT),* ISBN 3-89653-797-0, Aachen, Germany, 14-15 September 2000

Poon DM & Hui-Chan CW (2009) Hyperactive stretch reflexes, co-contraction, and muscle weakness in children with cerebral palsy. *Dev Med Child Neurol.* Vol. 51, No. 2 (Feb, 2009) pp. 128-35, ISSN: 0012-1622.

Prosser LA, Lee SC, Barbe MF, VanSant AF & Lauer RT (2010) Trunk and hip muscle activity in early walkers with and without cerebral palsy--a frequency analysis. *J Electromyogr Kinesiol.* Vol. 20 No. 5 (Oct, 2010) pp. 851-9, ISSN: 1050-6411.

Raez MBI, Hussain MS, & Mohd-Yasin F. (2006) Techniques of EMG signal analysis: detection, processing, classification and applications. *Biol Proced Online.* (Aug 2006) ISSN: 1480-9222.

Rechtien JJ, Gelblum JB, Haig AJ, & Gitter AJ. (1999) Guidelines in electrodiagnostic medicine. Technology review: dynamic electromyography in gait and motion analysis. *American Association of Electrodiagnostic Medicine, Muscle Nerve Suppl.* Vol. 8 (1999) pp. S233-8, ISSN: 0148-639X.

Ronager J, Christensen H, & Fuglsang-Frederiksen A. (1989) Power spectrum analysis of the EMG pattern in normal and diseased muscles. *J Neurol Sci,* Vol. 94, (1989) pp. 283–94, ISSN: 0022-510X.

Sadeghi H, Allard P, Shafie K, Mathieu PA, Sadeghi S, Prince F, et al. (2000) Reduction of gait data variability using curve registration, *J. Gait Posture,* 2000 Dec; Vol. 12 No. 3 (Dec, 2000) pp. 257-64, ISSN: 0966-6362.

Staude GH (2001) Precise onset detection of human motor responses using a whitening filter and the log-likelihood-ratio test. *IEEE Trans Biomed Eng,* Vol. 48 (2001) pp. 1292–305, ISSN: 0018-9294

Staude GH & Wolf W (1999) Objective motor response onset detection in surface myoelectric signals, *Med. Eng. Phys.,* v Vol. 21 (1999) pp. 449–467, ISSN: 1350-4533.

Wakeling J, Delaney R, & Dudkiewicz I (2007) A method for quantifying dynamic muscle dysfunction in children and young adults with cerebral palsy. *Gait Posture* 2007; Vol. 25, No. 4 (Apr, 2007) pp. 580–9, ISSN: 0966-6362.

2

Electromyography in Myofascial Syndrome

Juhani Partanen
University Hospital of Helsinki
Department of Clinical Neurophysiology
Finland

1. Introduction

Myofascial syndrome is a muscular pain syndrome with regional symptoms, often in limb girdle or neck and back area. It is common and causes much disability and inability to work. Myofascial pain may be activated by precision work, repetitive strain or recent injury. Typical findings in symptomatic muscles are taut bands and painful trigger points (TrPs), where pressure elicites a typical spreading of pain (Cummings & Baldry, 2007). Microdialysis of TrPs has detected local elevation of contraction, and inflammatory and pain metabolites (Shah et al., 2008). Reduced high-energy phosphate levels but no signs of myositis have observed in painful muscles in histological studies (Bengtsson et al., 1986).

2. Electromyography of trigger points

There are several studies of EMG in TrPs. There is no sustained spontaneous activation of motor unit potentials (MUPs) (spasticity) or any signs of denervation i.e. fibrillation potentials or motor unit potential alterations typical for nerve sprouting (Couppé et al., 2001).

2.1 Spontaneous electrical activity at the endplate

When EMG in TrPs is compared to EMG in painless points of the same or other muscle, there are some differences. TrPs show more numerous local findings of spontaneous electrical activity (SEA) than control points (Couppé et al., 2001). SEA may consist of endplate activity which is reflected in two forms, often activated together: endplate noise (EPN) (miniature end plate potentials MEPPs) and end plate spikes (EPS). In EPN there are either small, discrete high-frequency depolarizations rarely exceeding 100 μV (MEPPs) or just "sea shell" noise, depending on the orientation and localization of the needle electrode with respect to the source (Wiederholt, 1970). It was also claimed that EPN is more prevalent in TrPs within the end plate zone and more prevalent in active than latent TrPs (Simons et al., 2002). End plate spikes are larger in amplitude than MEPPs, exceeding even several hundred microvolts. EPSs are usually observed together with EPN (Fig. 1).

EPSs have a characteristic irregular firing pattern with numerous short intervals less than 30 ms. Thus it is easy to distinguish EPSs from other spontaneous EMG patterns or MUPs. In addition, EPSs have a characteristic wave form with initial negativity or with a short (less than 0,3 ms) initial positivity. Rarely, EPSs with a typical firing pattern but a large polyphasic waveform may be observed (Partanen, 1999).

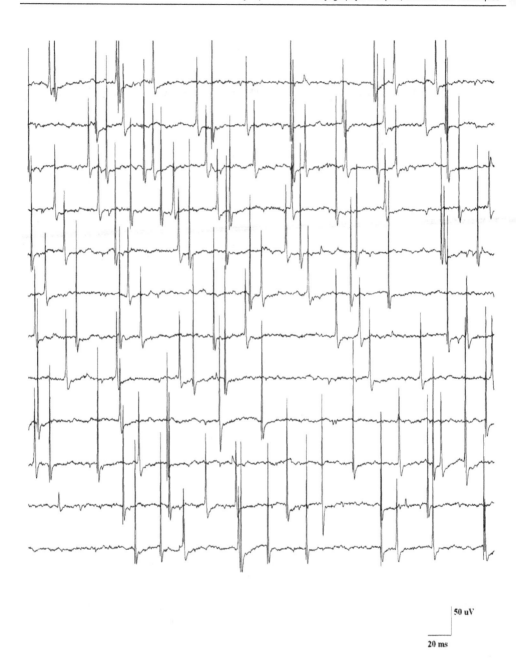

50 uV

20 ms

Fig. 1. Several sequences of end plate spikes in an active spot of a normal relaxed muscle. Most of them have a negative onset but some have a short initial positive component. Observe also the end plate noise in the background. From Pathophysiology, with permission.

2.2 Complex repetitive discharge

Another spontaneous waveform, which is repeatedly found in taut bands is complex repetivite discharge (CRD) (Fig. 2). It was originally described by Janet Travell in TrPs

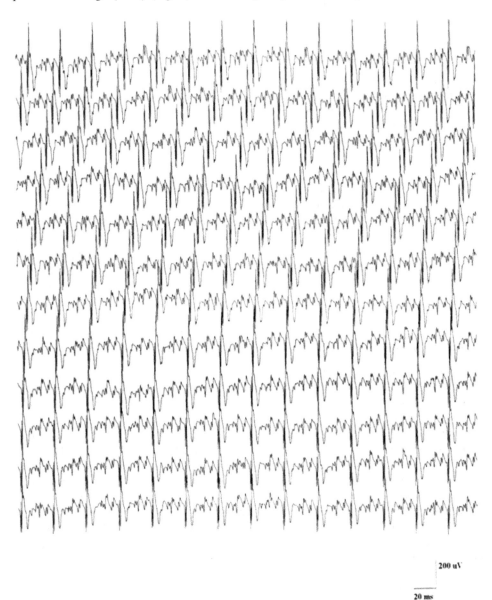

200 uV

20 ms

Fig. 2. Complex repetitive discharge (33 Hz) in a taut band of the levator scapulae muscle of a patient suffering from myofascial syndrome. Otherwise the needle EMG was normal. From Pathophysiology, with permission

(Travell, 1957) but later on it was depicted in about 15% of patients suffering from myofascial syndrome (Ojala et al., 2006). CRD has been observed in several types of chronic neuropathy or myopathy (Emeryk et al., 1974a), but in these cases CRD is accompanied by other pathological alterations in EMG. In myofascial syndrome CRD is observed in muscles with otherwise normal EMG (Ojala et al., 2006).

3. Prevailing hypotheses of the origin of EPN, EPS and CRD

EPN and MEPPs are observed to originate from the postsynaptic surface of the neuromuscular junction. MEPPs are activated by spontaneous leakage of small amounts of acetycholine (exocytosis) from the nerve terminal. MEPPs are local, non-propagated discrete depolarizations of muscle membrane. MEPPs should be found mainly at the end plate zone of the muscle, where neuromuscular junctions are localized. EPSs are supposed to be elicited by summation of a number of MEPPs, if the sum potential exceeds the critical level to fire an action potential (Buchthal & Rosenfalck, 1966). Another explanation is a nerve potential activated by the irritation caused by the EMG needle electrode. The nerve potential then travels to the nerve terminal and activates a postsynaptic action potential which is recorded with the same EMG needle as an EPS (Dumitru, 1995). CRD is supposed to arise when an action potential is circulating in muscle fibres, leaping from one fibre to another with ephaptic conduction, forming eventually a vicious cycle with sustained circulation of action potentials (Trontelj & Stålberg, 1983). The participation of motor neurone and even "spindelisation" of extrafusal muscle fibres due to changed innervation was also discussed (Emeryk et al., 1974b).

4. Discussion of the discrepancies of prevailing hypotheses for EPS and CRD and suggestions for new explanations

Even if mechanical irritation of nerve terminal may cause marked increase of the frequency of MEPPs, there are no data demonstrating that this may cause activation of postsynaptic action potentials of the muscle fibre, recorded as EPSs. The mechanical irritation of the terminal motor nerve branch by the needle electrode may cause injury potential and rarely rhythmic spontaneous activity but sustained irregular firing has not been described in experimental studies (Wall et al., 1974). Thus the firing pattern of EPSs clearly differs from the known patterns of injury potentials (Macefield, 1998). CRDs are not found in totally denervated muscles (personal observation). Thus, evidently CRD needs the presence of intramuscular motor axons. In fact, CRD in myofascial syndrome may represent activation of a spinal reflex arch, instead of an ephaptic circuit of muscle fibres (see Heading 7).
The third explanation for EPSs is that they are action potentials of intrafusal muscle fibres. There are several points which suggest this possibility, for example activation of EPSs by passive stretching of the muscle (Partanen, 1999; Partanen & Nousiainen, 1983).

5. Multi-channel recordings of EPSs

Different patterns of propagation of EPSs may be observed with multi-channel recording of EPSs in relaxed human muscles, using 3-5 EMG needles in parallel with the muscle fibres (Fig 3).

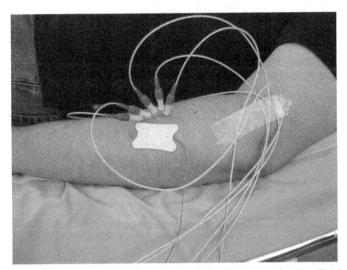

Fig. 3. A five-channel recording of the extensor carpi radialis muscle. The EMG needles are lying in parallel with the muscle fibres and the interelectrode distance is 3 mm.

The first type of EPSs does not propagate at all: there are local large potentials (Fig. 4). The second type of EPSs propagates for a short distance (a few mm) (Fig. 5) and third type propagates like a motor unit potential (Fig. 6-7). The first type may reflect activity of intrafusal nuclear bag fibres, which show this non-propagating junctional potential pattern in experimental recordings (Barker et al., 1978). The second type of EPS with a short propagation

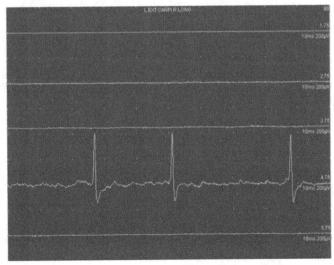

Fig. 4. An end plate spike sequence in channel 4. It does not propagate at all. It was not possible to find synchronous potentials in any of the other channels. End plate spikes may represent activation of a nuclear bag muscle fibre. Calibration 10 ms, 200 µV.

distance is in concert with the activity of nuclear chain fibres (Barker et al., 1978) and the third type corresponds to the activity of beta motor units (Partanen, 1999; Partanen & Palmu, 2009).

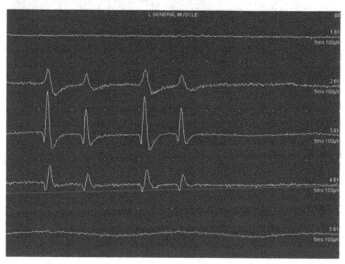

Fig. 5. Sequence of end plate spikes propagating from channel 2 to channel 4 (note the development of positive onset). This sequence may represent activation of nuclear chain muscle fibres. Calibration 5 ms, 100 μV.

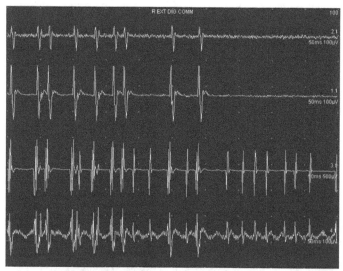

Fig. 6. Two sequences of end plate spikes. One is propagating to all channels and may represent beta motor unit potentials. The other propagates only from channel three to channel four and may represent activation of nuclear chain fibres. Calibration 50 ms, 100 μV, except Ch 3, 500 μV.

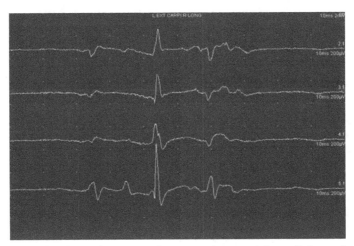

Fig. 7. Propagation of voluntarily activated motor unit potentials to all channels. Because of the slow firing of motor unit potentials compared to end plate spikes, they do not recur in this time window. Calibration 10 ms, 200 μV.

6. The "integrated hypothesis" for myofascial syndrome

The "integrated hypothesis" for myofascial syndrome comprises a local energy crisis of muscle tissue caused by strain. This leads to accumulation of irritative metabolites and thus activation of local nerve terminals with sustained contraction of postsynaptic muscle fibre. This is followed by rigor and a contraction knot, and development of a taut band, as well as activation of pain and sympathetic nerve fibres (Simons et al., 1999; Cummings & Baldry, 2007).

7. Discussion of the discrepancies of "integrated hypothesis" and suggestion of a new explanation for myofascial syndrome

The capillaries of extrafusal muscle tissue offer an effective perfusion, which is able to transport all irritative metabolites out of the muscle tissue. Thus the local inflammation of muscle without any signs of myositis seems improbable. On the other hand the capillaries of muscle spindles are different. There is a blood/spindle barrier and a non-permeable capsule around the spindle (Banks & Barker, 2004). Thus metabolites released into the capsular periaxial space of muscle spindle are readily concentrated. Sustained fusimotor activation of muscle spindle caused by for example precision work may achieve increased release of contraction metabolites intrafusally. This may activate release of inflammatory metabolites and finally pain metabolites. Only Ia-afferents of the muscle spindle activate alpha motor neurons (myotatic reflex). II- III- and IV-afferents activate intrafusal muscle fibres via gamma- and beta efferent pathways. III- and IV-afferents have been observed inside the muscle spindle (Paintal, 1960, Stacey, 1969). If inflammatory and pain metabolites are concentrated intrafusally, III- and IV-afferents, which comprise also chemical and pain receptors, may activate gamma- and beta-efferent activity via spinal reflex pathway. Beta efferent activation may be seen as CRD in EMG of taut bands for a limited time. Thus taut bands may be formed by extrafusal muscle fibres of beta motor units in metabolic exhaustion and rigor. Myotatic reflex (twitch) is present in taut bands (Shah et al., 2008) and this reflex is evidently activated by intact Ia afferent- alpha efferent reflex arch (Partanen et al., 2010).

8. Final comments

Needle EMG in myofascial syndrome is usually normal. In 15 % of patients CRD may be observed in some of the trigger points in taut bands (Ojala et al., 2006). This finding seems to be specific for myofascial syndrome, if there are no other EMG alterations. It remains to be seen if a thorough study of as many trigger points as possible increases the possibility to find CRD in a greater percentage of patients. The search may be justified because dry needling is also one of the treatments of myofascial syndrome (Cummings & Baldry, 2007). Incidence of end plate activity is increased in trigger points but this fact is not useful for diagnostics, because end plate activity is often observed in painless points as well. MEPPs with EPSs may represent intrafusal activity. In neuromuscular junctions of alpha motor units only MEPPs but not EPSs may be seen (Partanen et al., 2010). The different hypotheses discussed here can be tested and they help to comprehend the context "myofascial syndrome", which is not accepted by all physicians. At present the diagnosis of myofascial syndrome is clinical: there are no specific laboratory or imaging studies or other means to confirm the diagnosis (Dommerholt & Huijbregts, 2011).

9. References

Banks, R. W., & Barker, D. (2004). The muscle spindle, In: *Myology* (3rd edition), Engel, A., & Franzini-Armstrong , C., pp. 489-509, McGraw-Hill, Medical Publishing Division, New York

Barker, D., Bessou P., Jankowska, E., Pagès, B., Stacey, M.J. (1978). Identification of intrafusal muscle fibres activated by single fusimotor axons and injected with fluorescent dye in cat tenuissimus spindles. *J. Physiol*, Vol 275, pp. 149-165

Bengtsson, A., Henriksson, K. G., & Larsson, J. (1986). Reduced high-energy phosphate levels in the painful muscles of patients with primary fibromyalgia. *Arthritis & Rheumatism*, Vol.29, No.7, (July 1986), pp. 817-821

Buchthal, F., & Rosenfalck, P. (1966). Spontaneous electrical activity of human muscle. *Electroencephalography and Clinical Neurophysiology*, Vol.20, No.4, (April 1966), pp. 321-336

Couppé, C., Midttun, A., Hilden, J., Jørgensen, U., Oxholm, P., & Fuglsang-Frederiksen, A. (2001). Spontaneous needle electromyographic activity in myofascial trigger points in the infraspinatus muscle: a blinded assessment. *Journal of Musculoskeletal Pain*, Vol.9, No.3, pp. 7-17

Cummings, M., & Baldry, P. (2007). Regional myofascial pain: diagnosis and management. *Best Pract Res Clin Rheumatol.*, Vol.21, No.2, (April 2007), pp. 367-387

Dommerholt, J., & Huijbregts, P. (2011). *Myofascial trigger points: pathophysiology and evidenceinformed diagnosis and management*, Jones and Bartlett Publishers, Sudbury, Mass.

Dumitru, D. (1995). *Electrodiagnostic Medicine*, pp. 29-64, 218-221, Hanley & Belfus, Philadelphia

Emeryk, B., Hausmanowa-Petrusewicz, I., & Nowak, T. (1974a). Spontaneous volleys of bizarre high-frequency potentials (b.h.f.p.) in neuro-muscular diseases. Part 1. Occurrence of spontaneous volleys of b.h.f.p. in neuro-muscular diseases. *Electromyogr Clin Neurophysiol*, Vol.14, No.3, (June-July 1974), pp. 303-312

Emeryk, B., Hausmanowa-Petrusewicz, I., & Nowak T. (1974b). Spontaneous volleys of bizarre high-frequency potentials (b.h.f.p.) in neuro-muscular diseases. Part II. An analysis of the morphology of spontaneous volleys of bizarre high-frequency potentials in neuro-muscular diseases. *Electromyogr Clin Neurophysiol*, Vol.14, No.4, (August-September 1974), pp. 339-354

Macefield, V. G. (1998). Spontaneous and evoked ectopic discharges recorded from single human axons. *Muscle & Nerve*, Vol.21, No.4, (April 1998), pp. 461-468

Ojala, T. A., Arokoski, J. P. A., & Partanen, J. V. (2006). Needle-electromyography findings of trigger points in neck-shoulder area before and after injection treatment. *J. Muskuloskel. Pain*, Vol.14, pp. 5-14

Paintal, A. S. (1960). Functional analysis of group III afferent fibres of mammalian muscles. *J Physiol* Vol.152, pp. 250-270

Partanen, J. (1999). End plate spikes in the human electromyogram. Revision of the fusimotor theory. *J Physiol*, Paris, Vol.93, No.1-2, (January-April 1999), pp. 155-166

Partanen, J. V., & Nousiainen, U. (1983). End-plate spikes in electromyography are fusimotor unit potentials. *Neurology*, Vol.33, No.8, (August 1983), pp. 1039-1043, Cleveland

Partanen, J. V., Ojala, T. A., & Arokoski, J. P. A. (2010). Myofascial syndrome and pain: A neurophysiological approach. *Pathophysiology*, Vol.17, (February 2010), pp. 19-28

Partanen, J. V., & Palmu, K. (2009). Different ways of propagation of human end plate spikes in electromyography. *Muscle Nerve*, Vol.40, (2009), pp. 720-721

Shah, J. P., Danoff, J. V., Desai, M. J., Parikh, S., Nakamura, L. Y., Phillips, T. M., & Gerber, L. H. (2008). Biochemicals associated with pain and inflammation are elevated in sites near to and remote from active myofascial trigger points. *Arch Phys Med Rehabil*, Vol.89, No.1, (January 2008), pp. 16-23

Simons, D. G., Hong, C. Z., & Simons, L. S. (2002). Endplate potentials are common to midfiber myofascial trigger points. *Am J Phys Med Rehabil*, Vol.81, No.3, (March 2002), pp. 212-222

Simons, D. G., Travell, J. G., & Simons, L. S. (1999) *Myofascial Pain and Dysfunction: The Trigger Point Manual*, Vol.1, *Upper Half of Body*, (2nd edition), Williams & Wilkins, Baltimore

Stacey, M. J. (1969). Free nerve endings in skeletal muscle of the cat. *J Anat*; Vol.105, pp. 231-254.

Travell, J. (1957). Symposium of the mechanisms and management of pain syndromes. *Proc Rudolf Virchow Med Soc*, Vol.16, pp. 128-136

Trontelj, J., & Stålberg, E. V. (1983). Bizarre repetitive discharges recorded with single fibre EMG. *J Neurol Neurosurg Psychiatry*, Vol.46, No.4, (April 1983), pp. 310-316

Wall, P. D., Waxman, S., & Basbaum, A. I. (1974). Ongoing activity in peripheral nerve: injury discharge. *Exp Neurol*, Vol. 45, pp. 576-589

Wiederholt, W. C. (1970). End-plate noise in electromyography. *Neurology*, Vol.20, No.3, (March 1970), pp. 214-224, Minneapolis

3

Location of Electrodes in Surface EMG

Ken Nishihara[1] and Takuya Isho[2]
[1]Department of Physical Therapy, School of Health and Social Services
Saitama Prefectural University
[2]Department of Rehabilitation
National Hospital Organization Takasaki General Medical Center
Japan

1. Introduction

Motor unit action potentials (MUAPs) from motoneurons are transmitted to muscles through end-plates and then propagated to the tendons. These bioelectrical signals are detected via electromyography (EMG), which is performed using electrodes.

The electrodes used in EMG are primarily surface electrodes and inserted (wire or needle) electrodes, of which surface and wire electrodes are mainly used for kinesiological studies. Surface electrodes are widely used because of noninvasive attachment, painless usage, suitability for detecting muscle activation by generation of EMG signals and simplicity, although detection is usually limited in surface muscles. Surface EMG is a practical and noninvasive procedure that has potential usage in sports and rehabilitation medicine.

The signal amplitude of surface EMG is analyzed to estimate the level of muscle contraction, while the frequency component is used to estimate performance of muscle activation. For example, a change in EMG signal amplitude is regarded as a change in the strength of muscle activation, and a shift of the surface EMG signal towards a lower mean frequency is correlated with decreasing muscle fiber conduction velocity due to muscle fatigue. However, the detected EMG signal amplitude and mean frequency are influenced by the location of surface electrodes, although the action potentials in a muscle are generated at the same time. For these reasons, the location of surface electrodes is very important for accurate evaluation of muscle activation.

In this chapter, the propagation or conduction of action potentials is illustrated to understand the EMG signal recorded by surface electrodes. Proper electrode locations are suggested with theoretical and practical methods.

2. Surface EMG signals according to the propagation of action potentials

EMG can explain the superimposed waveform of MUAPs, which are detected by electrodes. The EMG signal can be prepared by the summation of theoretically generated MUAP waveforms. The EMG signal observed by electrodes can also be estimated.

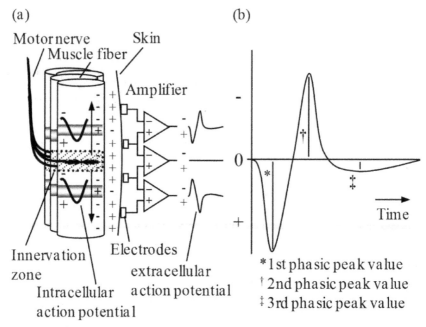

Fig. 1. Theoretical waveform of an MUAP measured using a surface electrode.
The action potential from the innervation zone (IZ) is propagated bilaterally along the
muscle fibers. The direction of the waveform will reverse depending on whether the surface
electrode is proximal or distal to IZ (a). The normal MUAP is triphasic, consisting of larger
first- and second-phase peaks and a smaller third phase peak (b; Nishihara et al., 2010).

2.1 Detection of MUAP waveform with surface electrodes

Rosenfalck recorded action potentials during muscle contraction in individual muscle fibers
of frogs, rats and humans, and performed a detailed calculation of the predicted action
potentials when the signals were detected by bipolar electrodes placed on the skin surface
(Rosenfalck, 1969). In humans, the basic action potential is triphasic; the first two phases are
similar in amplitude, whereas the terminal phase has a peak-to-peak amplitude, which is
only 5%–10% of those of the first two phases (Fig. 1).

If only a single MUAP is generated, whether the peak in each phase starts in a positive or
negative direction theoretically depends on whether the recording bipolar electrode is
proximal or distal to IZ (Hilfiker & Meyer, 1984; Zalewska & Hausmanowa-Petrusewicz,
2008).

The waveform of an MUAP is propagated from the end-plate to the muscle tendons. If the
end-plates are concentrated in one location, then the direction of the positive or negative
side of the MUAP waveform will reverse depending on whether the position of the
electrode that is recording muscle activity is proximal or distal to IZ (Masuda & Sadoyama,
1991). The waveform of a MUAP will be canceled or attenuated in IZ.

When measuring a surface EMG signal during voluntary contraction, many MUAPs can
interfere with each other, thus making it more complicated to identify a single whole MUAP
from a raw waveform display.

2.2 Relationship between the direction of electrodes and muscle fibers

Action potentials from motoneurons are propagated along muscle fibers. Bipolar surface electrodes are usually placed in the approximated direction of muscle fibers and used with a differential amplifier, which suppresses signals common to both electrodes.

The potential at one electrode is subtracted from that at the other electrode, and then the difference is amplified. Subsequently, the common noise of both electrodes is eliminated.

Multichannel electrodes arranged along the direction of muscle fibers can be used to investigate the muscle fiber conduction velocity or propagation of the action potentials. However, many EMG channels must be used for a single muscle (Nishizono et al., 1979). Multichannel surface array electrodes or grid electrodes would facilitate the stable observation of action potentials because these electrodes are attached to a plate that fixes the electrodes in close proximity to each other (Fig. 2; Zwarts & Stegeman, 2003).

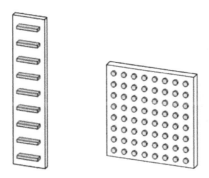

Fig. 2. Multichannel surface array electrodes (left) and grid electrodes (right). The gray rectangles and circles represent electrodes attached to the boxes.

The propagated MUAPs are attenuated depending on their distance from the surface electrodes, the location of subcutaneous tissue, and the electrical impedance of the skin (Fig. 3). Usually, MUAPs generated at a distance from the electrode are greatly attenuated. The higher frequency components of the interfered waveform are more difficult to detect when surface electrodes are placed over subcutaneous tissue; in addition, it is difficult to identify the propagation of MUAPs. The propagation pattern from raw EMG signals may be observed during lower level of voluntary muscle contraction (Fig. 4).

The propagations are estimated by detecting time shifts of pulses, which are considered as one MUAP although they appear across EMG signals of several channels (Fig. 4). The time shifts of pulses indicate that the surface electrodes are approximately located along the direction of muscle fibers. The pulses shift maximally when the electrodes are placed along the direction of muscle fibers that are anatomically arranged in the same direction. Close to the tendons of a muscle, however, the amplitude of the EMG signal is reduced and the time shifts of pulses are unidentifiable.

Appropriate analysis techniques are needed to estimate the propagation of EMG signals in higher level of muscle contraction because many motor units are activated and the generated MUAPs interfere with the observed raw waveforms of EMG.

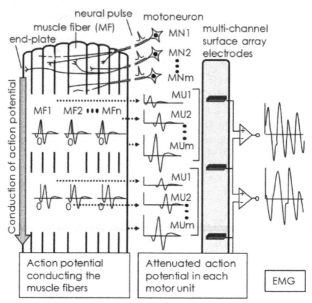

Fig. 3. Theoretical EMG signal from action potentials propagated along muscle fibers. The action potentials propagated along muscle fibers are attenuated according to the distance between the muscle fibers and the surface electrodes and are superimposed in surface EMG (Nishihara et al., 2003).

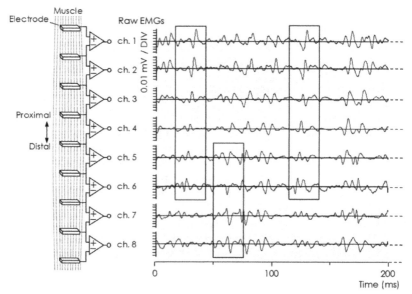

Fig. 4. Example of raw EMG signals detected by multichannel surface array electrodes. The propagations are estimated by detecting the continuous time shifts across several channels (rectangular boxes).

2.3 Cross-correlation method to estimate the propagation of action potentials

The cross-correlation method has been widely applied to estimate action potential propagation by multichannel surface EMGs using automated computer programs (Yaar & Niles, 1991). The correlation coefficient ($R\tau$) used to calculate the time shift is calculated from the reference EMG (X) and comparison EMG (Y) using the following equation (1):

$$R\tau = \frac{\displaystyle\sum_{i=0,j=i+\tau}^{N,N+\tau} (X_i - \overline{X}) \cdot (Y_j - \overline{Y})}{\sqrt{\displaystyle\sum_{i=0}^{N}(X_i - \overline{X})^2 \cdot \sum_{j=i+\tau}^{N+\tau} (Y_j - \overline{Y})^2}} \tag{1}$$

where $R\tau$ is a normalized value ranging from −1 to +1. The peak value of $R\tau$ displaced from time 0 is the time shift reflecting the conduction time between the two EMG signals (Fig. 5). A time shift could be assumed to occur according to the muscle fiber conduction. If the surface electrodes were attached in the proper direction, the peak value of $R\tau$ would be close to 1, which is relatively high.

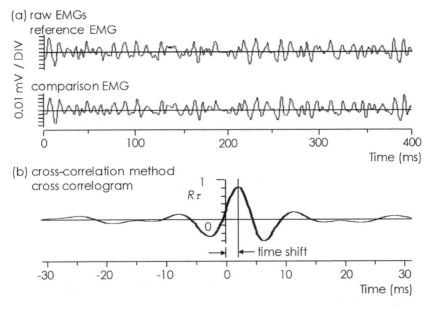

Fig. 5. Sample records of raw EMG signals (a) and the time shift estimated by the cross-correlation method (b).
The time shift estimated using the cross-correlation method by calculating the time between zero and the peak of the cross-correlogram of an EMG signal (Nishihara et al., 2003).

2.4 Peak averaging method to estimate the propagation of action potentials

The propagation pattern from a raw surface EMG signal can be observed by detecting the peaks in a surface EMG and averaging them using computer programs (Nishihara et al., 2003; Isho et al., 2011).

The smallest value at which the pulses were not detected from resting muscle EMGs was set as the threshold to avoid the detection of a noise component. When a positive peak value was larger than the set threshold in the EMG signals, the amplitude and time were registered as the peak of positive pulse. The negative peak value of the EMG signals is processed as the peak of negative pulse using the same method.

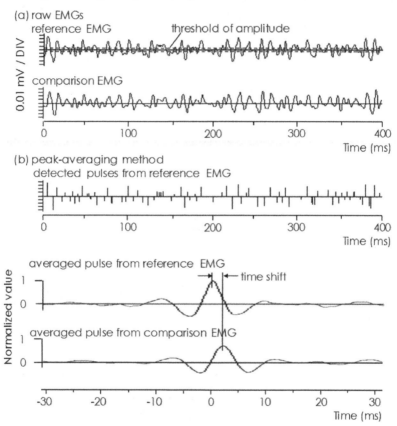

Fig. 6. Sample records of raw EMGs (a) and action potentials estimated using the peak averaging method (b).
The time shift is the time difference between the peak averaged pulses obtained using the peak averaging method (Nishihara et al., 2003).

Pulses from a reference EMG were superimposed at time 0 and averaged to minimize the irregular components of other interfering action potentials and noises. The value of the averaged pulse (PAi) at the point i on the reference EMG is obtained using the following equation (2):

$$PA_i = \frac{\sum_{j=1}^{N} \frac{1}{A_j} \cdot X_{T_j+i}}{N} \tag{2}$$

where N is the number of detected pulses in EMG with the reference electrodes, X is the reference EMG, Aj is the peak value of a detected pulse j in X, and Tj is the time at which a peak detected pulse j is obtained in X.

The peak value of PAj is 1, and its peak point of time is 0.

An averaged pulse is obtained simultaneously from a comparison EMG with an averaged time delay. The waveform of the comparison EMG is averaged with the same Aj and Tj of the detected pulse j in the reference EMG (not in the comparison EMG). Thus, the averaged pulse PBi at point i from the comparison EMG is obtained using the following equation (3):

$$ PB_i = \frac{\sum_{j=1}^{N} \frac{1}{A_j} \cdot Y_{T_j+i}}{N} \tag{3} $$

where Y is the comparison EMG.

The time shift estimated by investigating the time difference between PAi and PBi is calculated from the time difference between the peaks or cross-correlation of PAi and PBi (Fig. 6).

This method permits simple observation of the propagation of action potentials across multichannel array electrodes.

3. Surface EMG signals in IZ

Action potentials were generated in the end-plates used for signal transmission from motoneurons. These end-plates are usually concentrated in areas such as IZ. The propagation pattern was investigated using the peak averaging method, and the location of IZ was also estimated by analyzing this propagation pattern.

3.1 EMG recording

Multichannel array electrodes were attached to the medial aspect of the belly in the direction of fibers of the biceps brachii muscle and the array was secured to the skin with surgical tape. The array electrodes comprised nine wires (material: silver/silver chloride, width: 1 mm, length: 10 mm) attached at 5-mm intervals to a transparent acrylic resin box.

A weight band was attached to the wrist of the subject. Isometric elbow flexion was performed for one second to the extent of <10% maximum voluntary isometric contraction, and an EMG signal was recorded. The adequacy of the distance between the array electrodes and the tendons was checked by palpation.

3.2 Estimation of IZs

The averaged pulses from the recorded EMG signal were calculated as shown in Fig. 7. If the array electrodes are shifted towards the adjacent muscles, the time shifts are not clear, and hum components, which are easily mixed if the reference electrode is incompletely attached, are detected as pulses. This results in many dummy averaged pulses appearing in each channel. In that case, the locations of electrodes must be corrected.

The origin of the propagation is considered as IZ. If the directions of electrodes and muscle fibers are substantially different, these time shifts of averaged pulses would not be clearly shown, or the peak correlation coefficient obtained would be of a relatively low value (equation (1)).

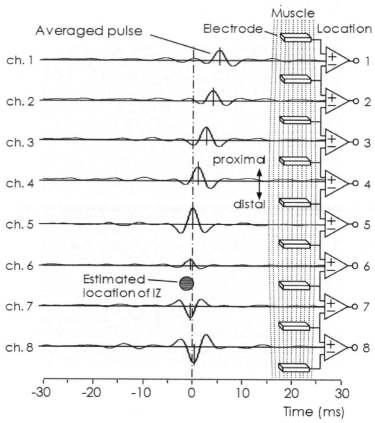

Fig. 7. Example of the generation of averaged pulses.
The EMG signal is the same as that in Fig. 4. Channel 5 was selected as the reference EMG. Detected pulses from the EMG signal are averaged, and these averaged pulses indicate the direction of propagation in muscle fibers. In this subject, the estimated location of IZ is between channels 6 and 7 (Nishihara et al., 2009).

4. IZ locations and directions of muscle fibers across several muscles

IZs are usually located around the muscle belly, or in other words, around the center of muscle fibers. However, determining the locations of IZs is difficult by the muscles. The muscles have been classified by the structures.

4.1 The structure of muscles according to the direction of muscle fibers

Muscles are classified on the basis of the direction of muscle fibers rather than the overall direction of the muscle (Fig. 8). The biceps brachii muscle is a typical example of a fusiform muscle, because it has a relatively uniform direction of muscle fibers with IZ located around its center in most cases. However, IZs were dispersed in many cases in spite of the biceps brachii muscle being used for the study in all cases (Fig. 9).

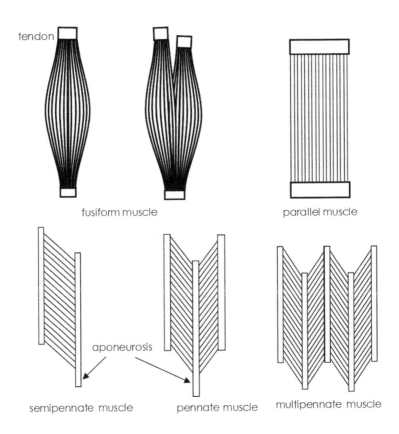

Fig. 8. Classification of muscles based on the directions of muscle fibers.

The direction of fibers is irregular in many muscles; consequently, IZs of these muscles are scattered around them (Saitou et al., 2000). Therefore, it is very difficult to attach surface electrodes in the exact direction of the muscle fibers of such muscles. In this case, the EMG signal does not comprise the waveform of generated MUAPs as illustrated in Fig. 1. The time shifts of averaged pulses from the gluteus medius muscle are not very clear compared to those from the biceps brachii muscle (Fig. 10). Clear time shifts do not appear even when the directions of array electrodes are rotated up to 30° (not shown in this figure).

The deltoid muscle is divided into three sections: anterior, intermediate, and posterior. In particular, the intermediate section of the deltoid muscle has a typical pennate structure. The direction of the muscle fibers in this section of the deltoid muscle are irregular compared to that of the biceps brachii muscle. The time shifts across the channels of the averaged pulses are not very clear; therefore, it is difficult to investigate the location of IZ (Fig. 11; Nishihara et al., 2008).

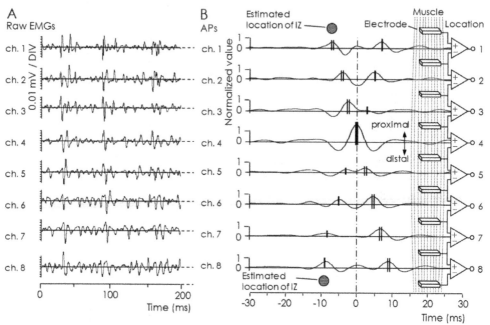

Fig. 9. An example of dispersed IZs in the biceps brachii muscle.
The calculation method is same as that described in Fig. 7. (A) Channel 4 is selected as the reference EMG. (B) The estimated locations of IZs are proximal at location 1 and distal at location 8 in this subject.

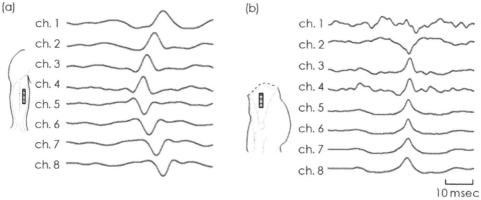

(a) The time shifts of averaged pulses across the various channels are revealed in the biceps brachii muscle. (b) However, the time shifts of averaged pulses are not revealed in the gluteus medius muscle. The gray rectangles demonstrate the locations of array electrodes, which were attached at 10-mm intervals.

Fig. 10. An example of calculating the averaged pulses of different muscles.

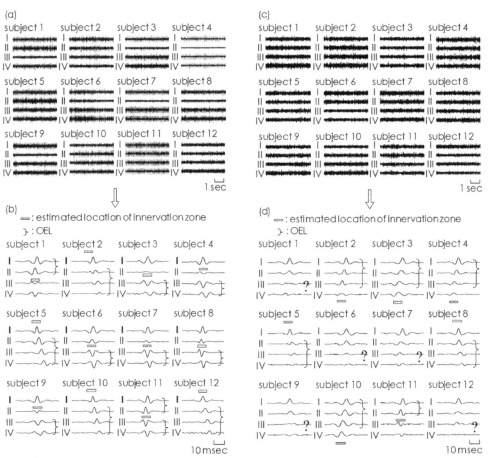

(a) Raw EMG signals of the biceps brachii muscle are shown. Particularly small amplitudes are exhibited in channel 3 in subject 1 and channel 2 in subjects 3, 4, 7, 8 and 9. (b) Calculated averaged signals of the muscles with pulse detection in EMG for channel 1 (shown in bold). (c) Raw EMG signals of the intermediate section of the deltoid muscle are shown. (d) Propagation patterns are shown for seven subjects. The propagation patterns of the other five subjects were not estimated because central peaks in the averaged signals could not be obtained for all four channels, or peaks in the averaged signals of neighboring channels did not exhibit time differences in the propagation of action potentials along electrodes. The optimum electrode location (OEL) is investigated on the basis of the location of IZ (Nishihara et al., 2008). Note the lower amplitudes of the raw EMG signals around channels of IZ locations.

Fig. 11. Analysis of EMG signals for the biceps brachii muscle (left) and deltoid muscle (right).

4.2 EMG signals near IZ

The changes in EMG signal amplitudes near IZs can be estimated if multichannel electrodes are used. For example, EMG signals with smaller amplitudes are observed using the raw EMG signals of the biceps brachii muscle as shown in Fig. 11, and the data for these channels agree with those of the channels near estimated IZs. The EMG signal amplitude can be calculated from the root mean square (RMS) of the EMG signal. The RMSs of EMG signals are obviously attenuated near IZ as shown in Fig. 12. Sufficiently large RMS values can be obtained at locations far from IZs.

IZs of the deltoid muscle are not very clear compared to those of the biceps brachii muscle (Fig. 11, d). However, this does not imply that the EMG signal of the deltoid muscle more correctly reflects the level of muscle activation than that of the biceps brachii muscle. Small RMS values are shown in some channels of subjects, although the locations of IZs are not estimated in the deltoid muscle (Fig. 12, right half). The EMG signal amplitudes may be attenuated by the different electrode directions relative to the axes of the muscle fibers rather than the small, scattered IZs in the deltoid muscle.

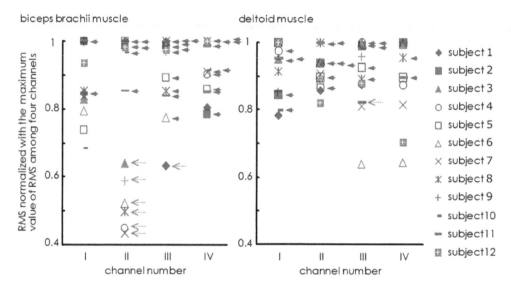

◄ : subject's channel of estimated OEL

◄⋯ : subject's channel of estimated location influenced by innervation zone

Fig. 12. RMSs of raw EMG signals for the subject channels depicted in Fig. 11. The EMG signals shown in Fig. 11 a and c are used. The subject's channel of estimated location, which was influenced by IZ, gave particularly small values (indicated by the large arrow with dotted line) compared with the subject's channel of estimated OEL (indicated by the small arrow with solid line). Small values were recorded in the channels of subjects whose deltoid muscle was not evaluated (channels 3 and 4 of subject 6 and channel 4 of subject 12).

5. Conclusion

These results demonstrate that EMG signals are affected by location of electrodes. Proper location of electrodes can be suggested by these findings.

5.1 Identification of targeted muscle

The location of electrodes has to be carefully determined for the targeted muscle. Superficial muscle could be identified with manipulation. When the electrodes were shifted towards the adjacent muscles, the unassumed action potentials from different muscles were mixed with the EMG signal. The electrodes were also easy to place on the tendon of the muscle. In that case, low-amplitude EMG signals that do not reflect muscle activity could be observed. Muscle and tendons can be distinguished by palpation.

5.2 Identification of the direction of muscle fibers

The direction of electrodes affects the EMG signal when the direction is differing from the directions of muscle fibers. The direction of the electrodes must align with that of muscle fibers. An ideal situation would be when one whole MUAP is detected by one electrode and the next one by the other electrode. The muscle fibers need not always be in the direction of the muscle. However, if muscle fibers are diagonally directed, obtaining sufficient space to attach bipolar electrodes may prove difficult.

5.3 Attaching the reference electrode

The reference electrode must be attached firmly to eliminate noise components such as hum. The reference electrode has to be located on electrically neutral tissue such as a bony prominence. The propagation pattern is not revealed by the peak averaging method (Fig. 7) if large noise components are included in the EMG signal.

5.4 The relationship between electrode and IZ locations

Propagation has to be regarded relative to the location of electrodes because their placement can affect the signal amplitude and frequency components in surface EMG. As previously mentioned, to correctly quantify muscle activity, electrodes must be placed along the course of muscle fibers between tendons in the targeted muscle. The cutaneous area, which is useful for observing the surface EMG signal, could be very limited in this restricted rule. For this reason, the electrodes should be located near the muscle belly. However, the EMG signal is easily affected when the electrodes are located near IZs, which are concentrated in the muscle belly (Fig. 11). A stable EMG signal is necessary for the reliable investigation of voluntary muscle activation.

The channels located near the estimated IZs agree with the channels of the smallest amplitude or RMS of the EMG signals (Fig. 12). As a result, it is suggested that electrodes should be placed at a sufficient distance from IZ for detection of the surface EMG signals during voluntary muscle contraction.

Moreover, IZ is known to shift with changes in muscle length due to muscle activity. In other words, when electrodes are attached to the skin and EMG for muscle activity is recorded, the positional relationship between the surface electrodes and IZ can shift markedly. Electrodes must also be attached after considering the moving IZ during EMG recording (Nishihara et al., 2010).

5.5 Effect of muscle structure

The aforementioned rules are based on the assumption that all muscle fibers are aligned in the same direction and IZs are concentrated in the muscle belly of the targeted muscle. The anatomical structure of the targeted muscle must be investigated before attaching the electrodes. However, in muscles with irregularly oriented muscle fibers, such as pennate muscles, the proper direction of electrodes could be not determined. There are limitations to consider regarding the optimum surface electrode locations while investigating the activity of these muscles using EMG signals.

6. References

Hilfiker, P., & Meyer, M. (1984). Normal and myopathic propagation of surface motor unit action potentials. *Electroencephalography and Clinical Neurophysiology*, Vol.57, No.1, pp. 21-31, ISSN 0013-4694

Isho, T., Nishihara, K., Gomi, T. (2011). Inter-method measurement variability of muscle fiber conduction velocities during isometric fatigue contraction. Proceedings of *16th International Congress of the World Confederation for Physical Therapy*, Amsterdam, The Netherlands, June, 2011

Masuda, T., & Sadoyama, T. (1991). Distribution of innervation zones in the human biceps brachii. *Journal of Electromyography and Kinesiology*, Vol.1, No.2, pp. 107-115, ISSN 1050-6411

Nishihara, K., Hosoda, K., & Futami, T. (2003). Muscle fiber conduction velocity estimation by using normalized peak-averaging technique. *Journal of Electromyography and Kinesiology*, Vol.13, No.6, pp. 499-507, ISSN 1050-6411

Nishihara, K., Kawai, H., Gomi, T., Terajima, M., & Chiba, Y. (2008). Investigation of optimum electrode locations by using an automatized surface electromyography analysis technique. *IEEE Transactions on Biomedical Engineering*, Vol.55, No.2, pp. 636-642, ISSN 0018-9294

Nishihara, K., Chiba, Y., Moriyama, H., Hosoda, M., Suzuki, Y., & Gomi, T. (2009). Noninvasive estimation of muscle fiber conduction velocity distribution using an electromyographic processing technique. *Medical Science Monitor*, Vol.15, No.9, pp. MT113-120, ISSN 1234-1010

Nishihara, K., Chiba, Y., Suzuki, Y., Moriyama, H., Kanemura, N., Ito, T., Takayanagi, K., & Gomi, T. (2010). Effect of position of electrodes relative to the innervation zone on surface EMG. *Journal of Medical Engineering & Technology*, Vol.34, No.2, pp. 141-147, ISSN 0309-1902

Nishizono, H., Saito, Y., & Miyashita, M. (1979). The estimation of conduction velocity in human skeletal muscle in situ with surface electrodes. *Electroencephalography and Clinical Neurophysiology*, Vol.46, No.6, pp. 659-664, ISSN 0013-4694

Rosenfalck, P. (1969). Intra- and extracellular potential fields of active nerve and muscle fibers. A physico-mathematical analysis of different models. *Acta Physiologica Scandinavica*, S321, pp. 1-168, ISSN 0001-6772

Saitou, K., Masuda, T., Michikami, D., Kojima, R., & Okada, M. (2000). Innervation zones of the upper and lower limb muscles estimated by using multichannel surface EMG. *Journal of Human Ergology*, Vol.29, No.1, (May , 2000), pp. 35-52, ISSN 0300-8134

Yaar, I., & Niles, L. (1991). Muscle fiber conduction velocity Dip analysis versus cross correlation techniques. *Electromyography and Clinical Neurophysiology*, Vol.31, No.8, pp. 473-482, ISSN 0301-150X

Zalewska, E., & Hausmanowa-Petrusewicz, I. (2008). Approximation of motor unit structure from the analysis of motor unit potential. *Clinical Neurophysiology*, Vol.119, No.11, pp. 2501-2506, ISSN 1388-2457

Zwarts, M., & Stegeman, D. (2003). Multichannel surface EMG: basic aspects and clinical utility. *Muscle & Nerve*, Vol.28, No.1, (January, 2003), pp. 1-17, ISSN 0148-639X

4

The Relationship Between Electromyography and Muscle Force

Heloyse Uliam Kuriki, Fábio Mícolis de Azevedo,
Luciana Sanae Ota Takahashi, Emanuelle Moraes Mello,
Rúben de Faria Negrão Filho and Neri Alves
Univ. Estadual Paulista
Univ. de São Paulo
Brazil

1. Introduction

The generation of physical movement in animals involves the activation and control of muscle forces. Understanding the mechanisms behind force generation and control is essential for professionals who work to promote health. The human body can be represented as a system of articulated segments in static or dynamic balance. Within this system, movement can arise from internal forces acting outside the joint axis, causing angular displacement of these segments, or by forces external to the body. Knowledge of the contribution of muscle forces to joint position and movement is of great importance for the study of muscle activity during exercise and also for understanding the coordination of muscle activities during functional movement. However, muscles forces cannot be easily measured in vivo; rather, they must be assessed, calculated or modeled (Amadio & Duarte, 1996; Amadio & Barbanti 2000).

Closely associated with the generation of force by a muscle, is the generation of an electrical signal that can be observed by placing electrodes on the skin surface to detect underlying electrical activity displaying the associated waveform on a computer monitor. This process is called electromyography (EMG) and the waveform is the electromyogram. The assumption that there is an association between EMG and underlying muscle forces is the basis for many applications of EMG, allowing inferences regarding various aspects of muscle physiology. However, it is not possible to measure muscle force directly using EMG. Since 1952 there have been studies that show some cases where there is a linear relationship between force and EMG (Lippold, 1952), however this relationship is not always simple and linear. In recent years methods for detecting and processing EMG signals have been refined considerably, with the availability of better equipment, tools, mathematical, statistical and computational techniques. Although the determination of muscle strength using EMG measurements has also evolved, it has not yet fully exploited the technological potential available. In this chapter, we describe a practical approach to the quantitative evaluation of muscle force through analysis of the EMG signal.

2. Muscle strength

Force is a fundamental concept, understood as an agent capable of modifying the state of rest or motion of a body. Force can be defined as:

$$F=m.a \tag{1}$$

where m is mass and and a, acceleration.

Animals move and interact with the environment generating muscleforce, either voluntarily or passively. Biomechanics is a field of science dedicated to understanding human movement and the study of the muscular forces involved in human movement. It is the application of mathematical principles, laws and concepts to mechanical, biological systems. It studies the generation and performance of internal and external forces on these systems and the effects of these forces on each part of the body. These forces can be calculated indirectly by parameters of kinematics and dynamics of movement or based on the mechanical characteristics of the locomotor system and its functional structures. External biomechanics refers to externally observable characteristics of the body studied, for example, its movement in space: position, velocity, acceleration, externally applied forces, reaction forces and muscle electrical activity (Amadio & Duarte, 1996; Amadio & Barbanti, 2000).

The muscle behavior approach to biomechanics uses analytical methods that include anthropometry, kinemetry, dynamometry and electromyography. The EMG is the method of recording the electrical activity of a muscle, including information about the physiological processes that occur during muscle contraction. The biological structure of the body, movement dynamics and characteristics of the measurement techniques complicate the analysis of the motion variables and indicators of internal phenomena. The assessment of muscle strength, in particular, becomes more complex due to the mechanisms of controlling dosage or magnitude, enabling the execution of movements or of achieving internal and external balance amongst body elements. Thus, direct measures of muscle strength and interaction forces between segments are not viable. Assessments of internal forces are based on models built from the parameters of motion of the body or its segments, measures of external linkages, or both. Understanding the relationships between internal forces and movement is one of the major methodological challenges for biomechanics (Amadio & Duarte, 1996).

3. Determinant factors for the generation of muscle strength

The term muscle strength refers to the ability of a muscle to generate tension. For the generation of muscular force that produces mechanical work, the first necessary condition is nerve stimulation that triggers the process. Sensory input from muscles travels via afferent pathways to the central nervous system (CNS), where it promotes the recruitment of motor neurons that stimulates muscle fibers and results in the generation and demonstration of muscle strength. These muscle forces act through a bone system that depend on nervous, muscular, and biomechanical factors, as shown in Figure 1.

The functional unit of muscle is the motor unit (MU), which consists of an alpha motor neuron and all fibers innervated by it. Muscle fibers are the structural unit of contraction. One UM can have from 3 to 2000 muscle fibers, depending on the degree of control and strength required by the muscle: muscles that control fine movements and require precise but low strength have fewer fibers per MU, whereas the large muscles that control larger movements requiring greater strength, may contain 100 to 1000 fibers per MU (Rash, 2002).

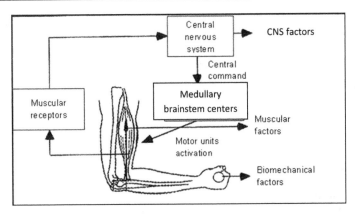

Fig. 1. Diagram illustrating the factors associated with muscle force generation.

The contraction of muscle fibers occurs when action potentials are generated in the motor neuron that supplies them. When the action potential reaching the motor neuron and axon terminal exceeds the threshold of depolarization in the postsynaptic membrane of the neuromuscular junction, it becomes a muscle action potential. Different from nerve action potentials, the muscle action potential is propagated in both directions of the muscle fiber, triggering the process of the sliding of actin filaments on myosin, the major contractile proteins of the myofibrils, thus, promoting muscle contraction (Fox & Keteyian, 2000).

During voluntary contractions, muscle force is modulated by the central nervous system, which combines recruitment with the frequency of MU activation and synchronization. MU recruitment involves the control of the number and type of fibers activated. The frequency of activation of MUs refers to the fact that the fibers do not remain contracted, relaxing after each activation, and therefore reflects the repeatability of activation. The synchronization of activation refers to the temporal coincidence of the pulses of two or more MUs firing in combination. The greater the ability to recruit MUs simultaneously, the greater the force produced by the muscle (Barbanti et al., 2002; Fox & Keteyian, 2000). These mechanisms operate in different proportions depending on the muscle. Relatively small muscles, such as those of the hand; and big muscles, like those of the legs and arms are controlled by different schemes of recruitment and activation (Basmajian & De Luca, 1985).

Muscle fibers are classified either as type I or type II, according to their metabolic and functional capabilities. As the number of MUs per muscle is variable, the ratio of fiber types varies among individuals (Rash, 2002; Fox & Keteyian, 2000). Type I fibers are recruited first during muscle contraction, and are always active regardless of exercise intensity.Type IIA fibres are recruited next, and, with higher levels of exercise demand, type IIB are recruited. Type II fibers are typically recruited during tasks involving rapid effort, high power and high intensity (Fox, Keteyian, 2000; Gerdle et al., 1991).

Muscle strength is also influenced by the contractile and elastic structure of the muscle itself. The contractile units refer to the proteins of the functional units of the muscle, the sarcomeres, containing filaments of actin and myosin. An elastic component is present in the connective tissue sheaths surrounding the muscle (epimysium), the bundles of muscle fibers (perimysium) and the interior of the muscle fiber (endomysium), which join at their ends to form tendons. During concentric muscle contraction, there is a slip of actin filaments on the myosin filament; the filament length remains constant, but the muscle length decreases.

Instead, during the eccentric contraction, muscle length is increased. And during an isometric contraction, slippage of the contractile elements occurs and elastic strain arises, i.e., muscle work is performed, although there is no movement observed (Fox & Keteyian, 2000; Nordin & Frankel, 2001). Muscle strength depends on the length of the muscle. When the actin and myosin overlap along their entire lengths, the number of crossbridges reaches its maximum, allowing the muscle to generate maximum tension. The length at which force is produced with the greatest intensity varies between different muscles within a single individual, but does not change in the same muscle across different individuals (Mohamed et al., 2002; Nordin & Frankel, 2001).

In addition to the generation ofactive tension through the sliding of the filaments, there is the phenomenon of passive tension, which arises from the stretch of connective or elastic tissue (or elastic. As muscle length shortens, these passive elements become "loosened" and their contribution to muscle tension decreases gradually as tension subsides (Mohamed et al., 2002).

In addition to neural and muscular components there are biomechanical factors, which can influence muscle action of muscle without direct relationship to power generation. Such factors include angular variations of the joint and different types and levels of resistance that may be applied. In a biomechanical system involving two muscle segments and a joint, variation of joint angle determines the degree of mechanical advantage that a limb has when generating force. The perpendicular distance between the axis of the joint and tendon line of action defines this mechanical advantage. The outer lever refers to the distance between the joint axis and the point at which resistance is applied, and changes when the joint angle is modified. There are different types of overload that can be applied to a limb such as those produced by fixed weight, elastic resistance and isokinetic [isokinetic WHAT?]. The action of a muscle, of course, responds differently to each overload imposed. This answer depends on the multiplier or reducing effect of the internal and external lever system, as well as the speed of the gesture in question. These factors are all interconnected. The angular variation of the limb is directly related to the change in muscle length.

Knowing all the variables that can influence muscle strength, we are able to propose a model for its calculation. In this chapter we base the calculation of muscle strength to the quadriceps muscle during isometric and isotonic exercises, in the position showed in figure 2.

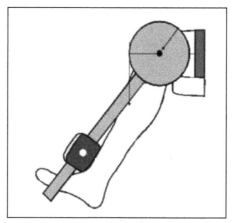

Fig. 2. Schematic diagram of the exercise. For the isometric contraction the movement occurs against a fixed resistance and for the isotonic the knee is able to execute the extension.

4. Experimental protocol

We will illustrate the lever model using the example of the quadriceps muscle. To calculate the strength of the quadriceps muscles, three steps are needed: i) a theoretical simulation of muscle force based on biomechanical models, ii) experimental testing to determine the curve of maximal isometric strength of knee extension as a function of joint angle, and iii) analysis of the internal relationship between muscle strength and the EMG signal during isometric and isotonic exercises. These steps will be detailed below:

4.1 Simulation of muscle strength

The adoption of an appropriate biomechanical model of the knee joint is essential to measure the forces transmitted by these muscles to the skeletal system. In the muscle model of Hill (Hof & Van Den Berg, 1981) force is described to be made up of three components: i) a parallel elastic component (PEC), which represents the elasticity of the passive elements of the muscles and ligaments ii) a contractile component (CC), which determines the behavior of active elements of the muscle, and iii) elastic components connected in series (SEC). These components should not be construed as if each one corresponds to a separate constituent of the muscle structure. Figure 3 shows a representation of the Hill model. The length of the elements is expressed by the relation:

$$x = l l 0 \tag{2}$$

where l is the length at a given moment, and l_0 is the length in the resting position.

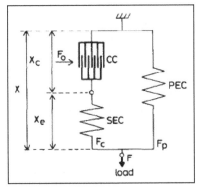

Fig. 3. Schematic diagram of Hill model.

The modeling of the motor unit will be discussed in a later section of this chapter. First we describe the contribution of contractile and passive components to force generation. The intensity of each component depends on the length of the muscle in a non-linear and non-monotonic way, as shown in Figure 3. Passive elastic force (curve 1, fig. 4) is exerted by the elastic components and contractile force is generated by the contractile proteins (curve 2, fig. 4). The sum of these two components produces the curve 3, which represents the overall strength of the muscle as a function of its length. The curve illustrates that maximum force is generated when the muscle is stretched to approximately 1.2 to 1.3 times its resting length. This position often coincides with the length of the muscle in a relaxed state. It appears that the anatomical architecture of the musculoskeletal system is organized for the benefit of the force-length relationships of the muscular system (Basmajian & De Luca, 1985).

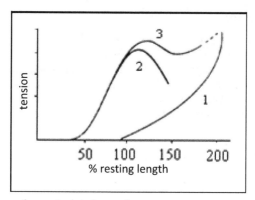

Fig. 4. Force-length curve for an isolated muscle.

In addition to length-dependent characteristics of strength, there are also speed-dependent properties. The ability to generate muscle force depends on the speed and type of contraction. Thus, movements in concentric, eccentric and isometric contractions illustrate important differences in force behavior (Figure 5) (Barbanti et al., 2002). The ability of a muscle to generate force is higher in an isometric situation (contraction velocity equal to zero) than in a concentric contraction, and this capacity decreases as the speed of contraction increases. The velocity of shortening that a muscle can produce is at its maximum when the external load is zero, but as the load increases, muscle shortening slows until the external load is equal to the maximum force that the muscle can exert (isometric contraction). If the load continues to increase even more, the muscle will contract eccentrically. During an eccentric contraction, the muscle can develop tension higher than in isometric contraction, and in this case the force increases with speed of muscle contraction (Barbanti et al., 2002; Nordin & Frankel, 2001).

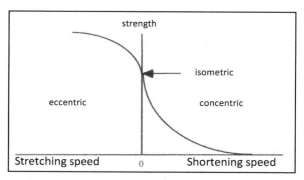

Fig. 5. Force-velocity curve for an isolated muscle.

An equation that describes the curves shown in figures 3 and 4 can be derived from the Hill model shown in figure 3. The force F that represents the total force generated by the muscle is given by:

$$F = Fc + Fp \qquad (3)$$

where F_c is the contractile component in series and in the passive state (CC and SEC) and F_P is the force provided by parallel components (PEC).

As previously discussed, the force generated by the parallel components grows exponentially, so can be expressed by:

$$Fp(x) = Fpoep(x-1) \qquad (4)$$

where x is the total length of the muscle, F_{Po} and p the parameters of the exponent.

This relationship represents the properties of muscle, tendon, ligament and joint when a muscle is not active. Normally passive forces have significant values when the muscle is close to the greatest or smallest possible length . Contractile force, as discussed, depends on speed, and can be described by the following equations:

$$Fc= F0fxc-nvcb1+vcb, \text{ for } v_c 0 \qquad (5)$$

$$Fc \leq (1+c)F0f(xc), \text{ for } v_c < 0 \qquad (6)$$

where v_c is the velocity of shortening of the muscle and x_c is the length of the contractile component shown in Figure 3, $f(x_c)$ is a function of normalization to values between 0 and 1 and F_0 is the F_c value when $f(x_c)$ is maximum. The F_c values decrease with increasing v_c for $v_c > 0$ and the rate of decrease depends on the parameter b, while n defines the concavity of the curve. For values of $v_c > 0$, the force F_c is greater than in the isometric case, where the difference is given by the parameter c.

Through these equations, it can be seen that the Hill model provides a very close representation of experimentally observed muscle behavior.

The muscle strength in the isometric activity, that is, when v_c is equal zero, can be seen from equations 4, 5 and 6. These equations can then be rewritten to reflect isometric contraction.

$$Fc = F0f(xC) \qquad (7)$$

Then

$$F= F0fxC+ Fpoep(x-1) \qquad (8)$$

In this last equation it can be observed that in isometric activity, muscle strength depends on the length of the muscle, and that the diagram from figure 2 is represented by $x = x_e + x_C$. Thus, it can be appreciated that during so-called isometric contractions there is actually considerable variation in the lengths of the contractile elements of the muscle(x_C).

4.2 Calculation of muscle strength (biomechanical models)

Several biomechanical models have been constructed to represent the performance of the musculoskeletal system in various situations of interest to sports, clinicians or others. The representations include two-dimensional approaches, to complex computer simulations that produce quantitative and three-dimensional visual representations. Currently available computing resources, including those intended for graphic animation, allow for the development of powerful tools for motion analysis. There are softwares that enable the user to develop detailed musculoskeletal models with representations of bones, muscles, ligaments and other structures. It is also possible to input experimental data regarding motion to some of these softwares, through direct or inverse dynamics, and to calculate muscle forces and visualize the geometric changes of the musculoskeletal system.

The relation between strength applied externally by a limb and the muscle strength is, however, not obvious. To illustrate, we will consider the calculation of quadriceps strength during leg extension (concentric contraction) in the sitting position, with an external resistance applied perpendicular to the leg. To calculate the strength, we use a simple two-dimensional model of the quadriceps. The free body diagram is shown in figure 6, where L_p is the length of the leg, L_{cm} the longitudinal position of the center of mass, F_{pl} the force applied to the tibial tuberosity through the patellar ligament, F_c the contact tibio-femoral force, γ the angle between the patellar ligament and the axis of the leg, θ the angle of the knee joint, W_p the weight of the leg and F_a the external force applied perpendicular to the limb.

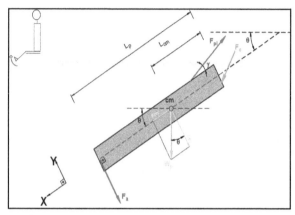

Fig. 6. Free body diagram representing the leg of a sitting person in a movement of concentric contraction of the quadriceps.

Through geometrical considerations illustrated in the free body diagram and calculation of torque, in which $\Sigma\tau=I\alpha$, and τ the torque, I the moment of inertia and α the angular acceleration, an equation can be written that defines the strength of the quadriceps muscle as a function of joint angle θ.

$$Fq=LpFa+LcmWpcos\theta+I\alpha RBm \qquad (9)$$

In this equation, Fq is the force exerted by the quadriceps, I is the moment of inertia of the leg, α is the angular acceleration during exercise and Bm is the moment arm of force of the patellar ligament in relation to the point of tibiofemoral contact, around which the femur rotates. It must be recognizeded that the point of rotation changes as a function of the angle θ, and consequently the moment arm also changes. The relationship between the strength of the patellar ligament and the force exerted by the quadriceps is called R ($R= F_{pl}/F_q$) and also varies with the joint angle θ.

Figure 7 shows the strength of the quadriceps calculated for different forces applied perpendicular to the leg, considering a female individual, typical for the anthropometric model adopted (De Leva, 1996), with mass of 61.9 kg and height of 1.73 m. In these simulations using the values of R and Bm obtained by Van Eijden et al. (1986) and Kellis and Baltzopoulos (1999), respectively, the experimental condition assumed that the angular velocity was constant - W = ct and α = 0. The model was developed considering that the external force is always applied perpendicular to the limb and, therefore, remains constant. It can be observed that, while the leg moves a certain weight through the range of motion, the quadriceps displays variable strength. With this simple model, it is only possible to assess the strength of the muscle group, not each component part, (in this case, the vastus medialis, vastus lateralis, vastus intermedius and rectus femoris muscles).

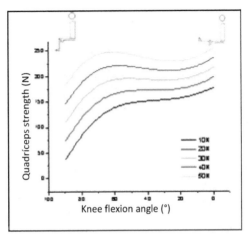

Fig. 7. Simulation of the quadriceps muscle strength in knee extension exercise in sitting position.

The maximum force that a limb is able to apply externally varies with angular position. This is because the geometrical arrangement determines the degree of mechanical advantage, and also because changes in muscle length alter the efficiency of muscle force generation, in addition to the the different contributions of different components of the muscle group.

Figure 8 shows the maximum force applied externally by a leg during isometric contraction of the quadriceps. In the same graph the corresponding force generated by the quadriceps

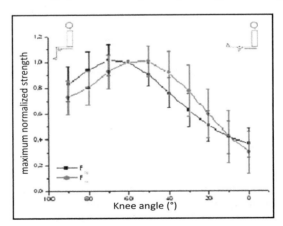

Fig. 8. Values of the applied force and muscle strength normalized as a function of the knee joint angle (average of 10 individuals).

muscle group is shown, calculated by the model (equation 9). The values are normalized by the strength at a 60° angle and were obtained from 10 female volunteers, with a mean age of 20.4 ± 1.6 years, mean weight of 51.15 ± 6.72 kg and mean height of 1.66 ± 0.05 m, during cued isometric contractions, with the maximum force defined as the greatest force exerted across three repetitions.

4.3 General considerations on the assessment of muscle strength

In the preceding sections, we have discussed aspects related to muscle force generation, presenting briefly the main factors - nerve, muscle and biomechanical - that determine the ability to generate muscle force. We have qualitatively discussed the participation of active and passive elements of muscle and shown that the force generated by a muscle can be represented by the Hill model. To understand the role of muscle force generation in movement, it is necessary to refer to biomechanical models. This was then demonstrated using a simple model of the quadriceps, in which we calculated the force exerted by this muscle when the leg applies an external force. Then, results were presented showing the maximum strength of the quadriceps as a function of joint angle in isometric contractions.

Starting from the theories of force generation in muscle fibers, it is not easy to understand the internal force exerted by a muscle, when it involves a complex articulation, such as the quadriceps. One very important consideration for health professionals involves the participation of each portion of the muscle in force generation as a function of angular position. For example, figure 9 shows how the different portions of quadriceps acting on the knee extension.

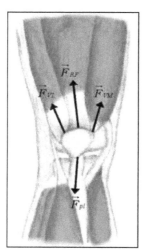

Fig. 9. Illustrative schema of how the forces of each portion of the quadriceps acts during the contraction.

The EMG signal is recorded by electrodes in response to muscle activity. As previously mentioned, skeletal muscle cells are formed by the muscle fibers, which constitute the structural contractile units. Each fiber, if excited, has the ability to stretch or contract. The activation of the muscle fiber by nerve endings induces two waves of depolarization that travel at a speed of 3 to 6m/s. The internal tissue is electrically conductive. Thus, electrical signals related to depolarization of the fiber can be recorded by electrodes on the skin or muscle.

Two events occur simultaneously during muscle contraction: one electrical and one mechanical. Depolarization releases calcium ions, which starts the process of contraction in the main body of the muscle fiber. But this contraction is much slower than the cycle of depolarization, which occurs over approximately 2 ms. Maximum forces are achivved between 20 to 150ms after depolarization and then decaying gradually due to reabsorption of calcium. Consequently, it cannot be said that there is a direct relationship between EMG and force.

In muscle contraction, the degree of force can be controlled by changes in the number of recruited MUs or by changes in the frequency of recruitment. To increase the strength of a muscle the number of fibers recruited must increase one by one in order of size (size principle). After recruitment of all fibers, force can be further increased by increasing the frequency of activation. The EMG signal is a record of action potentials produced during a muscle contraction. The action potential motor unit (APMU) is the temporal and spatial summation of individual action potentials of all fibers of a MU. However, the catchment area of an electrode will often include more than one MU, because the muscle fibers of different MUs are interwoven throughout the muscle. Any portion of the muscle may contain fibers belonging to 20-50 MUs. An electrode located in this field will detect the algebraic sum of several APMUs within its catchment area. In order to maintain muscle contraction, the nervous system sends a sequence of stimuli, so that the MUs are activated repeatedly, resulting in a train of APMUs. The EMG signal is the superposition of the resulting space-time relationship of these trains, considering the number of MUs involved for maintenance and activation of muscle contraction.

4.4 Relationship between EMG and force

The relationship between force and surface EMG during voluntary contractions is not well understood. Some authors have concluded , for various muscles, that the magnitude of the EMG signal is directly proportional to muscle strength for isometric and/or isotonic contractions with constant speed, but others claim that this relationship is not linear (Bilodeau et al., 2003; Gerdle et al., 1991; Gregor et al., 2002; Herzog et al., 1998; Karlsson & Gerdle, 2001; Moritani & Muro, 1987; Onishi et al., 2000). In most cases, the EMG increases non-linearly with increasing force of muscle contraction (Guimaraes et al., 1994; Madeleine et al., 2000; Lawrence & De Luca, 1983; Solomonow et al., 1990). Theoretical analyses suggest that the amplitude of the signal in isometric contraction should increase with the square root of the force generated if the motor units are activated independently (Basmajian & De Luca, 1985; Lawrence & De Luca, 1983). This variety of different interpretations among researchers not surprising, given the inherent limitations of surface EMG. The measured force of muscle contraction is a result of the global activity of the underlying muscle fibers, and surface EMG provides information about the electrical activity of motor units located in the region near the electrode; in most experiments, the catchment area of the electrode does not extend sufficiently to detect the signal generated across the entire muscle volume (De Luca, 1997; Siegler et al., 1985).

Factors that prevent the direct quantification of muscle force from EMG signals include cross-talk, variations in the location of the recording electrodes and the involvement of synergistic muscles in force generation.

The electrical cross-talk of adjacent muscles is often considered as a possible factor that complicates the determination of the relationship between EMG and force. Its influence would manifest most prominently when the measured strength of the muscle increases. The presence of cross-talk is more dominant in smaller muscles where the electrodes (especially the surface) must be placed close to the adjacent musculature. The complexity of cross-talk is also determined by the anisotropy of muscle tissue and homogeneity of the tissues adjacent to the muscle. Often it is not possible to identify precisely the source of contamination of the physiological signal.

The degree of synergistic action of other muscle groups and the amounts of co-contraction between antagonistic muscle groups can change the contribution of muscle strength in research on the net force measured in the joint (Lawrence & De Luca, 1983). Ideally, in order to improve the EMG-force relationship, the muscle chosen should be the muscle uniquely responsible for generating the force measured (Bigland-Ritchie, 1981).

The relative location of fast and slow muscle fibers inside the muscle, and their distribution and location relative to the electrode are also factors to be considered. The amplitude of the action potential generated by a single muscle fiber is proportional to its diameter. Fast fibers generally have larger diameters and display a greater range of action potentials than slow fibers, and consequently generate a higher signal amplitude. However, the amplitude of the action potential, is a function of the distance between the active fibers and the recording electrodes, and the greater the distance, the lower the measured amplitude. The largest motor units, containing the largest diameter of fast twitch fibers are preferentially recruited at high force levels, according to the size principle (Henneman et al., 1965; Henneman & Olson, 1965). Thus, the relative location of fast muscle fibers in relation to the electrodes, determines how the electrical activity of these motor units affects the surface EMG signal (Basmajian & De Luca, 1985). It has been reported that muscles with homogeneous composition of fibers, such as the soleus of the cat, display a linear force-EMG relationship (Guimarães, 1994).

Figure 10 shows, as an example, an EMG signal picked up during a ramp isometric contraction (with slow growth to isometric force) in the vastus lateralis (VL), vastus medialis (VM) and rectus femoris (RF) muscles. The EMG signal shown –was passed through a third-order Butterworth filter, and band passed between 20 to 500 Hz during signal acquisition – but was otherwise unprocessed and therefore, it is called raw. The load shown in the figure refers to the external resistance applied to the leg. The signal intensity in the three muscles clearly increases with increasing external force. The questions that arise are: What is the relationship between force and EMG signal for each muscle? What treatment should be given to the EMG signal? What is the involvement of each muscle to form the resultant force? The following discussion seeks to bring some clarity to these issues.

In general, most studies involving the relationship between EMG and force aim to develop a noninvasive method to measure muscle strength during different actions. In experimental biomechanics there are different ways process of raw EMG signal and thus extract parameters related to the level of muscle contraction. Debate continues regarding the best signal processing techniques to use (Siegler et al., 1985). For example, one can find examples in the literature, in which strength has been related to the intensity, or to the median or mean frequency of the EMG signal.

Among the most used EMG parameters for such analysis, is the time series analysis, in which the the effective value of the signal, is derived from the root mean square - RMS (Basmajian & De Luca, 1985; Bigland-Ritchie, 1981; Bilodeau et al. 2003; Gerdle et al. 1991;

Gregor et al. 2002; Guimaraes et al. 1994; Herzog et al. 1998; Lawrence & De Luca, 1983; Madeleine et al., 2000; Onishi et al., 2000; Solomonow et al., 1990). This is a method to quantify the signal amplitude, recommended to assess the level of muscle activity, since the parameter is not affected by the superposition of APMU (Acierno et al., 1995; Basmajian & De Luca, 1985; De Luca, 1997). We have reported a positive correlation between this approach to parameter analysis and the strength of the quadriceps muscle in an isometric ramp task, suggesting that the coinciding increase in RMS and strength reflects two main mechanisms: the recruitment of new motor units and an increase in the frequency of active units firing (Bilodeau et al. 2003; Karlsson & Gerdle, 2001; Gerdle et al., 1991).

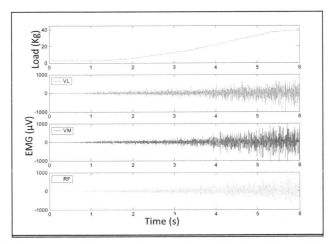

Fig. 10. EMG of the vastus medialis (VM), vastus lateralis (VL) and rectus femoris (RF) during a ramp contraction.

The normalization of the signal is a very important aspect in signal analyses displaying this relationship. A prominent feature of signal RMS is its variability, which makes it inherently difficult to compare signal amplitude across different individuals or even across different sessions within the same individual. To enable these comparisons, normalization processes are needed. The normalization process can be accomplished using a variety of reference methods. The most common example, which is standard in isometric exercises, is to express muscle contractions as a percent of the EMG amplitude observed in maximal voluntary isometric contraction (MVIC). It should however, be noted that in isotonic exercises, this process may lead to distortions, given that the muscle acts differently when changing the angular position of the limb, especially during maximal contraction. It is therefore essential to remember, that during isotonic exercise, there is an effect of changes in muscle length in electromyographic activity, as pointed out by Mohamed et al. (2002).

5. EMG x force analysis for the quadriceps

In this section we present an analysis of the EMG-force relationship for the quadriceps. This muscle is composed of four portions: rectus femoris (RF), vastus medialis (VM), vastus lateralis (VL) and vastus intermedious (VI); and the force applied to the patella is the result of the forces generated by each portion, therefore:

$$FVL+FVM+FRF+FVI=Fq \tag{10}$$

Where FVL is the force exerted by the VL, FVM is the force of VM, FRF is the force of RF, FVI is rhe force of VI and Fq is the resultant force of the quadriceps muscle group.

In figure 11 the forces that act on the quadriceps are illustrated. FVI is not presented because it is a deep muscle. (fig. 11.b).

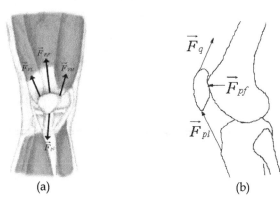

(a)   (b)

Fig. 11. a) schematic representation of the forces involved in quadriceps action. b) Forces acting on the patella, whose fixation point varies with the knee angle. Fpl is the patellar tendon force, Fq is the resultant quadriceps force and Fpf is the tibiofemoral contact force.

Each muscle's contribution is different and depends on various factors. The EMG assessed during voluntary contractions provides a way to verify differences in the activation behavior of the different quadriceps portions (Pincivero et al., 2003). Studies have demonstrated that contraction of different muscle portions contraction is dependent on the contraction intensity. During isometric contractions of low to moderate intensity, the VL recruitment is significantly higher than VM and RF; the highest activation of the VM occurs close to maximum force levels, when EMG becomes equivalent to that of the VL and RF (Pincivero et al., 2003). However, we highlight that different studies show methodological variations, so it is difficult to compare results. It should be also considered that each muscle has distinct physiological and structural properties, and these morphological characteristics are altered with changes in muscle length. Each portion can present its greater length (where the greater force is generated) at different joint angles.

The physiological and structural properties and the morphological characteristics, altered with the change in muscle length, differ for each of the agonist muscles, in this case, the four portions that make up the quadriceps muscles. Taking into account that the magnitude of the overall strength of the quadriceps is the sum of the contribution of each component muscle, we can define an α relationship between the strength modules of each muscle and the overall strength of the muscle group.

$$\alpha VL=FVLFq \rightarrow FVL=\alpha VLFq \tag{11}$$

$$\alpha VM=FVMFq \rightarrow FVM=\alpha VMFq \tag{12}$$

$$\alpha RF=FRFFq \rightarrow FRF=\alpha RFFq \tag{13}$$

$$\alpha VI=FVIFq \rightarrow FVI=\alpha VIFq \tag{14}$$

It can be assumed that the intensity of EMG is related to the magnitude of the force generated (F), because the EMG signal is generated regardless of the direction and sense of strength. You can also define a function β representing the relationship between EMG and F for any muscle, such as:

$$\beta\theta,F,v,w=EMGF \tag{15}$$

Where $\beta(\theta, F, v, \omega)$ is the function that correlates EMG with the quadriceps total force.
In this expression we consider the explicit dependence of β with four variables: θ, the angular position; ω, the angular displacement speed of the member, given by $w=d\theta dt$; F, the intensity of muscle strength; and v, the velocity contraction which is related to the temporal variation of force ($v \propto dFdt$). The dependence on these variables was noted in the previous discussions, experimental verification of the authors and the literature studies. The ability to generate muscle force depends on its length, and it varies with the angular position, justifying the dependence on θ and ω. The experimental results show that, even holding other variables constant, there is a dependence on the level of force F. It is also noted that the contraction velocity v is an important factor. The speed of contraction is related to the time necessary for the force range up to the level considered.
Based on the above discussion, it can be said that in an experimental situation in which the quantities θ, F, v and ω are known and held constant, there is a direct relationship between EMG and force given by β. Thus, for example, to the VL, we have:

$$EMGVL=\beta VL(\theta,F,v,w)FVL \tag{16}$$

Substituting eq.(16) in eq.(11):

$$EMGVL=\beta VL(\theta,F,v,w)\alpha VLFVL \tag{17}$$

Defining the product by α per $\beta(\theta, F, v, \omega)$ as $r(\theta, F, v, \omega)$, this product represents the function that correlates the overall strength of the quadriceps with the EMG signal portion of each muscle. Thus, to the VL, we have:

$$EMGVLFq=rVL(\theta,F.v,w) \tag{18}$$

In the same way, we can definethe r_{VM}, r_{RF} and r_{VI} for the other muscles. Although already discussed, it is important to emphasize that the angle θ is the variable that dependes on the initial condition of the muscle, including both length and tension. The value of the function r depends on the level of force, and this reflects recruitment strategies and types of fiber used by the muscle during low and high levels of force. Also very important are the dependencies of this function on muscle velocity and angular velocity of the limb. The first is related to the temporal variation of the force, while the second is related to the temporal variation of the angle.

5.1 Force and EMG in isometric contraction
The study of muscle strength using EMG has been applied more frequently and with greater success in isometric or in limited sectors of dynamic contractions that approximate the isometric condition (De Luca, 1997; Herzog et al. 1998 ; Lloyd & Besier, 2003).

In the particular case of isometric exercise, the function that correlates the overall strength of the quadriceps with the EMG signal can be expressed by equation 19, when the angle θ is constant and consequently $w=d\theta dt=0$. Thus, for the VL, we have:

$$EMGVLFq=rVL(\theta cte, F, v) \tag{19}$$

Although θ does not vary in the isometric case, the relationship between EMG and force must be different for each angle, and depends on the level of strength and speed of contraction. It is well documented that in isometric conditions the magnitude of EMG provides a reasonable estimate of the force exerted by the muscle. Basmajian and De Luca (1985) concluded that the relationship between the intensity of EMG signal and muscle force measured during an isometric contraction has considerable inter-subject variation and, moreover, the dependence of the type of muscle is almost linear for the small muscles of the hand and non-linear for larger limb muscles - this distinction in behavior may possibly reflect the difference in the properties of firing rate and recruitment of small and large muscles, as well as other anatomical and electrical considerations, including a dependence on the level of training.

The examples showed in this text are result of an evaluation with ten female subjects with no history of pain in the knee joint, 20.4 ± 1.6 years, 51.15 ± 6.72 kg and 1.66 ± 0.05 m. For the experiment was used a leg extension chair, a system of surface EMG with Ag/AgCl electrodes placed in the bellies of the VMO, VL and RF, with a gain of 20 times, CMRR greater than 80dB and impedance of 1012 Ω. Were also used a load cell type strain-gauge with a capacity of 5000N and an electrogoniometer.

Figure 12 shows a normalized EMG signal as a function of force. EMG data are normalized by the value obtained at maximal contraction and the force is normalized by the maximum

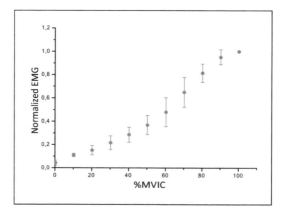

Fig. 12. Normalized EMG values of the vastus lateralis, measured isometrically in ramp at 20° of knee flexion.

force (MVIC). The illustrated values are the average of 10 subjects, and the EMG was obtained from the VL muscle. There is a positive correlation between EMG and force, as noted by Karlsson and Gerdle (2001), Gerdle et al. (1991) and Bilodeau et al. (2003). There are two regions that are clearly close to linear. A change in the slope of the force-EMG relationship is associated with a change in recruitment strategy; after full recruitment the frequency of activation is varied (Merletti & Parker, 2004).

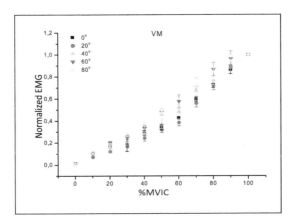

Fig. 13. Normalized EMG values of the vastus medialis, assessed isometrically in ramp at 0, 20°, 40°, 60° and 80° of knee flexion.

The same behavior is observed across different angles and muscles, but with different slopes, as shown in figure 13. In this figure, the data are for the VM muscle of a single volunteer. Although there is great variability, the dependence of the EMG values on the joint angle is clearly illustrated. This same behavior, with the same curves is observed in all subjects studied. Even in isometric exercise, keeping θ constant and $\omega=0$, and the experimental care to keep v constant, the function $r(\theta_{ct}, F, v_{ct}, \omega=0)$ which relates the force with EMG still varies with the level of strength, which in fact can be seen in figure 12.

5.2 EMG in MVIC

The maximum isometric contraction is always taken as an individual reference, especially for the normalization of EMG signals. In Figure 8, we showed that the maximum force that the individual can exert with the leg, in isometric contractions of the quadriceps, as well as the maximum force of quadriceps, varies with joint angle. Figure 14 shows the corresponding normalized EMG signal from an individual, for the three portions analyzed. It appears that the EMG signal as well as the relationship between EMG and force, when the individual generates full force, and the maximum force all change as a function of joint angle. Therefore, the results of studies in which normalization has been performed at different angles are not easily comparable.

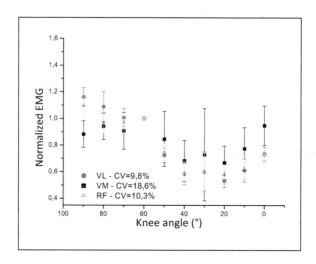

Fig. 14. EMG values during MVIC as a function of joint angle, for an individual, where VL: vastus lateralis, VM: vastus medialis and RF: rectus femoris.

5.3 Comparison of EMG with the force calculated by the model

As shown in the Hill model, even when there is an isometric contraction, there is a change in muscle length. This is important; in equation 20, it can be seen that there is a dependency between the EMG-force relationship and contraction velocity. These two aspects are equivalent, because the change in muscle length predicted by the Hill model in the isometric case, has a direct correlation with contraction velocity. The results presented in this section were all obtained at about the same rate of growth of the force ramp, i,e., at the same contraction velocity, so the function β for each angle is the same.

The graphs in figures 12 and 13 show EMG normalized according to MVIC versus isometric force normalized across the maximum force. Here we can see that force is that which was applied externally, that is, the force that the leg applies in the experimental system, rather than the quadriceps force, as shown in equation 19. Although a linear relationship is shown, this is not a causal relationship. When considering the strength of the quadriceps as the model predicts, we must also consider individual variations such as size and weight of the leg, and these may be more or less significant for the different component muscles.

The same EMG data from figures 12 and 13, when plotted as a function of the quadriceps muscle strength normalized by the maximum - as shown in Figures 15 and 16, show a change in slope, which differs from angle to angle. This is because, for the same applied force, the force that develops in the quadriceps is different for every angle, as already mentioned.

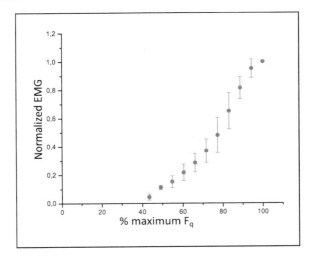

Fig. 15. Normalized EMG values of vastus lateralis in function of the percentage of quadriceps force, asssessed isometrically in ramp, in 20° of knee flexion.

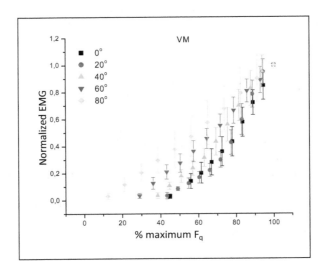

Fig. 16. Normalized EMG values of vastus medialis in function of the percentage of quadríceps force, assessed isometrically in ramp, in 0, 20°, 40°, 60° and 80° of knee flexion.

In the literature, the EMG has been compared to the applied force or torque. As in the preceding discussion, even if a coherent relationship is shown, it cannot be considered causal, because the EMG is generated by the muscle strength and is not related to the biomechanical parameters of the joint.

5.4 Isotonic contractions

In dynamic contractions, the relationship between EMG and force has a greater complexity due to experimental and physiological characteristics. A movement implies change in joint angle over which the muscle acts. Angular displacement can change the muscle geometry, and then the relative positions between the active motor units and surface electrodes may change (Basmajian & De Luca, 1985; Doorenbosch & Harlaar, 2004).

The complexity of the EMG-force relationship in an isotonic contraction can be understood through the function $r(\theta, F, v, \omega)$, where θ, F, v e ω are varied simultaneously. Therefore, to quantitatively assess the strength of isotonic contractions, in addition to the experimental care with the placement of the electrodes and movement of the skin, should be restricted to the situation that is closest to an isometric contraction. In fact, it is desirable to minimize the effect of each variable. Thus, we recommend the use of low levels of force, and control of the application of force during movement in order to limit variation in this parameter ($F{\sim}ct$), which is important to v exert little influence on r, and impose a lower angular velocity ($w{\sim}0$).

6. Other instrumental tools and applications

To obtain the data presented in this chapter, the relationship between electromyography and strength in the quadriceps muscle was evaluated through conventional measures, using a differential EMG electrode placed on the skin. As discussed above, there is a limitation in these measures arising from the fact that the EMG signal recorded is the sum of action potentials occurring in the area of the electrode.. Studies show that the use of electrode arrays significantly improves the ability to estimate force with EMG measures. An interesting example of such analysis can be seen in Staudenmann et al. (2006) who employed multivariate statistical analysis of principal components.

Although this chapter has discussed the measurement of muscle strength by measuring EMG, it can be said that most applications of EMG are related to some aspect of muscle force generation, because the signal is generated when muscle contractile elements are activted. In this respect, it is pertinent to mention other methods, such as: i) the use of PCA (principal component analysis) to identify the pulse trains of action potentials on a surface electromyography signal collected with multiple electrodes (Nakamura et al., 2004); ii) application of multivariate statistical techniques and multidimensional visualization in 3D space - Viz3D (Artero, 2005), to identify differences between isometric activities carried out against a rigid obstacle and with a weight of equivalent inertial load (Mello, 2007); iii) applications in studies of muscle coordination, techniques that allow, through measures of EMG, set parameters for determining the action of various muscles; and iv) studies of the relationship between force sensation and muscle stretching (Branco et al., 2006).

The magnitude of force or torque has also been compared with the spectral variables of the EMG signal (Bernardi et al., 1996, Bilodeau et al., 2003; Gerdle et al., 1991; Hermans et al., 1999; Karlsson & Gerdle, 2001; Moritani & Muro, 1987; Onishi et al., 2000). The calculation of these parameters should involve the application of appropriate techniques to obtain the power spectrum of the EMG signal. The parameters obtained in the frequency domain involves more complex procedures than those for the time domain, being the spectral distribution obtained by the fast Fourier transform or discrete Fourier transform (Bendat Piersol, 1986). Recent studies show the technique of wavelet transform as a very interesting tool for analysis in the frequency domain.

7. Conclusion

In this chapter, we have explored the relationship between EMG signals and muscle strength calculated using biomechanical models. In the literature, a common approach has been to adjust the intensity of EMG using equations derived from the Hill model. It has also been shown that the application of EMG to measure the force requires a process of calibration parameters for each individual. This process of calibration and standardization should be conducted having enough control of the variables that influence the relationship between EMG and force, as specified in equation 13.

The relationship between electrical activity and isometric muscle strength has been the focus of research since the 1950s. However, we still lack consensus regarding a precise methodology that can be widely used to quantify muscle strength based on EMG. The use of EMG as a metric for determining the force is both fascinating, and challenging. It is fascinating because of the possibilities for making a quantitative measure of strength in an individual while performing a gesture, through noninvasive surface electrodes. It is challenging in view of the complexity and variability inherent in biological signals, especially in dynamic situations. However, the application of current equipment for collecting and processing the signal remains the motivation for the use of EMG as a metric measure of force. The study of this issue, using methodologies that combine calibration processes or normalize instrumental resources, including arrays of electrodes, and signal processing using multivariate statistical techniques (PCA), can provide great advances.

8. References

Acierno, SP; Baratta, RV; Solomonow, M. (1995). *A practical guide to electromyography for biomechanists*, Bioengineering Laboratory/LSUMC Department of Orthopaedies, Louisiana.

Amadio, AC, Duarte M. (1996). *Fundamentos biomecânicos para análises do movimento humano*. Laboratório de Biomecânica/EEFE-USP, São Paulo.

Amadio, AC, Barbanti, VJ. (2000). *A biodinâmica do movimento humano e suas relações interdisciplinares*, Estação Liberdade, ISBN 85-7448-019-3, São Paulo.

Artero AO. (2005). *Estratégias para apoiar a detecção de estruturas em visualizações multidimensionais perceptualmente sobrecarregadas*, Instituto de Ciências Matemáticas e de Computação/ICMC, USP, São Carlos.

Barbanti, VJ et al. (2002). *Esporte e atividade física: interação entre rendimento e saúde* (1), Manole, ISBN 8520413889, São Paulo.

Basmajian, JV; De Luca, CJ. (1985). *Muscles alive: their functions revealed by electromyography* (5), Williams and Wilkins, ISBN 068300414X, Baltimore.

Bendat, JS; Pierson, AG. (1986). Decomposition of wave-forces into linear and nonlinear components. *Journal of Sound and Vibration*, Vol.106, No.3, May.1986, pp.391-408, ISSN 0022-460X.

Bernardi, M et al. (1996). Motor unit recruitment strategy changes with skill acquisition. *European Journal Applied Physiology*, Vol. 74, No. 1, Aug. 1996, pp. 52-59, ISSN 1439-6319.

Bigland-Ritchie, B. (1981). EMG/force relations and fatigue of human voluntary contractions. *Exercise Sport and Science Reviews*, Vol.9, pp.75-117, ISSN 1538-3008.

Bilodeau, M. et al. (2003). EMG frequency content changes with increasing force and during fatigue in the quadriceps femoris muscle of men and women. *Journal of Electromyography and Kinesiology*, Vol.13, No.1, Feb. 2003, pp.83-92, ISSN 1050-6411.

Branco VR. Et al. (2006). relação entre a tensão aplicada e a sensação de desconforto nos músculos isquiotibiais durante o alongamento. Revista Brasileira de Fisioterapia, Vol.10, No.4, Dez.2006, pp.465-472, ISSN 1413-3555.

De Leva, P. (1996). Adjustments to Zatsiorsky-Seluyanov's segment inertia parameters. *Journal of Biomechanics*, Vol.29, No.9, Sept. 1996, pp.1223-1230, ISSN 0021-9290.

De Luca, CJ. (1997). The use of surface electromyography in biomechanics. *Journal of Applied Biomechanics*, Vol.13, No.2, May. 1997, pp.135-163, ISSN 1065-8483.

Doorenbosch, CAM.; Harlaar, J. (2004). Accuracy of practicable EMG to force model for knee muscles: short communications. *Neuroscience Letters*, Vol.368, No.1, Sept. 2004, pp.78-81, ISSN 0304-3940.

Fox, E.; Foss, ML.; Keteyian, SJ. (2000). Bases fisiológicas do exercício e do esporte (6), Guanabara-Koogan, ISBN 8527705303, Rio de Janeiro.

Gerdle, B. et al. (1991). Dependence of the mean power frequency of the electromyogram on muscle force and fibre type. *Acta Physiologica Scandinavica*, Vol.142, No.4, Aug. 1991, pp.457-465, ISSN 0001-6772.

Gregor, SM. et al. (2002). Lower extremity general muscle moment patterns in healthy individuals during recumbent cycling. *Clinical Biomechanics*, Vol.17, No.2, Feb. 2002, pp.123-129, ISSN 0268-0033.

Guimarães, AC. et al. (1994). EMG-force relationship of the cat soleus muscle studied with distributed and non-periodic stimulation of ventral root filaments. *Journal of Experimental Biology*, Vol.186, No.1, Jan.1994, pp.75-93, ISSN 0022-0949.

Hermans, V.; Spaepen, AJ.; Wouters, M. (1999). Relation between differences in electromyographic adaptations during static contractions and the muscle function. *Journal of Electromyography and Kinesiology*, Vol.9, No.4, Aug. 1999, pp.253-261, ISSN 1050-6411.

Henneman, E.; Somjen, G.; Carpenter, DO. (1965). Functional significance of cell size in spinal motoneurons. *Journal of Neurophysiology*, Vol.28, May. 1965, pp.560-580, ISSN 0022-3077.

Henneman, E.; Olson, CB. (1965). Relations between structure and function in the design of skeletal muscles. *Journal of Neurophysiology*, Vol.28, May. 1965, pp.581-598, ISSN 0022-3077.

Herzog, W. et al. (1998). EMG-force relation in dynamically contracting cat plantaris muscle. *Journal of Eletromyography and Kinesiology*, Vol.8, No.3, June 1998, pp.147-155, ISSN 1050-6411.

Hof, AL.; Van Den Berg, JW. (1981). EMG to force processing I: an electrical analogue of the hill muscle model. *Journal of Biomechanics*, Vol.14, No.11, pp.747-758.

Karlsson, S.; Gerdle, B. (2001). Mean frequency and signal amplitude of the surface EMG of the quadriceps muscles increase with increasing torque – a study using the continuous wavelet transform. *Journal of Eletromyography and Kinesiology*, Vol.11, No.2, Apr. 2001, pp.131-140, ISSN 1050-6411.

Kellis, E.; Baltzopoulos, V. (1999). The effects of the antagonist muscle force on intersegmental loading during isokinetic efforts of the knee extensors. *Journal of Biomechanics*, Vol.32, No.1, Jan. 1999, pp.19-25, ISSN 0021-9290.

Lawrence, JH.; De Luca, CJ. (1983). Myoelectric signal versus force relationship in different human muscles. *Journal of Applied Physiology*, Vol.54, No.6, June. 1983, pp.1653-1659, ISSN. *8750-7587*.

Lippold, OCJ. (1952). The relation between integrated action potentials in a human muscle and its isometric tension. *The Journal of Physiology*, Vol. 117, pp. 492-499, ISSN *1469-7793*.

Lloyd, DG.; Besier, TF. (2003). An EMG-driven musculoskeletal model to estimate muscle forces and knee joint moments in vivo. *Journal of Biomechanics*, Vol.36, No.6, June 2003, pp.765-776, ISSN 0021-9290.

Mohamed, O.; Perry, J.; Hislop, H. (2002). Relationship between wire EMG activity, muscle length and torque of the hamstrings. *Clinical Biomechanics*, Vol.17, No.8, Oct. 2002, pp.569-576, ISSN 0268-0033.

Moritani, T.; Muro, M. (1987). Motor unit activity and surface electromyogram power spectrum during increasing force of contraction. *European Journal of Applied Physiology*, Vol.56, No.3, May 1987, pp.260-265, ISSN 1439-6319.

Madeleine, P. et al. (2000). Mechanomyography and electromyography force relationships during concentric, isometric and eccentric contractions. *Journal of Electromyography and Kinesiology*, Vol.10, No.1, Feb. 2000, pp.33-45, ISSN 1050-6411.

Mello EM. (2006). *Estudo da atividade mioelétrica em exercícios isométricos com diferentes contrações*, Programa de Pós-Graduação Interunidades Bioengenharia, USP, São Carlos.

Merletti, R.; Knaflitz, M.; De Luca, CJ. (1990). Myoelectric manifestations of fatigue in voluntary and electrically elicited contractions. *Journal of Applied Physiology*, Vol.69, No.5, Nov. 1990, pp.1810-1820, ISSN *8750-7587*.

Nakamura H. et al. (2004). The application of independent component analysis to the multi-channel surface electromyographic signals for separation of motor unit action potential trains: part I - measuring techniques. *Journal of Electromyography and Kinesiology*, Vol.14, No.4, Aug. 2004, pp. 423-432, ISSN 1050-6411.

Nordin, M.; Frankel, VH. (2001). *Biomecânica básica do sistema musculoesquelético (3)*, Guanabara-Koogan, ISBN 852770823X, Rio de Janeiro.

Onishi, H. et al. (2000). Relationship between EMG signals and force in human vastus lateralis muscle using multiple bipolar wire electrodes. *Journal of Electromyography and Kinesiology*, Vol.10, No.1, Feb.2000, pp.59-67, ISSN 1050-6411.

Pincivero, DM. et al. (2003). Knee extensor torque and quadriceps femoris EMG during perceptually-guided isometric contractions. *Journal of Electromyography and Kinesiology*, Vol.13, No.2, Apr. 2003, pp.159-167, ISSN 1050-6411.

Rash, GS. (2002). *Electromyography fundamentals*. Gait and Clinical Movement Analysis Society. Disponível em:<www.gcmas.org>. Acesso em: 17/10/05.

Siegler, S. et al. (1985). Effect of myoeletric signal processing on the relationship between muscle force and processed EMG. *American Journal of Physical Medicine*, Vol.64, No.3, pp.130-149, ISSN 0002-9491.

Solomonow, M. et al. (1990). The EMG-force relationship of skeletal muscle dependence on contraction rate, and motor units control strategy. *Electromyography and Clinical Neurophysiology*, Vol.30, No.3, Apr. 1986, pp.141-152, ISSN. 0301-150X.

Staudenmann D. et al. (2006). Improving EMG-based muscle force estimation by using a high-density EMG grid and principal component analysis. IEEE TRANSACTIONS

ON BIOMEDICAL ENGINEERING, Vol.53, No.4, Apr. 2006, pp.712-719, ISSN 0018-9294.

Van Eijden, TMGJ. et al. (1986). A mathematical model of the patellofemoral joint. *Journal of Biomechanics*, Vol.19, No.3, pp.219-229, ISSN 0021-9290.

Whiting, WC.; Zernicke, RF. (2001). *Biomecânica da lesão muscuesquelética* (1). Guanabara-Koogan, ISBN 852770630X, Rio de Janeiro.

5

Clinical Implications of Muscle-Tendon & -Force Interplay: Surface Electromyography Recordings of *m. vastus lateralis* in Renal Failure Patients Undergoing Dialysis and of *m. gastrocnemius* in Individuals with Achilles Tendon Damage

Adrian P. Harrison[1], Stig Molsted[1], Jessica Pingel[2],
Henning Langberg[2] and Else Marie Bartels[3]
[1]*IBHV, Faculty of Life Sciences, Copenhagen University*
[2]*Institute for Sports Medicine, Bispebjerg Hospital, Copenhagen NV*
[3]*The Parker Institute, Frederiksberg Hospital, Frederiksberg*
Denmark

1. Introduction

The Surface Electromyography (sEMG) technique offers a safe, quick, pain-free, non-invasive and repeatable means of assessing the important physiological processes that cause muscles to generate force and produce movement, yet it has many limitations that must be understood, considered, and removed where possible (Hermens et al., 1999). Thus, it has been said of electromyography that;

> "*EMG is a tempting muse .. it is too easy to use and consequently too easy to abuse*"
> *(De Luca CJ 1993 – Wartenweiler Memorial Lecture).*

An sEMG signal comprises what is otherwise termed a compound muscle action potential (CMAP) being the sum of any number of motor unit action potentials within a given recording area. However, just such an sEMG signal, which provides an insight into the level of activity of a given skeletal muscle, can be altered/affected in many ways by what have been defined as causative, intermediate and deterministic factors (De Luca, 1997). The causative factors include such parameters as the configuration of the recording electrodes (size, distance apart etc.), skin thickness and subcutaneous tissue composition and depth, blood flow, muscle fibre diameter and orientation as well as the number of active motor units within the muscle of choice and their firing rate one with another, that is to say their synchronization (De Luca, 1997). Added to these parameters are the intermediate factors which include the choice of using a differential electrode filter, the risk of cross-talk from adjacent muscles or underlying tissue, the occurrence of spatial filtering as a consequence of fibre depth, the volume of the muscle that is detectable, and the conduction velocity of muscle fibres. Finally, there are the deterministic factors which comprise the number of active motor units within a muscle as well as their detectability, their recruitment and stability, plus the action potentials resulting from such active motor units and their amplitude and duration. These then, when combined, give rise to an sEMG or compound muscle action potential which has a given amplitude and any number of spectral variables. It is the analysis of such sEMG signal data and its interpretation in terms of muscle force (RMS conversion), the activation of a muscle (On *versus* Off), any signs of fatigue and hints relating to the biochemical processes in a muscle that make this such a tempting, yet complex field to study (see Fig. 1 & 2).

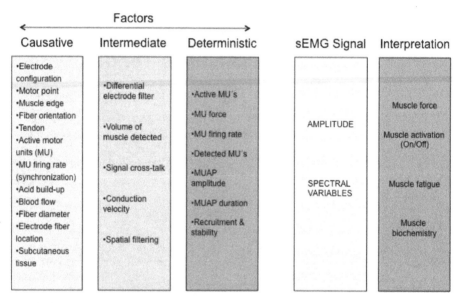

Fig. 1. The factors "causative", "intermediate" and "deterministic" and their effect on both sEMG signal amplitude and spectral variables, and the interpretation one can make of a recorded sEMG signal (after De Luca, 1997).

In spite of the large number of variables that influence the sEMG signal (De Luca,1997; Farina et al., 2004; Hogrel, 2005), studies on correlations between intrinsic muscle parameters and recorded signals are becoming more numerous (Gerdle et al., 1997; Karlsson & Gerdle, 2001; Kupa et al.,1995; Larsson et al., 2002 & 2006; Tygesen & Harrison, 2005).

In rats, EMG parameters have been shown to be a useful tool to predict muscle excitability (Harrison & Flatman, 1999), and in sheep the technique has been used to follow postnatal muscle development (Tygesen & Harrison, 2005). sEMG recordings have also been related to the morphological state of muscles, for example i) muscle fibre composition (identified using MHC isoforms or mATPase activity)in humans (Gerdle et al., 1997; Larsson et al., 2002 & 2006) and in rats (Kupa et al., 1995) and, ii) muscle fibre diameter in humans (Gerdle et al., 1997; Larsson et al., 2006) and in rats (Kupa et al., 1995).

With the non-invasiveness of sEMG recordings comes the possibility, for clinicians and physiologists alike, to determine whether structural and functional changes have occurred in muscles over a period of time.

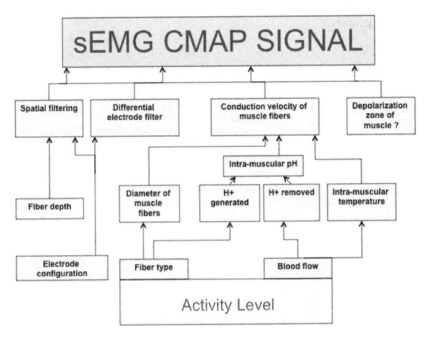

Fig. 2. Factors affecting the sEMG signal during a period of sustained contraction. In the case of "conduction velocity", "intramuscular pH" and "H+ generated" a clear association between changes in these parameters over time during a period of sustained contraction has been established. It is less clear, however, as to whether and with what degree "depolarization zone of muscle" is changed during a period of sustained contraction (after De Luca, 1997).

Recorded parameters such as signal Area and Corrected Peak relate to muscle force production, and over time they can be used to give an idea of an individual's fatigue resistance, along with an RMS analysis of the recorded signal, whereas Leading Slope and Trailing Slope are more closely related to the speed of contraction and relaxation in a given muscle, providing information about an individual's physical capabilities, as well as the fibre-type composition of specific muscles (De Luca, 1997).

It is relevant to measure sEMG prior to and after strength training. An increase in muscle strength after a period of strength training can be due to an improvement in neuro-muscular communication and/or an increase in the cross-sectional area of muscle fibres. In cases where no response to strength training is observed, the limiting factor may be due to affected neuro-muscular function. Indeed, CKD are associated with neuropathies (Krishnan et al., 2005), which could well affect the sEMG signal and any response to strength training. Thus the sEMG serves as a control/explanatory factor together with muscle strength measurements and CSA fibre measurements when looking for an indicator of strength training success in individuals.

The sEMG of a person with good muscle function would therefore be characterized by a signal with the following characteristics; relatively high frequency, large corrected peak, relatively stable RMS – at least initially, and fast leading and trailing slopes.

1.1 Understanding & interpreting sEMG signals
1.1.1 sEMG parameters

sEMG signals can be characterized either by temporal analysis (e.g. peak amplitude, root mean square or average rectified values), by spectral analysis (e.g. mean frequency, median frequency), or by propagation analysis (e.g. muscle fibre conduction velocity).

Amplitude estimations are used frequently in sEMG research. The amplitude of a voluntary signal is stochastic (random) and can therefore be reasonably represented by a Gaussian distribution function. The amplitude of a sEMG signal is highly influenced by the distance and the conductivity of the tissue between the active fibres as well as the recording electrodes, their properties and placement. The root mean square, that is to say the square root of the average power of the sEMG signal for a given period of time, is a technique that allows for rectification of the raw "bipolar" signal, converting it to a "monopolar" amplitude that is easier to present and interpret (Hermens et al., 1999). The average rectified value takes the rectified signal one step further and represents the area under the rectified sEMG signal over a period of time. It is generally thought that the root mean square is more appropriate when assessing voluntary contractions as it represents the signal power, unlike the average rectified value, which has no specific physical meaning (De Luca, 1997).

1.1.2 sEMG issues

As motor units are recruited and potentially increase their firing rate during sustained muscle activation, increasing numbers of motor unit action potentials (MUAP's) may contribute to an sEMG signal at any one point in time. It would be logical then to predict that the magnitude of the sEMG signal should increase almost linearly with activation rate. However, the sEMG signal underestimates the actual activation signal sent from the spinal cord to a particular muscle since increasing MUAP overlap and signal cancellation typically occurs, and this reduces the sEMG signal. This loss of sEMG signal has been shown to arise from the linear summation of overlapping positive and negative phases of motor unit potentials which serve to cancel one another out and thereby reduce the amplitude of the signal (Day & Hullinger, 2001; Keenan et al., 2005; Keenan et al., 2006).

In general terms, the sEMG parameters "area" and "amplitude" relate to the force of contraction, yet no simple equation exists to describe their relation. Indeed, the fact that the amplitude increases as muscle force increases only serves to provide a qualitative indicator. Quantitatively, exactly how much the force varies between two tasks cannot at present be answered with any certainty. One should be very cautious then when using the sEMG signal as an absolute measure of the force developed by a muscle as there are occasions when this relation can become non-linear (De Luca, 1997; Turker, 1993). Apart from the fact that the amplitude is highly influenced by both extrinsic and intrinsic parameters, two other factors have an enormous effect on the relation between force and amplitude. The first is that of the number of motor units detected by the recording electrodes is almost always less that the number of active motor units in an active muscle. The second is the issue of relative placement of active motor units with regard to the recording electrodes, such that if a newly recruited motor unit is located in close proximity to a recording electrode, that motor unit will contribute more than an average unit of energy to the recorded signal. Conversely, if a newly recruited motor unit is located at a distance from the recording electrode, the force in that muscle will most likely increase whilst the amplitude of the sEMG signal will not alter dramatically (De Luca, 1997).

Clinical Implications of Muscle-Tendon & -Force Interplay: Surface Electromyography Recordings of
m. vastus lateralis in Renal Failure Patients...

69

Spectral analysis of the sEMG signal has been used to study muscle fatigue (Komi & Tesch, 1979; Linssen et al., 1991; Milnerbrown & Miller, 1986; Moritani et al., 1982), and changes in motor unit recruitment (Bernardi et al., 1996; Bernardi et al., 1999; Solomonow et al., 1990). Spectral analyses have also been used to estimate the activation of type I and type II muscle fibres during a contraction (Gerdle et al., 1988; Gerdle et al., 1991; Tesch et al., 1983), as well as to predict the actual muscle fibre type composition (Kupa et al., 1995). Interpretation of the most commonly used spectral descriptors (mean frequency and median frequency) is facilitated by the use of the power spectral density function. The mean frequency has a smaller estimation of variance than the median frequency, yet the median frequency is less sensitive to noise and more sensitive to fatigue (Hermens et al., 1999; Merletti et al., 1992). Thus these different characteristics should be considered when analyzing an sEMG signal. For example, under conditions of a high signal:noise ratio the mean frequency is preferable due to the low variance, but under conditions where the signal:noise ratio is low, one should consider using the median frequency because of its relative insensitivity to noise (Hermens et al., 1999).

In propagation analysis, the muscle fibre conduction velocity is measured using two electrodes with the same alignment as the muscle fibres. By measuring the inter-electrode distance, the muscle fibre conduction velocity can be calculated as the ratio between the distance and the time delay between the two recorded signals. In most cases the underlying tissue poses very little local variation, so in terms of both detected signals the filtering effects can be assumed to be similar. This gives the muscle fibre conduction velocity parameter an advantage compared to temporal and spectral analysis, where the filtering effect of underlying tissue may distort the travelling signal (Hermens et al., 1999; Hogrel, 2005). The muscle fibre conduction velocity is to some degree proportional to the muscle fibre diameter. Thus in general muscles with large diameter fibres, such as those belonging to higher threshold motor units, will possess a greater average muscle fibre conduction velocity, which will in turn shift the frequency spectrum towards the high frequency range (De Luca, 1997).

To illustrate use of sEMG in a clinical setting, we will give an account of two chosen studies which together will show where sEMG has its strength and which considerations have to be made when using sEMG in these settings.

2. Uremic study

2.1 Introduction

Patients with end-stage renal disease (ESRD; uremia) have limited physical fitness, which can lead to subsequent problems, namely cardiac dysfunction and depression (Gutman et al., 1981; Painter, 1988, Kouidi et al., 1997; Shalom et al., 1984), as well as muscle abnormalities, which severely affect their daily life, whether it be work- or recreation-related (Nakao et al., 1982). Yet, whilst muscle weakness is a common complaint amongst dialysis patients, it remains an unexplained phenomenon.

Muscle atrophy with uremia has been shown to be fibre-specific, in that the disease is mainly associated with a loss of type II fibres and predominantly the type IIB fibres, which are fast-twitch and glycolytic in nature (Fahal et al., 1997). Atrophy of type I (slow-twitch, oxidative fibres) also occurs in some patients (Molsted et al., 2007; Moore et al., 1993). Yet despite these changes, exercise training has been shown to significantly alleviate the loss of physical capacity that occurs in dialysis patients with end-stage renal disease (Shalom et al., 1984; Painter, 1988; Eidemak et al., 1997; Kouidi et al., 1998; Molsted et al., 2004).

Whilst these patients suffer an array of medical problems that plagues them and the quality of their life (QoL), they are interested in receiving any form of help that will improve their condition and help them to lead a more normal life. It is for this reason that studies have been attempted to assess the causes behind the observed muscle atrophy and physical weakness that they incur. It should be mentioned though that these studies are not without problems. Patients arriving for a period of dialysis are usually very weak and can become easily confused, and after their dialysis most cannot wait to get out into the World and use the time and energy they have had temporarily restored upon them. This necessitates that any experimental design must be simple and easy to understand, it should not be painful, and most of all it must be relatively quick – time being of the essence after a period of dialysis. Thus it has been our experience that whilst studies of nerve conduction have not been accepted by patients with end-stage renal disease, being seen as both time consuming and painful, our sEMG recordings have been well tolerated.

2.2 Patients
Patients were recruited from Rigshospitalet, Denmark. Inclusion criteria were; ages above 18 years, undergoing haemodialysis for a minimum of three months, and being able to climb stairs. Exclusion criteria were inability to participate in the intervention due to physical health, blindness, lower limb amputation, diabetic retinopathy, severe cognitive reduction, and treatment with the anti-coagulation drug Fondaparinux. All patients gave their informed consent and the protocol was approved by the local ethical committee (H-D-2008-124).

2.3 Training programme
The included patients participated in a training programme consisting of heavy load resistance training three times a week for a period of 16 weeks. The exercise sessions varied in time from the last dialysis, since some patients were dialyzed three times a week, others only twice a week.
The exercise began with 5 minutes of warm-up. Three exercises were performed at each exercise session: leg press, leg extension and leg curl. During the intervention period the load was increased and repetition maximum (RM) decreased from 15 to 6 RM. An individual patient's progress during the interventions was adjusted according to changes of 1-6 RM.

2.4 sEMG recordings, measurements and analyses
The study used both a single and a double differential electrode configuration, with electrodes (N-00-S & R-00-S; Blue Sensor R, Medicotest A/S, Ølstykke, Denmark) configured as described previously (Harrison et al., 2006). sEMG recordings were taken *via* an ML 131 amplifier connected to a PowerLab 4/25T A/D converter (AD Instruments, Chalgrove, Oxfordshire, UK) with a further connection to a Mac PowerBook Air with Chart v. 5.5.6 Software, Peak Parameters, and Spike Histogram extensions. Input impedance was 200 MΩ differential, and a high- and a low-pass filter of 3 Hz and 500 Hz, respectively, were used. Sampling speed was set to 40,000 per second.
Recordings, which were taken from the vastus lateralis of the left leg, followed the guidelines laid out in the *European Recommendations for Surface ElectroMyoGraphy* as detailed by the SENIAM project (Hermens et al., 1999). Differential recordings of sEMG signals were made *via* surface electrodes from the *vastus lateralis*, as described in detail previously. Information of any expected electromyography performance results were not divulged, and

Clinical Implications of Muscle-Tendon & -Force Interplay: Surface Electromyography Recordings of
m. vastus lateralis in Renal Failure Patients...

71

patients were not allowed to follow their sEMG recordings on the computer screen in real
time. The recorded sEMG signal was assessed as described previously (Harrison et al., 2006)
in terms of signal frequency (Hz) and peak-to-peak amplitude (V), using Chart analysis
software (AD Instruments, Chalgrove, Oxfordshire, UK).

2.5 Statistics

Data distribution was tested using a Q-Q plot. Due to the discovery that the data was not
normally distributed, statistical analysis of any effects was performed using non-parametric
tests. A Wilcoxon Signed Ranks Test was applied to measure significant differences between
pre-training (Baseline) and post-training (Re-test) values. Data are presented as means plus
and minus the standard error of the means (SEM). All tests were two-tailed and significance
was deemed to be at $P \leq 0.05$.

2.6 Results

A clear and significant improvement in the amplitude of the recorded sEMG signal was
noted in the uremic patients when values taken pre-training were compared with those
obtained post-training (see Fig. 3).

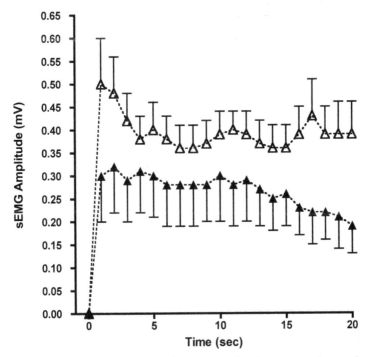

Fig. 3. The recorded sEMG signal from *m. Vastus lateralis* of uremic patients taken prior to
(▲) and after a 16 week programme of strength training (△). Recordings, which represent a
20 second period of sustained leg lift, were taken at a sampling rate of 40,000 data samples
per second, using an impedance of 200 MΩ and a high- and low-pass filter of 3 Hz and 500
Hz, respectively. Values represent the Mean ± SEM of 8 patients.

In contrast, to the sEMG amplitude values, measurements of the sEMG signal frequency from these uremic patients were not significantly altered by a 16 week period of strength training (see Fig. 4). Indeed, if anything one gets the impression, at least initially, that a lower firing frequency is employed by these patients during a period of sustained leg extension and contraction of *m. Vastus lateralis.*

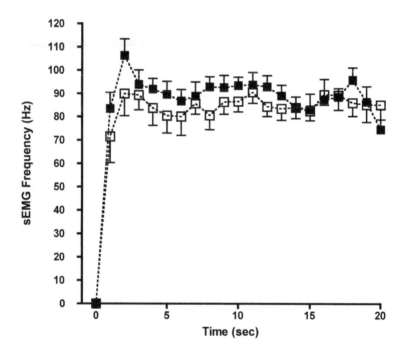

Fig. 4. The recorded sEMG signal from *m. Vastus lateralis* of uremic patients taken prior to (■) and after a 16 week programme of strength training (□). Recordings, which represent a 20 second period of sustained leg lift, were taken at a sampling rate of 40,000 data samples per second, using an impedance of 200 MΩ and a high- and low-pass filter of 3 Hz and 500 Hz, respectively. Values represent the Mean ± SEM of 8 patients.

Our investigation of muscle performance in the uremic patients also included a sEMG recording of *m. Vastus lateralis* taken during a period of dynamic contraction (see Fig. 5).

Clinical Implications of Muscle-Tendon & -Force Interplay: Surface Electromyography Recordings of
m. vastus lateralis in Renal Failure Patients...

73

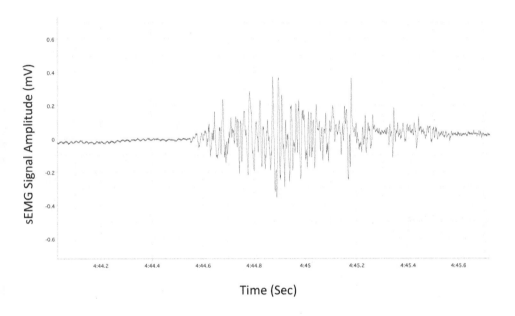

Fig. 5. The results of a dynamic muscle strength test involving a knee extension with 1 RM.
This figure illustrates a sEMG recording taken from *m. Vastus lateralis* at a recording speed of
40,000 data samples per second. Note the burst of power as the leg is extended. This sEMG
signal was analyzed in terms of its peak-to-peak amplitude (mV) and its inherent frequency
(Hz).

Both the dynamic and the isometric sEMG signal were analyzed in terms of their inherent
frequency and their amplitude. Recordings taken after a period of 16 weeks of strength
training "Re-test" were then compared with "Baseline" pre-training levels, and the results
are shown below in Table 1.

Dynamic 1RM 1. Sec			
Parameter	*Baseline*	*Re-test*	*P*
Frequency (Hz)	71 ± 11	71 ± 6	NS
Amplitude (mV)*	309 ± 81	571 ± 71	0.017
Dynamic 1RM 1. sec/kilo			
Frequency/kilo (Hz/Kg)	1.3 ± 0.2	0.9 ± 0.1	NS (0.093)
Amplitude/kilo (mV/Kg)*	6.2 ± 2.4	7.2 ± 1.1	NS

Isometric 50% 1RM 20 sec			
Parameter	*Baseline*	*Re-test*	*P*
Frequency Peak (Hz)	107 ± 6	102 ± 5	NS
Amplitude Peak (mV)*	350 ± 104	568 ± 86	NS
Frequency Mean (Hz)	89 ± 5	85 ± 5	NS
Amplitude Mean (mV)*	273 ± 83	396 ± 54	NS
Isometric 50% 1RM 20 sec/kilo			
Frequency Peak/kilo (Hz/Kg)	3.7 ± 0.5	2.6 ± 0.4	0.017
Amplitude Peak/kilo (mV/Kg)*	14.8 ± 6.6	14.2 ± 2.3	NS
Frequency Mean/kilo (Hz/Kg)	3.0 ± 0.3	2.2 ± 0.3	0.017
Amplitude Mean/kilo (mV/Kg)*	11.6 ± 5.2	10.1 ± 1.7	NS

Table 1. The response of *m Vastus lateralis* to a period of 16 weeks of strength exercise training in uremic patients. Data are presented as uncorrected values *versus* values corrected for the weight lifted (per kilo) by the patients. Note that sEMG correction for individual variation in terms of the weight lifted has a huge effect on the results, highlighting the fact that signal analysis can affect the interpretation of the recordings. Values represent the Mean ± SEM of n=8 haemodialysis patients. * indicates x 1000.

2.7 Discussion

The first large-scale studies of the physical capacity of patients with chronic renal failure were performed at the end of the 1970´s as reviewed by Laville & Fouque (1995). It was noted that 50% of patients requiring dialysis had stopped their professional activity as a result of chronic renal failure, attributed to coronary (15% of patients), cardiovascular (23%), and bone or muscle (24%) related conditions (Evans et al., 1985).

In a recent study involving patients on haemodialysis, *in vivo* measurements of muscle function were made using sEMG (Harrison et al., 2006). The sEMG frequency recorded prior to dialysis was generally found to be abnormal, when compared with a normal range of 2nd *dorsal interosseous* muscles of the hand and on the thigh *m. Vastus lateralis*. This study also revealed a clear benefit of haemodialysis in terms of sEMG frequency of the 2nd *dorsal interosseous* muscle (Harrison et al., 2006). Moreover, these authors found that the *in vivo* analysis of sEMG changes with a session of haemodialysis seemed to be limited to relatively fast-twitch muscles, a finding that was supported by a study of isolated rat *extensor digitorum longus* muscle, in which changes in the uremic environment were shown to exert a rapid loss of contractile force (Harrison et al., 2006).

In the present study, the combined graphs and table show that a period of exercise training results in an improved sEMG amplitude with very little change to the signal frequency. This finding, which indicates that a period of exercise training in these patients results in the ability to lift more weight (kilos), may be due to enhanced spatial summation (Henneman et al., 1965) - that is to say an increased and more synchronized recruitment of motor units. However, a considerable degree of individual variation is masked by this data set, and upon correction of the sEMG amplitude and frequency data for the weight in kilos used under training, a different interpretation is arrived at. Suddenly, signal analysis designed to remove an element of individual variation from the data now reveals that a period of exercise training induces an increase in sEMG signal frequency, and not an alteration in sEMG amplitude. It has to be said though, that this form of signal analysis reveals a finding that is more consistent with what is known to occur during the initial period following commencement of exercise training. What is observed is an improvement in neuro-muscular recruitment and activation "coordination" that typically precedes fibre and vascular changes "hypertrophy". Indeed, this conclusion is supported by the fact that looking at the histology of the fibres, we have not found any significant changes in fibre, cross-sectional area with the 16 week period of strength training in biopsies taken from *m. Vastus lateralis* in these patients (data not shown).

Of course recordings of sEMG from muscles of such patients are not without problem, and the interpretation of such data should not be made without careful consideration. In Figures 1 & 2 we identified a number of factors that can affect sEMG recordings, and in terms of uremic patients perhaps the most important would be as follows;

Fig. 1: **Causative** – active motor units, motor unit firing rate (synchronization) & fibre diameter

Intermediate – volume of muscle detected (fibre diameter) & conduction velocity

Deterministic – active motor units, detected motor units, motor unit action potential amplitude, motor unit action potential duration, recruitment & stability

Fig. 2: Diameter of muscle fibres, conduction velocity of muscle fibres & blood flow

In uremic patients one finds that ion imbalances and the build up of toxic compounds, confounded by other health issues and the effects of medication, affect neuro-muscular recruitment and activation. The effect is that neural conduction velocity is impaired, that fewer motor units tend to be active, and when active they often reveal action potentials that are of long duration and consequently of small amplitude. More long-term changes with uremia also include an atrophy of muscle fibres and a reduction in vascularisation, which will affect causative factors as well as intermediate factors, and furthermore reduce the blood flow to the contracting muscle fibres.

With strength training, it seems that a natural loss of synchronization and recruitment of motor units as the uremia progresses can be reversed. As mentioned earlier, we have not seen any changes in fibre size, and it therefore seems that the improved sEMG signal, which is supported by an improved physical function determined with a sit-to-stand test (data not shown), is due not to an increase in the number or size of active fibres, but rather a better control of those already working fibres.

3. Tendinopathy study

3.1 Introduction

The Achilles tendon is one of the most frequently injured tendons of the body due to trauma and overuse – very often in young or middle-aged, physically active subjects (Alfredson et al., 2000; Cook 2009). This arises, most likely, from muscle force in the gastrocnemius being trained to develop an extremely rapid and high level of force without being compensated by equally rapid changes in the Achilles tendon (Olesen et al., 2006; Holm et al., 2009). Although adaptation of tendons has been demonstrated (Langberg et al., 2007; Couppé et al., 2009), this adaption is slower than the development of a stronger muscle, and the tendon does not possess the dimensions necessary to accommodate such rapid increases in force production, and the result will very often be damage to the tendon structure or partial/complete rupture (Hess, 2010).

A number of systemic diseases are also known to be associated with general defects in matrix metabolism and structure that compromise tendon strength and elasticity, moreover the term 'spontaneous tendon rupture' is being used on a more regular basis in both the sports- and work-environments (Järvinen et al., 2001). Indeed, despite the fact that the Achilles tendon is the strongest tendon in the human body, there are increasing numbers of cases of overload of the Achilles tendon, both associated with sports as well as to work-related situations. It is estimated that the most common healthcare problem in Denmark is muscular-skeletal, accounting for approximately 15 % of all diseases (Ekholm et al., 2006). In spite of the extent of the problem not much is at present known about the etiology and pathogenesis of chronic tendon pain. The cause of the lack of knowledge within the area is primarily due to several limiting factors. First, that the early development of tendinopathy is unsymptomatic (Fredberg & Stengaard-Pedersen, 2008). Second, the establishment of a human tendinopathy model is deemed unethical. A few animal studies have been performed using an overuse protocol developed by Soslowsky and colleagues (Scott et al., 2007; Perry et al., 2005; Soslowsky et al., 2002), where rats ran with a velocity of 17m/minute, 5 days/week, 1 hour/day, either uphill or downhill for a period of between 2-16 weeks. In such experiments, a decreased collagen fiber organization and increased numbers of cell nuclei were observed (Soslowsky et al., 1996; Glazebrook et al., 2008). Yet, exactly how the tendon manages the active tension transfer from muscle to bone and if this tension transfer is affected by tendinopathy remains unclear. Thus, a form of assessment or a technique that could detect potentially damaging changes in a tendon very early on, and in so doing prevent muscle dysfunction, would be of great benefit.

It is with this point in mind, that we have investigated Achilles tendon parameters in combination with the contractile profile of *m. Gastrocnemius* in a number of healthy sports subjects, as a way of increasing the current knowledge of the ways in which tendon adapts to the mechanical loading associated with running/jogging. Our approach has been to better understand the active participation of tendons in the tension transfer from muscle to bone, and in order to achieve this goal we have returned to the topic of recording artefacts to see if they might not be used to some advantage.

3.2 Subjects

Healthy subjects were recruited from www.forsøgsperson.dk. Inclusion criteria were; no current tendon injury issues, regular training and ability to complete 60 minutes running on a treadmill. In total 8 subjects were examined (5 males; 3 females). The average age was 31

Clinical Implications of Muscle-Tendon & -Force Interplay: Surface Electromyography Recordings of
m. vastus lateralis in Renal Failure Patients...

77

years (24-40) and average weight of was 74 kg (54-85). All had a BMI between 19 and 25, i.e. normal weight. All participants gave their informed consent and the protocol was approved by the Copenhagen and Frederiksberg Municipalities ethical committee (H-2-2010-121).

3.3 sEMG recordings, measurements and analyses

The study used both a single and a double differential electrode configuration, with electrodes (N-00-S & R-00-S; Blue Sensor R, Medicotest A/S, Ølstykke, Denmark) configured as described previously (Harrison et al., 2006). sEMG recordings were taken *via* an ML 131 amplifier connected to a PowerLab 4/25T A/D converter (AD Instruments, Chalgrove, Oxfordshire, UK) with a further connection to a Mac PowerBook Air with Chart v. 5.5.6 Software, Peak Parameters and Spike Histogram extensions. Input impedance was 200 MΩ differential, and a high- and a low-pass filter of 3 Hz and 500 Hz, respectively, were used. Sampling speed was set to 40,000 per second.

Recordings were taken from the vastus lateralis of the left leg, following the guidelines laid out in the *European Recommendations for Surface ElectroMyoGraphy* as detailed by the SENIAM project (Hermens et al., 1999). Differential recordings of sEMG signals were made *via* surface electrodes from the *vastus lateralis*, as described in detail previously. Information of any expected electromyography performance results were not divulged, and subjects were not allowed to follow their sEMG recordings on the computer screen in real time. The recordings were carried out during 60 minutes treadmill running at a velocity of around 10 km/hour. The recorded sEMG signal was assessed as described previously (Harrison et al., 2006) in terms of signal frequency (Hz) and peak-to-peak amplitude (V), using Chart analysis software (AD Instruments, Chalgrove, Oxfordshire, UK).

3.4 Statistics

Data are presented as means plus and minus the standard error of the means (SEM). All tests were two-tailed and significance was deemed to be at $P \leq 0.05$.

3.5 Results

The results, (see Fig. 5 & 6), show that for lateral and medial *m.Gastrocnemius*, there is a pattern of sEMG signal parameter change over a 60 minute run/jog. After a few minutes of adjustment to a steady running/jogging rhythm, the sEMG mean amplitude becomes fairly stable, only showing signs of fatigue during the last ten minutes. It is likely that there is a fibre type distribution difference between the lateral and medial heads of *m.Gastrocnemius* as the lateral head increases slightly in sEMG frequency, while the amplitude decreases as the run/jog proceeds, whilst the medial head shows the reverse trend.

Of more importance from our perspective is the measurement of the sEMG to tendon artefact peak (ΔmSec), which remains very stable and uniform throughout the entire run/jog (see Fig. 6 & 7).

3.6 Discussion

In a recent paper written by De Luca and colleagues (2010) the authors address the issue of inevitable noise contamination of sEMG signals taken from muscles. Such noise originates from the skin-electrode interface, the electronics used to amplify the recorded signal, and a number of external sources (see Figs. 1 & 2). De Luca and colleagues focused on the low-frequency part of the recorded sEMG spectrum and proposed a number of approaches that can be taken to refine the recorded signal in a clinical setting (De Luca et al., 2010).

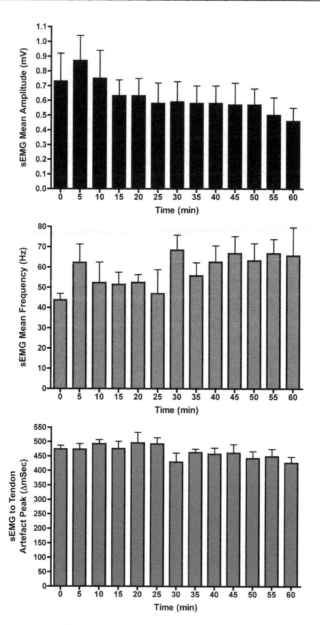

Fig. 6. The mean recorded sEMG signal from *m. Gastrocnemius* (Lateral Head) of healthy subjects – Upper Panel: Amplitude (mV), Middle Panel: Frequency (Hz) and Lower Panel: sEMG to Tendon Artefact Peak (ΔmSec). Recordings, which represent 5 minute interval means of a 60 minute run/jog at 11-13 km/hr, were taken at a sampling rate of 40,000 data samples per second, using an impedance of 200 MΩ and a high and low pass filter of 3 Hz and 500 Hz, respectively. Values represent the Mean ± SEM of 8 subjects.

Clinical Implications of Muscle-Tendon & -Force Interplay: Surface Electromyography Recordings of
m. vastus lateralis in Renal Failure Patients...

79

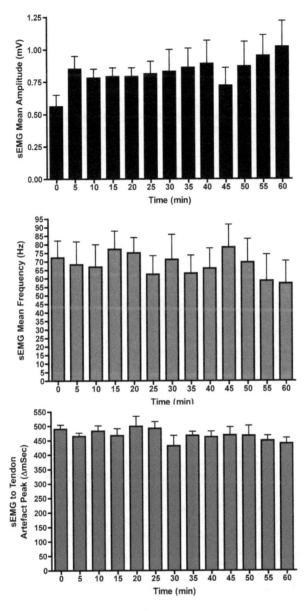

Fig. 7. The mean recorded sEMG signal from *m. Gastrocnemius* (Medial Head) of healthy
subjects – Upper Panel: Amplitude (mV), Middle Panel: Frequency (Hz) and Lower Panel:
sEMG to Tendon Artefact Peak (ΔmSec). Recordings, which represent 5 minute interval
means of a 60 minute run/jog at 11-13 km/hr, were taken at a sampling rate of 40,000 data
samples per second, using an impedance of 200 MΩ and a high and low pass filter of 3 Hz
and 500 Hz, respectively. Values represent the Mean ± SEM of 8 subjects.

However, a good working knowledge of the artefacts one can encounter when recording a sEMG signal in a clinical setting can also provide a recording opportunity, which researchers may wish to exploit rather than eradicate. Typically, one finds that movement artefacts represent a large proportion of the recorded signal at low spectrum frequencies (60% or more) (De Luca et al., 2010). Here, one may envisage that just such a movement artefact could be of importance and use when assessing muscle:tendon interactions. Indeed, our results, obtained with healthy controls, show that just such a recorded movement artefact taken from the Achilles tendon of individuals whilst running/jogging can be used successfully in connection with a sEMG signal recording from both heads of *m. Gastrocnemius*.

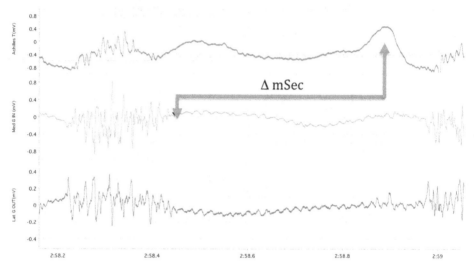

Fig. 8. The results of a 10 km/hr jog on Achilles tendon (upper panel) and both the medial head (middle panel) and lateral head (lower panel) of *m. Gastrocnemius*. The sEMG recording was from the right leg and at a recording speed of 40,000 per second per channel. Note, that after the synchronized bursts of power in the medial and lateral heads of Gastrocnemius a rise in the Achilles tendon signal to a maximum follows, after a delay of some 430 mSec, and this is again followed by a rapid fall back to resting levels. This deflection in the Achilles tendon trace is, however, merely a recording artefact representing the movement of the tendon under tension relative to the electrodes on the skin. The sEMG signal was analyzed in terms of its peak-to-peak amplitude (mV) and its inherent frequency (Hz).

The Achilles tendon is one of the most frequently injured tendons of the body due to trauma and overuse – very often in young or middle-aged, physically active subjects (Alfredson et al., 2000; Cook 2009). However, a recent study has shown that many inactive and often obese people develop tendinopathy (Gaida et al., 2008). Furthermore, one could easily imagine that tendinopathy in such individuals will result in these patients becoming even more inactive and therefore even more overweight. The question that then arises is how does muscle force affect the tendon tissue, when the tissue is overloaded either chronically as with obesity, or very frequently as with elite athletes. Muscle force in the gastrocnemius can be trained to develop an extremely rapid and high level of force, which may not always

Clinical Implications of Muscle-Tendon & -Force Interplay: Surface Electromyography Recordings of
m. vastus lateralis in Renal Failure Patients...

81

be met by equally rapid changes in the Achilles tendon (Olesen et al., 2006; Holm et al., 2009). Although adaptation of tendons has been demonstrated (Langberg et al., 2007; Couppé et al., 2009) the tendon does not possess the dimensions necessary to accommodate such rapid increases in force production, with the result that damage, often to the tendon structure or partial/complete rupture, occurs. Thus, an understanding of the active participation of tendons in the tension transfer from muscle to bone may lead to more optimal and effective treatment of tendinopathy – perhaps through further studies of the sEMG to tendon artefact peak.

Recent *in vivo* studies utilizing ultrasound imaging have shown that the human Achilles tendon undergoes a pattern of rapid lengthening and shortening during the stance phase of running (Lichtwark et al., 2007). Such a change in the tendon has a clear benefit in terms of the return of elastic energy stored in the Achilles tendon to the muscle, making the muscle:tendon unit largely free of metabolic costs. Another advantage of this change is that the Achilles tendon enables *m. Gastrocnemius* fascicles to remain nearly isometric for a large part of each stance (Ishikawa et al., 2007). Combined these changes greatly enhance the efficiency of this muscle:tendon interface.

Creep is defined as the lengthening of an elastic structure held under constant tension, or in other words an increasing lengthening per contraction cycle (Ker et al., 2000). To date, some scientists believe that tendon is capable of creep during periods of constant loading (Ker et al., 2000; Maganaris et al., 2002). However, increased lengthening for a given force as explained by creep would necessitate a reduction in tendon stiffness. Moreover, just such a creep, should it exist in human tendon, must most likely be detectable during the course of a run. In just such an experiment Farris and colleagues (2011) recently documented that the loading experienced during a single bout of running had no effect on the stiffness of the Achilles tendon, and that its properties remained stable throughout the period of activity – a finding that argues strongly against the existence of creep in loaded human tendons.

Looking at our results (see Fig. 6 & 7) for the sEMG to tendon artefact peak, we find that throughout a 60 minute run/jog there are no signs of a change in the time interval between the onset of muscle contraction with the initiation of the sEMG signal in both the lateral and medial heads of *m. Gastrocnemius* in healthy subjects. This confirms the findings of Farris et al., (2011), lending weight to the fact that Achilles tendon properties remain stable throughout a period of activity. Keeping this in mind, the tendon artefact would seem to be a useful tool, rather than something that should be filtered out of the recording, enabling the assessment of tendon inflammation and/or damage at an early stage, thus avoiding muscle dysfunction.

Indeed, the sEMG to tendon artefact peak has been found to be very consistent between individuals in the healthy subject group. The delta mSec value indicates the elasticity of the tendon as it interacts with the contracting muscle, absorbing the muscle force and transferring it gradually and smoothly over to the bone and the ankle joint. This should not be confused with creep, which is a change in tendon length once loaded. Rather the recorded artefact illustrates the development of tension/loading within a healthy tendon as muscle contraction proceeds and tendon loading approaches a maximum. Consequently, if an Achilles tendon is damaged and seriously inflamed, one would expect it to have less elasticity and a lower maximum load upon muscle contraction, which would be observed as a much lower delta value. Preliminary data with a few subjects with tendon injuries supports this idea (data not shown).

As stated earlier, recordings of sEMG from leg muscles of healthy subjects, as well as from injured individuals with tendinopathy, are not without problem, and the interpretation of such data should not be made without careful consideration. In Figures 1 & 2 we identified a number of factors that can affect sEMG recordings, and in terms of running/jogging and tendinopathy perhaps the most important would be as follows;

Fig. 1: **Causative** – motor point, tendon, active motor units, motor unit firing rate, acid build-up & blood flow
Intermediate – conduction velocity
Deterministic – active motor units, motor unit firing rate, detected motor units, motor unit action potential amplitude, motor unit action potential duration, recruitment & stability

Fig. 2: Intra-muscular temperature, conduction velocity of muscle fibres & blood flow

In the individuals examined in this section, without doubt the biggest issues to be addressed in terms of a stable sEMG recording are those of lead movement and the release of sweat, which affects electrode adhesion and stable localization. We have sought to reduce lead movement and signal noise arising from the recording cables swinging and moving during running/jogging by asking participants to wear net stockings which serve to hold the cables in place close to the leg and thereby prevent lead movement noise. The second issue of sweat accumulation under the recording electrodes as individuals begin to warm up during the 60 minute run/jog is not so easily solved. We have chosen to use a self-adhesive and elastic tape to ensure that the recording electrodes do not move appreciably, and have cooled the environment in which the run/jog takes place. Nevertheless, in some instances these precautions are not adequate and a degree of sEMG signal noise is unavoidable.

Among the other confounding factors affecting the sEMG signal are parameters closely associated with the level and duration of the exercise itself. As metabolites are used by contracting fibres there is an inevitable acidification close to the muscle membrane which has the advantage of initially improving blood flow through the displacement of K^+, which serves to induce vasodilatation. However, it is known that a build up of H^+ ions close to muscles results in a loss of excitability. Thus a period of exercise over time will affect such parameters as the number of active motor units, the blood flow, and the intra-muscular temperature – the later having an impact on the conduction velocity of muscle fibres.

4. General discussion

As already stated at the start of this manuscript, surface electromyography as a technique offers a safe, quick, pain-free, non-invasive and repeatable way of assessing the physiological processes which cause muscles to generate force and produce movement. It is for this reason that it must be seen as *"a tempting muse"*. As to the critique that *"it is too easy to use and consequently too easy to abuse"* this is surely unfair. It seems to us that if sEMG is being abused as a technique then it is because those using the technique do not fully understand the factors comprising the recorded signal and, as a consequence, do not take the time to assess their results in a critical fashion. One would rarely make a diagnosis of an illness based on just one symptom – the patient has a fever so it must be malaria – and in just the same way, sEMG should be used as a technique alongside other forms of assessing physical function e.g. circulation, muscle strength, Quality of Life etc.

The strength of ones scientific judgement lies surely with a detailed knowledge of any particular technique. In this way, a working understanding of the sEMG signal, its low and high frequency spectrum, and the causes of noise and artefacts, can only serve to reduce the

Clinical Implications of Muscle-Tendon & -Force Interplay: Surface Electromyography Recordings of
m. vastus lateralis in Renal Failure Patients...

83

risk of abuse of this technique. Used alongside other assessment tools for judgment of an individual's health, sEMG will support and help towards validation of a diagnosis, and hopefully give directions towards the optimal form of treatment. In the case of tendinopathy, the described tendon artefact suddenly changes from being an artefact – which is something often considered as disturbance – to becoming the reliable measure for tendon condition.

One should not, however, ignore the fact that surface electromyography has a number of limitations that must be understood and corrected for, if meaningful measurements are to be obtained (De Luca, 1993; Hermens et al., 1999, Seniam 1999). In a memorial lecture at the International Society for Biomechanics in 1993, Carlo J. De Luca clearly outlined the inherent problems associated with surface electromyography and provided recommendations for electrode configuration, placement, signal sampling and recording (De Luca, 1993). Later a complete set of guide lines were given by the SENIAM initiative (Hermens et al., 1999). In the examples given here, these guidelines were followed closely in both studies.

Besides the technical aspects of ensuring an accurate sEMG signal recording from a muscle, one should also consider the biological aspects that affect signal parameters, most of which are beyond the recorders control. Here one should pay particular attention to factors that might cause muscle fatigue/weakness as a result of a progressive illness (e.g. uremia) or as the consequence of a period of exercise (e.g. running/jogging).

The aetiology of muscle fatigue is a particularly important question, as the losses in force, velocity and power that define fatigue often lead to serious limitations in muscle and whole body performance (Fitts, 1994). Fatigue results from the effects of multiple factors, which makes unequivocal identification of causative agents a difficult task. It is, however, known that force production is inhibited by a build-up in both P_i and H^+, two products that are known to change with a period of intense exercise with P_i increasing from 5 to 30 or 40 mM, and intracellular pH declining from 7.0 to 6.2 (Thompson & Fitts 1992; Fitts, 1994). Moreover, such changes not only affect force production in fast-twitch muscles, they also reduce cross-bridge interactions due to a changed ionic environment (Metzger & Moss, 1990), leading to a fatigue-induced drop in tension. In uremic patients, a clear reduction in phosphate is often noted after dialysis (48% reduction $P<0.01$) from a value of 1.85 mmol/l (normal adult range of 0.8-1.5 mmol/l). It is also known that alterations in sarcolemma function induce muscle fatigue by preventing cell activation (Sjøgaard, 1990). Indeed, it has been shown that exposure of muscles to a high extracellular K^+ concentration gives rise to depolarization of muscle fibres and results in a loss of contractility (Fitts, 1994), particularly when this is associated with a simultaneous reduction in extracellular Na^+ concentration (Nielsen & Overgaard, 1996).

In an earlier study by the authors investigating recorded interference EMG signals in the hand muscle *2nd dorsal interosseous* of uremic patients under a period of voluntary contraction, it was shown that a significant increase in the deterministic factor "mean signal frequency" occurred when one compared post- to pre-dialysis values (Harrison et al., 2002). These findings, which indicate an inhibitory effect of the uremic state prior to dialysis on the number of recordable events from this particular muscle, are unlikely to be affected by such problems as detection volume of the recording electrodes or by cross-talk from adjacent muscles, as the size and position of this muscle would exclude such issues. It therefore seems realistic to assume, that a haemodialysis session removes some form of inhibition at the level of; 1) the motor nerve e.g. K^+ or so called "middle molecules" with a molecular weight range of 500-2000 Daltons (Bostock et al., 2004), 2) the motor endplate, and 3) the muscle fibre, or any combination of these three. Moreover, the aforementioned study found that one of the largest changes in plasma values in patients undergoing dialysis was that of inorganic phosphate.

The exact mechanism of P_i on force production remains to be elucidated but one might speculate that the increased myoplasmic P_i may decrease force production by direct action on cross-bridge function, or change the distances in the filament lattice due to different ion binding to the filaments (Naylor et al., 1985; Bartels et al., 1985), alternatively increased P_i may inhibit the ATP driven sarcoplasmic Ca^{2+} uptake, such that less Ca^{2+} would be available for release, leading to a decline in force (Duke & Steele, 2000).

In the case of studies involving uremic patients this change in distribution of ions over the cell membrane between dialyses may very well affect the measured sEMG, showing most effect of training right after dialysis. Since each patient is assessed against themselves, this should not affect the overall effect of training, although the true maximal effect may be higher than that seen here.

Likewise, the changes seen in the runners/joggers over a 60 minute exercise period may very well be due to changes in ion balance over the muscle cell membrane. However, whilst this is a valid point with regard to muscle measurements, it has no importance in terms of the use of bipolar recording electrodes to assess tendon function, since this constitutes an artefact, which is independent of a change in frequency and/or amplitude.

5. Conclusions

What can be safely concluded from these results are that direct sEMG recordings can be used as part of an assessment package for weak patient groups with musculo-skeletal problems due to the following two facts. First, that sEMG is quick and painless, making the method well tolerated by weaker patient groups like the uremic patients. Although the method at present is not very specific, it may still be preferential if a clear procedure for measurements and interpretation of data can be set up. The areas to consider are the noise issues, cross-talk between fibres and muscle selection, electrode placement etc. Second, that sEMG is cheap and easily available in a clinical setting, as long as clear guidelines about measurements, data handling and interpretation for the selected setting are available.

Moreover, sEMG represents a trustworthy and reliable means of gaining an insight into muscle function/dysfunction, particularly when used in conjunction with other diagnostic tools.

In the case of uremic patients, sEMG correlates well with such forms of functional assessment as the "stand chair test" and the "Quality of Life Questionnaire – KDQOL-SF-36" (Heaf et al., 2010), and during periods of exercise training there is a significant effect on sEMG frequency and amplitude, indicating a clear improvement in coordination.

As for tendinopathy, it can be concluded from the present results that the application of non-invasive surface electromyography on both heads of *m. Gastrocnemius* during a period of jogging on a treadmill not only shows the initial phase of muscle synchronization as an athlete warms up, and the relative contributions made by the medial and lateral heads of this muscle, it also gives an insight into Achilles tendon activity when combined with a differential recording above the point of insertion to the calcaneous. Furthermore, used with understanding and alongside other diagnostic tools, this technique has the potential to extend our understanding of the active participation of tendons in the tension transfer from muscle to bone.

6. Acknowledgement

We thank Birgitte Holle for her skilled technical assistance in connection with the sEMG recordings, and Prof. Per Aagaard, the Institute of Sports Science and Clinical Biomechanics,

Clinical Implications of Muscle-Tendon & -Force Interplay: Surface Electromyography Recordings of
m. vastus lateralis in Renal Failure Patients...

85

University of Southern Denmark for his most valuable critique of our clinical data. We are also most grateful to the Oak Foundation in terms of the financial support offered (EMB) in connection with this work.

7. References

Alfredson, H.; Ljung, B.O.; Thorsen, K. & Lorentzon, R. (2000) In vivo investigation of ECRB tendons with microdialysis technique – no signs of inflammation but high amounts of glutamate in tennis elbow. *Acta Orthopedica Scandinavica,* Vol. 71, pp. 475-479.

Allison, G.T. & Purdam, C. (2009). Eccentric loading for Achilles tendinopathy – strengthening or stretching? *British Journal of Sports Medicine,* Vol. 43, pp. 276-279.

Bartels, E.M. & Elliott, G.F. (1985). Donnan potentials from the A- and I-bands of glycerinated and chemically-skinned muscles, relaxed and rigor. *Biophysical journal,* Vol. 48(1), pp. 61-76.

Bernardi,M.; Solomonow,M.; Nguyen, G.; Smith, A & Baratta, R. (1996). Motor unit recruitment strategy changes with skill acquisition. *European Journal of Applied Physiology and Occupational Physiology,* Vol. 74, pp 52-59.

Bernardi, M.; Felici, F.; Marchetti, M.; Montellanico, F.; Piacentini, M.F. & Solomonow, M. (1999). Force generation performance and motor unit recruitment strategy in muscles of contralateral limbs. *Journal of Electromyography and Kinesiology,* Vol. 9, pp. 121-130.

Cook, J. (2009). In search of the tendon holy grail: predictable clinical outcomes. *British Journal of Sports Medicine,* Vol. 43, p. 235.

Couppé, C.; Hansen, P.; Kongsgaard, M.; Kovanen, V.; Suetta, C.; Aagaard, P.; Kjaer, M. & Magnusson, S.P. (2009) Mechanical properties and collagen cross- linking of the patellar tendon in old and young men. *Journal of Applied Physiology,* Vol. 107, pp. 880-886.

Day, S.J. & Hullinger, M. (2001). Experimental simulation of cat electromyogram: Evidence for algebraic summation of motor-unit action-potential trains. *Journal of Neurophysiology,* Vol. 86, pp. 2144-2158.

De Luca, C.J. (1997). The use of surface electromyography in biomechanics. *Journal of. Applied Biomechanics,* Vol. 13, pp. 135–163.

De Luca, C.J.; Gilmore, L.D.; Kuznetsov, M. & Roy, S.H. (2010). Filtering the surface EMG signal: Movement artifact and baseline noise contamination. *Journal of Biomechanics,* Vol. 43, pp. 1573-1579.

Ekholm, O.; Kjøller, M.; Davidsen, M.; Hesse, U.; Eriksen, L.; Christensen, A.I. & Grønbæk, M. (2006). Sundhed og sygelighed i Danmark 2005 & udviklingen siden 1987. *København: Statens Institut for Folkesundhed.*

Farina, D.; Merletti, R.; Enoka, R.M. (2004). The extraction of neural strategies from the surface EMG. *Journal of Applied Physiology,* Vol. 96, pp. 1486–1495.

Farris, D.J.; Trewartha, G. & McGuigan, M.P. (2011). The effects of a 30-min run on the mechanics of the human Achilles tendon. *European Journal of Applied Physiology.* DOI: 10.1007/s00421-011-2019-8.

Fredberg, U. & Stengaard-Pedersen, K. (2008). Chronic tendinopathy: tissue pathology, pain mechanisms, and etiology with a special focus on inflammation. *Scandinavian Journal of Medicine and Science in Sports,* Vol. 18(1), pp. 3-15.

Gaida, J.E.; Cook, J.L. & Bass, S.L. (2008). Adiposity and tendinopathy. *Disability and Rehabilitation,* Vol. 30(20-22), pp. 1555-1562.

Gerdle, B.; Karlsson, S.; Crenshaw, A.G. & Friden, J. (1997). The relationships between EMG and muscle morphology throughout sustained static knee extension at two submaximal force levels. *Acta Physiologica Scandinavica,* Vol. 160:, pp. 341–351.

Gerdle, B.; Wretling, M.L. & Henriksson-Larsen, K. (1988). Do the fibre-type proportion and the angular velocity influence the mean power frequency of the electromyogram. *Acta Physiologica Scandinavica* Vol. 134, pp. 341-346.

Gerdle, B.; Henriksson-Larsen, K., Lorentzon, R. & Wretling, M.L. (1991). Dependence of the mean power frequency of the electromyogram on muscle force and fibre type. *Acta Physiologica Scandinavica,* Vol. 142, pp 457-465.

Glazebrook, M.A.; Wright, J.R. Jr; Langman, M.; Stanish, W.D. & Lee, J.M. (2008). Histological analysis of Achilles tendons in an overuse rat model. *Journal of Orthopedic Research* Vol. 26, pp. 840-846.

Harrison, A.P. & Flatman JA. (1999). Measurement of force and both surface and deep M wave properties in isolated rat soleus muscles. *American Journal of Physiology - Regulative Integrative and Comparative Phy*siology, Vol. 277, pp. R1646–R1653.

Harrison, A.P.; Flatman, J.A.; Nielsen, A.H.; Eidemak, I.; Mølsted, S. & Unmack, M.A. (2002). Integrated surface electromyography (EMG) analysis in m. vastus lateralis and m. 2. dorsal interosseous in uremic patients. *Journal of Muscle Research and Cell Motility,* Vol. 23, p. 29.

Harrison, A.P.; Nielsen, A.H.; Eidemak, I.; Molsted, S. & Bartels, E.M. (2006). The uremic environment and muscle dysfunction in man and rat. *Nephron Physiology* , Vol. 103(1), pp. 33-42.

Heaf, J.G.; Mølsted, S.; Harrison, A.P.; Eiken, P.A.; Prescott, L. & Eidemak, I. (2010). Vitamin D, Surface Electromyography and Physical Function in Uraemic Patients. *Nephron,* Vol. 115, pp. c244-c250.

Henneman, E.; Somjen, G. & Carpente, D.O. (1965). Functional significance of cell size in spinal motor neurons. *Electroencephalography and Clinical Neurophysiology,* Vol. 19, pp. 533-580.

Hermens, H.J.; Freriks, B.; Merletti, R.;, Stegeman, D.; Blok, J.;, Rau, J.,; Disselhorstklug, C. & Hâgg, G. (1999). SENIAM 8 - european recommendations for surface electromyography. *Roessingh Research and Develop*ment b.v., Enschede, The Netherlands, 1999.

Hess, G.W. (2010). Achilles tendon rupture: a review of etiology, population, anatomy, risk factors, and injury prevention. *Foot Ankle Speciality.* Vol. 3(1), pp. 29-32.

Hogrel, J,Y. (2005). Clinical applications of surface electromyography in neuromuscular disorders. *Clinical Neurophysiol*ology, Vol. 35, pp. 59–71.

Holm, L.; van Hall, G.; Rose, A.J.; Miller, B.F.; Doessing, S.; Richter, E.A. & Kjaer, M. (2009). Contraction intensity and feeding affect collagen and myofibrillar protein synthesis rates differently in human skeletal muscle. *American Journal of Physiology Endocrinology and Metab*olisme, Vol. 298, pp. E257-E269.

Ishikawa, M.; Pakaslahti, J. & Komi, P.V. (2007). Medial gastrocnemius muscle behavior during human running and walking. *Gait and Posture,* Vol. 25, pp. 380-384.

Järvinen, T.A.; Kannus, P.; Paavola, M.; Järvinen, T.L.; Józsa, L. & Järvinen, M. (2001). Achilles tendon injuries. *Current Opinion in Rheumatology,* Vol. 13(2), pp. 150-155.

Karlsson, S. & Gerdle, B. (2001). Mean frequency and signal amplitude of the surface EMG of the quadriceps muscles increase with increasing torque – a study using the continuous wavelet transform. *Journal of Electromyography and Kinesiology,* Vol. 11, pp. 131–140.

Clinical Implications of Muscle-Tendon & -Force Interplay: Surface Electromyography Recordings of
m. vastus lateralis in Renal Failure Patients...

87

Keenan, K.G.; Farina, D.; Maluf, K.S.; Merletti, R. & Enoka, R.M.(2005). Influence of amplitude cancellation on the simulated surface electromyogram. *Journal of Applied Physiology*, Vol. 98, pp. 120-131.

Keenan, K.G.; Farina, D.; Merletti, R. & Enoka, R.M. (2006). Amplitude cancellation reduces the size of motor unit potentials averaged from the surface EMG. *Journal of Applied Physiology*, Vol. 100, pp. 1928-1937.

Ker, R.F.; Wang, X.T. & Pike, A.V.L. (2000). Fatigue quality of mammalian tendons. *Journal of Experimental Biology*, Vol. 203, pp. 1317-1327.

Komi, P.V. & Tesch, P. (1979). EMG frequency-spectrum, muscle structure, and fatigue during dynamic contractions in man. *European Journal of Applied Physiology and Occupational Physiology*, Vol. 42, pp. 41-50.

Krishnan, A.V.; Phoon, R.K.S.; Pussell, B.A.; Charlesworth, J.A.; Bostock, H. & Kiernan, M.C. (2005). Altered motor nerve excitability in end-stage kidney disease. *Brain*, Vol. 128, pp. 2164-2174

Kupa, E.J.; Roy, S.H.; Kandarian, S.C. & Deluca, C.J. (1995). Effects of muscle-fiber type and size on EMG median frequency and conduction-velocity. *Journal of Applied Physiology*, Vol. 79, pp. 23–32.

Langberg, H.; Ellingsgaard, H.; Madsen, T.; Jansson, J.; Magnusson, S.P.; Aagaard, P. & Kjaer, M. (2007). Eccentric rehabilitation exercise increases peritendinous type I collagen synthesis in humans with Achilles tendinosis. *Scandinavian Journal of Medicine and Science in Sports*, Vol. 17, pp.61-66.

Larsson, B.; Andersen, J.L.; Kadi, F.; Bjork, J. & Gerdle, B. (2002). Myosin heavy chain isoforms influence surface EMG parameters: a study of the trapezius muscle in cleaners with and without myalgia and in healthy teachers. *European Journal of. Applied Physiology*, Vol. 87, pp. 481–488.

Larsson, B.; Kadi, F.; Lindvall, B. & Gerdle, B. (2006). Surface electromyography and peak torque of repetitive maximum isokinetic plantar flexions in relation to aspects of muscle morphology. *Journal of Electromyography and Kinesiology*, Vol. 16, pp. 281–290.

Lichtwark, G.A.; Bougoulais, K. & Wilson, A.M. (2007). Muscle fascicle and series elastic element length changes along the length of the human gastrocnemius during walking and running. *Journal of Biomechanics*, Vol. 40, pp. 157-164.

Linssen, W.H.J.P.; Stegeman, D.F.; Joosten, E.M.G.; Binkhorst, R.A.; Merks, M.J.H.; Terlaak, H.J. & Notermans, S.L.H. (1991). Fatigue in type-I fiber predominance – a muscle force and surface EMG study on the relative role of type-I and type-II muscle-fibers. *Muscle & Nerve*, Vol. 14, pp. 829-837.

Maffulli, N. & Longo, U.G. (2008). How do eccentric exercises work in tendinopathy? An Editorial. *Rheumatology*, Vol. 47, pp. 1444-1445.

Maganaris, C.N. & Paul, J.P. (2002). Tensile properties of the in vivo human gastrocnemius tendon. *Journal of Biomechanics*, Vol. 35, pp. 1639-1646.

Merletti, R.; Knaflitz, M. & De Luca, C.J. (1992). Electrically evoked myoelectric signals. *Critical Reviews in Biomedical Engineering*, Vol. 19, pp. 293-340.

Meyer, A.; Tumilty, S. & Baxter, G.D. (2009). Eccentric exercise protocols for chronic non-insertional Achilles tendinopathy: how much is enough? A Review. *Scandinavian Journal of Medicine and Science in Sports*, Vol. 19, pp. 609-615.

Milnerbrown, H.S. & Miller, R.G. (1986). Muscle membrane excitation and impulse propagation velocity are reduced during muscle fatigue. *Muscle & Nerve*, Vol. 9, pp. 367-374.

Molsted, S.; Eidemak, I.; Sorensen, H.T. & Kristensen, J.H. (2004). Five months of physical exercise in hemodialysis patients: Effects on aerobic capacity, physical function and self-rated health. *Nephron,* Vol. 96(3), pp. c76-c82.

Molsted, S.; Eidemak, I.; Sorensen, H.T.; Kristensen, J.H.; Harrison, A.P. & Andersen, J.L. (2007). Myosin heavy-chain isoform distribution, fibre-type composition and fibre size in skeletal muscle of patients on haemodialysis. *Scandinavian Journal of Urology and Nephrology,* Vol. 41(6), pp. 539-545.

Moritani, T.; Nagata, A. & Muro, M. (1982). Electro-myographic manifestations of muscular electromyography. *Medicine and Science in Sports and Exercise,* Vol. 14, pp. 198-202.

Morrissey, D.; Roskilly, A.; Twycross-Lewis, R.; Isinkaye, T.; Screen, H.; Woledge, R. & Bader, D. (2011). The effect of eccentric and concentric calf muscle training on Achilles tendon stiffness. *Clinical Rehabilitation* , Vol. 25, pp. 238-247.

Naylor, G.R.S.; Bartels, E.M.; Bridgman, T.D. &.Elliott, G.F (1985). Donnan potential changes in rabbit psoas muscle in rigor. *Biophysical Journal,* Vol. 48(1), pp. 47-60.

Olesen, J.L.; Heinemeier, K.M.; Langberg, H.; Magnusson, S.P.; Kjaer, M. & Flyvbjerg, A. (2006). Expression, content, and localization of insulin-like growth factor I in human achilles tendon. *Connective Tissue Research,* Vol. 47, pp. 200-206.

Perry, S.M.; McIlhenny, S.E.; Hoffman, M.C. & Soslowsky, L.J. (2005). Inflammatory and angiogenic mRNA levels are altered in a supraspinatus tendon overuse model. Journal of Shoulder and Elbow Surgery, Vol. 14(1 Suppl S), pp. 79S-83S.

Scott, A.; Cook, J.L.; Hart, D.A.; Walker, D.C.; Duronio, V. & Khan, K.M. (2007). Tenocyte responses to mechanical loading in vivo: a role for local insulin-like growth factor 1 signaling in early tendinosis in rats. *Arthritis and Rheumatology,* Vol. 56, pp. 871-881.

Simpson, M.R. & Howard, T.M. (2009). Tendinopathies of the Foot and Ankle. *American Family Physician,* Vol. 80, pp. 1107-1114.

Solomonow, M.; Baten, C.; Smit, J.; Baratta, R.; Hermens, H.; Dambrosia, R. & Shoji, H. (1990). Electromyogram power spectra frequencies associated with motor unit recruitment strategies. *Journal of Applied Physiology,* Vol. 68, pp. 1177-1185.

Soslowsky, L.J.; Carpenter, J.E.; DeBano, C.M.; Banerji, I. & Moalli, M.R. (1996). Development and use of an animal model for investigations on rotator cuff disease. *Journal of Shoulder Elbow Surgery,* Vol. 5, pp. 383-392.

Soslowsky, L.J.; Thomopoulos, S.; Esmail, A.; Flanagan, C.L.; Iannotti, J.P.; Williamson, J.D. 3rd & Carpenter, J.E. (2002). Rotator cuff tendinosis in an animal model: role of extrinsic and overuse factors. *Annals of Biomedical Engineering,* Vol. 30, pp. 1057-1063.

Tesch, P.A.; Komi, P.V.; Jacobs, I.; Karlsson, J. & Viitasalo, J.T. (1983). Influence of lactate accumulation on EMG frequency-spectrum during repeated concentric contractions. *Acta Physiologica Scandinavica,* Vol. 119, pp. 61-67.

Turker, K.S. (1993). Electromyography – some methodological problems and issues. *Physical Therapy,* Vol. 73, pp. 698-710.

Tygesen, M.P. & Harrison, A.P. (2005). Nutritional restriction in utero programs postnatal muscle development in lambs. *Animal Science Journal,* Vol. 76, pp. 261–271.

Van der Worp, H.; van Ark, M.; Roerink, S.; Pepping, G.-J.; van den Akker-Scheek, I. & Zwerver, J. (2011). Risk factors for patellar tendinopathy: a systematic review of the literature. *British Journal of Sports Medicine,* Vol. 45, pp. 446-452.

Part 2

Signal Processing

6

Nonlinear Analysis of Surface Electromyography

Paul S. Sung
Korea University, Seoul,
Republic of Korea

1. Introduction

Electromyography (EMG) detects electrically or neurogically activated muscle cells on the basis of waveform characteristics from a recorded signal. EMG is useful for evaluating and recording movement abnormalities. The EMG signals can also detect neuromuscular activation level and recruitment order in addition to analyze the biomechanics of human or animal movement (De Luca, 1984; Furey, 1963). The EMG signals are generated based on superimposed motor action potentials during active movement. The myoelectric signals are the instantaneous algebraic summation of all electrical discharges produced by a contraction of the muscle fibers. Muscle fatigue is quantified using surface EMG signals based on the power spectrum which is the Fourier transform of EMG time series (Knowlton *et al.*, 1951; Mannion & Dolan, 1994; Mannion *et al.*, 1997c). Normal electrical source is a muscle membrane potential of approximately -90 mV, and measured EMG potentials range between less than 50 µV and up to 20 to 30 mV, depending on the muscle under observation (Herzog *et al.*, 1987; Nigg *et al.*, 1988). Typical repetition rate of muscle motor unit firing is approximately 7–20 Hz, depending on the size of the muscle, previous axonal damage, and other factors (Hoffmann, 1968; Rack & Ross, 1975). Therefore, the EMG range can be utilized in many clinical and biomechanical applications as a diagnostics tool for identifying neuromuscular diseases, assessing low back pain (LBP), kinesiology, and disorders of motor control. EMG signals are also used as a control signal for prosthetic devices such as prosthetic hands, arms, and lower limbs. It is unknown how the median frequency (MF) of an individual depends on posture, extent of physical activity prior to measurements, and other attributing factors. Such factors may influence the shift of the MF in the fatigue measurement, which is not a consistent indicator for injuries to low back muscles. Subjects with LBP have less endurance and thus smaller MF during sustained muscle contractions (Mannion *et al.*, 1997a; Roy *et al.*, 1997). The MF of the EMG signal is used to characterize physiological aspects of skeletal muscles. The signal from surface EMG is the instantaneous algebraic summation of action potentials from muscle fibers, and its power spectrum can be estimated from a fast Fourier transform of the signal.

Fourier transform is a linear analysis of a signal and gives the power spectrum $P(f)$ (Hobbie, 1997). A linear system is described mathematically by equations with oscillatory or exponentially growing solutions. In contrast, EMG time series have an irregular pattern so that the signal must be interpreted as "noise." The noise is due to the interaction between a particular muscle and all other biomechanical "units" of the body. In many cases, the power spectrum follows an algebraic dependence $P(f) \sim 1/f\alpha$. The case $\alpha=0$ corresponds to "white noise" while $\alpha=2$ characterizes diffusive Brownian motion. Therefore, the MF of the EMG power spectrum is sensitive to physiological manifestations of muscular dysfunction as an alternative assessment tool to identify muscle fatigue (Mannion *et al.*, 1997b; Roy *et al.*, 1997). However, there is a lack of research that compares this tool with other nonlinear measurements based on pain level or dysfunction.

During a fatiguing contraction, a compression of the power spectrum of the EMG signal to lower frequencies is typically observed (Lindstrom *et al.*, 1974). This phenomenon is measured during a contraction as a decrease in the MF of the EMG signal. Individuals with better endurance than others exhibit a less precipitous decay rate of the MF (Mannion *et al.*, 1997b). Thus, it would be necessary to compare the results between Shannon entropy levels of the EMG and MF of the spectral quantities following intervention to enhance outcome measurements.

Other results indicated that subjects with LBP show less fatigue than healthy subjects (Humphrey *et al.*, 2005; Mannion *et al.*, 2001). Thus, despite considerable efforts by many researchers, a link between MF and musculoskeletal pain/dysfunction remains elusive. Moreover, the surface EMG is not a scientifically acceptable tool for the diagnosis of pain/dysfunction, and further studies are recommended to assess the specificity and sensitivity of surface EMG (Pullman *et al.*, 2000). Therefore, a clinical diagnosis and evaluation of LBP is still elusive, and the efficacy of therapeutic intervention and assessment for LBP cannot be tested reliably.

The power spectrum analysis provides an objective and noninvasive assessment of muscle function since EMG changes are associated with fatigue (De Luca, 1984; Mannion *et al.*, 1997a). However, contradictory results have been reported in studies using EMG as an outcome measure. The power spectrum has a limited dynamic range, and the change of the MF does not reflect such long-time correlations. New methods must be designed to capture biologically important characteristics from noisy time series. Researchers using nonlinear time series analysis have developed several mathematical tools to reveal the presence of power-law time correlations.

Investigations of physiologic time series have led to the understanding that some degree of noise is necessary for the proper functioning of biological systems (Belair *et al.*, 1995b; Glass, 2001; Strogatz, 2001). These systems must respond to external stimuli that may vary both in strength and time scale by many orders of magnitude. The "degree of irregularity" of time series can be quantified by computing the (information) entropy of the signal. The time-dependent entropy from the surface EMG signal and the entropy of the signal is lower for subjects with LBP than for healthy subjects. Furthermore, the entropy increases rapidly for short times [$t < 10$ ms], reaches a plateau value for intermediate times [10ms $< t < 500$ ms], and then increases diffusely for long times [approximately 500 ms] (Belair *et al.*, 1995a). This behavior suggests that the plateau value is relevant for the physiology of skeletal muscles (Chialvo, 2002; Goldberger *et al.*, 2002a). In this chapter, some of these methods to surface EMG time series are discussed, and the potential use of these methods as a diagnostic tool for LBP are explored.

Therefore, the purpose of this chapter is to explore the potential use of nonlinear time series analysis as a tool for the clinical diagnosis of LBP or neuromuscular dysfunction, especially low back muscle fatigue. Of particular interest is a comparison between methods based on the power spectrum and nonlinear time series analysis of EMG signals. In order to compare quantities derived from the EMG signals, it is important to compare the different types of analyses including nonlinear time series between subjects with and without musculoskeletal dysfunction/pain. Specifically, it is important to record and analyze the EMG signals for a group of subjects with LBP and a control group of healthy subjects using spectral analysis and methods from nonlinear time series analysis. Secondly, the reliability of the results based on power spectrum analysis and nonlinear time series analysis of EMG signals for subjects with and without LBP needs to be investigated. Thirdly, it is necessary to determine the sensitivity of the analyses and the distribution of the values of the entropy for a group of subjects with and without LBP.

2. Clinical assessment of LBP

A clinical assessment of LBP is important as a diagnostic tool since we cannot distinguish subjects with genuine pain from those who fraudulently claim to suffer from pain (Chaffin, 1969). The potential cost to society from malingerers could be quite high. Additionally, the effectiveness of various rehabilitation interventions is difficult to assess without a clinical diagnosis of LBP. The interpretation of surface EMG data is not as reliable as that from needle EMG, for example. A clinical diagnosis based on surface EMG is desirable since it is widely accepted by the general population.

A clinical diagnosis of LBP using EMG should be based on properties of the signal that change drastically in the presence of pain/dysfunction. If this is the case, the observed quantities from subjects with LBP are expected to be different than those from subjects without LBP. Because a shift in the MF of the spectrum is explained by the change in the velocity of the action potential, it reflects a quantitative change of the signal during a fatiguing exercise. On the other hand, a change in the entropy of the signal reflects a qualitative change in the physiologic system.

Subjects with LBP often have reduced muscle strength and endurance, which compromises the functional capacity of the spine and increases the likelihood of re-injury (Cholewicki & VanVliet, 2002; Wilder et al., 1996). In most cases, a compression of the power spectrum of the EMG signal to lower frequencies is observed during a fatiguing contraction. This compression is the result of slower muscle fiber action potential propagation and an alteration in shape due to changes in the excitability of the muscle cell membrane (Lindstrom et al., 1974; Panjabi, 1992). These phenomena are referred to as "myoelectric manifestations of fatigue" and are typically seen during a prolonged muscle contraction. Individuals with better endurance are expected to exhibit a smaller shift of the MF (Mannion et al., 1997b; Mannion et al., 2001). It has been reported that subjects with LBP exhibit a larger shift of the MF than subjects without LBP (Mayer et al., 1989; Roy et al., 1989).

2.1 Noise in biological systems

The characterization of the power spectrum with a single frequency indicates that the time dependence of the signal is approximated by a simple oscillatory behavior. In contrast, the EMG signal looks irregular to the naked eye, and thus cannot be approximated by a periodic behavior. Seemingly irregular time series have been observed in many biological systems such as the electrocardiography signal of the human heartbeat, the electroencephalogram signal in instances of epilepsy and human gait, and others (Costa et al., 2003; Costa, 2002; Goldberger et al., 2002a).

It has recently been suggested that physiological time series contain "hidden information" (Goldberger *et al.*, 2002a). A biomechanical model of the human body emerges in which individual "units" interact in a nonlinear fashion such that feedback loops operate over long temporal and spatial ranges. This self-regulation leads to reduced variability which is important for maintaining physiological control of biological systems. For example, the prediction of homeostasis reveals that the output of a wide variety of systems, such as the normal human heartbeat, fluctuates in a complex manner even under resting conditions.

It is generally believed that the irregularity of the signal allows biological systems to respond to external disturbances that vary over a wide range of time scales. The velocity of the action potential determines the short-time behavior of the surface EMG signal. In contrast, the physiologic origin of its long-time behavior is unknown. It is not even clear whether observed fluctuations ("noise") in the signal are external or are intrinsic to the physiologic system. Intrinsic noise can be explained by the combined action of inhibitory and excitatory "units" or components of the system (Koppell, 2000). The presence of external fluctuations can have important consequences for complex systems. It has been shown, for example, that a system of oscillators can become synchronized, which may then explain the combined action of the entire system (Costa *et al.*, 2003).

It is not known which model of skeletal muscles explains the presence of intrinsic noise in the EMG signal. This is a common situation encountered in many studies of complex systems. Nonlinear time series analysis has developed numerous tools to distinguish nonlinear or chaotic behaviors within the system from external noise. For chaotic systems, the number of dynamic degrees of freedom can be determined from the signal that is (roughly) equal to the number of inhibitory and excitatory units in the system.

In nonlinear time series analysis, the characteristic behavior of a system is extracted from a mathematical analysis of the signal. The behavior of the signal is quantified using concepts and ideas borrowed primarily from statistical physics and signal processing. In particular, the information entropy has been proposed as a measure of the irregularity of the signal (Costa *et al.*, 2003; Costa, 2002; Goldberger *et al.*, 2002b; Pincus, 2001). A periodic signal and a complete irregular signal (or "white noise") have zero entropy. A random (or stochastic) signal with long-time correlations is characterized by a finite entropy, $S>0$. For a large variety of physiologic systems, it has been shown that dysfunction is associated with a decrease in the entropy of the time series. This suggests that physiological dysfunction leads to either complete order or excessive disorder.

2.2 Entropy of electromyography

In a mathematical description, the signal at (discrete) "time" n, x_n, is treated as a random, or stochastic, variable (Kantz, 2003; Sprott, 2003). It is assumed that the signal is "stationary," i.e., the quantity $\sum_{i=1}^{t} x_{n-1+i}$ does not depend on the initial time n. The mean-square displacement is then defined by $\Delta(t) = \langle [\sum_{i=1}^{t} x_{n-1+i}]^2 \rangle$, where the average is taken with respect to the n. If the signal at time n is uncorrelated with the signal at a different time m, $\langle x_n x_m \rangle = 0$, the mean-square displacement increases diffusively, $\Delta(t) \sim t$. This case is generally referred to as "white noise." In the presence of long-time correlations, $\langle x_n x_m \rangle \sim 1/|n-m|^\nu$ for some exponent $\nu>0$, fractional Brownian walk follows $\Delta(t) \sim t^{2H}$ (Mandelbrot, 1983). Here, the Hurst exponent is $H=2\nu+1$ with $0<H<0.5$ for sub-diffusive and $0.5<H<1$ for super-diffusive "behavior". The presence of long-time correlations implies that the signal has no characteristic time scales and looks the same on all time scales. In a certain mathematical limit, the mean-square displacement and the entropy are related to each other $S \sim \ln \Delta$.

The entropy reflects properties of the signal on many different time scales and, therefore, does not have a simple relationship with the velocity of the action potential. It follows that properties of the surface EMG signal obtained via nonlinear time series analysis are complementary to the analysis of the power spectrum. Entropy has many interdisciplinary applications as in aging psychology or macromolecular engineering (Allen *et al.*, 1998; Allen *et al.*, 2004). Regarding time series applications, biological time series are complex data that need to be distilled to useful information such as assessing an illness. Nonlinear analysis using fractal geometry and random walks theory proved to be useful in the analysis of a variety of time series such as correlations between global temperatures and solar activity (Scafetta & West, 2003), earthquake statistics (Scafetta & West, 2004), human heartbeat (Ivanov *et al.*, 1999), and shapes of red cells under flow stress (Korol & Rasia, 2003). Recently, nonlinear time series generated by the back muscles' electrical activity was investigated between subjects with and without LBP motivated by the need to develop an evaluation tool for LBP (Lee *et al.*, 2010; Sung *et al.*, 2005; Sung *et al.*, 2007a; Sung *et al.*, 2010).

Using random walk concepts, Collins and De Luca have studied the erratic motion of the center of pressure of a standing human body (Collins & De Luca, 1994; Collins & De Luca, 1995). They found a crossover from superdiffusive random walks for short times to subdiffusive random walks for longer times. In our entropic analysis of EMG time series from back muscles, we observed a crossover from subdiffusive, Hurst exponent $H \leq 0.5$, to self-organization, Hurst exponent $H \approx 0$. The Renyi entropy associated with diffusive processes grows linearly with the logarithm of time, and the rate of growth is independent of the Renyi parameter (Kaufman, 1985; Kaufman, 2007). The entropy is the rigorous measure of lack of information. The information, or Shannon, entropy for a particular experimental condition with a set of M possible outcomes is (Gage, 1992; S. Shannon, 1997):

$$S_{\text{information}} = -\sum_{j=1}^{M} p_j \ln(p_j) \tag{1}$$

where pj is the relative frequency of outcome #j. It is uniquely determined from the Khinchin axioms: (I) it depends on the probabilities p only; (II) the lowest entropy ($S = 0$) corresponds to one of the p's being 1 and the rest being zero (i.e., total information); (III) the largest value for the entropy is lnM and is achieved when all p's are equal to each other (i.e., the absence of any information); and (IV) S is additive over partitions of the outcomes. If the last axiom is relaxed to consider only statistically independent partitions, Renyi found that the information entropy is replaced by a one-variable function (Cybulski *et al.*, 2004):

$$S(\beta) = \frac{1}{1-\beta} \ln(\sum_{j=1}^{M} p_j^\beta) . \tag{2}$$

For $\beta = 1$, the Renyi entropy equals the Shannon entropy. The Renyi entropy is related to the Tsallis entropy which is central to the current massive research effort in nonextensive statistical mechanics (Vinga & Almeida, 2004).

In the continuum limit: $p_j \approx \rho(x,t)\Delta x$, where x is the random variable, e.g. displacement for random walker, and ρ is the probability distribution function. The actual experiment was conducted for measuring the electrical signal from back muscles (Sung *et al.*, 2005). Consider a time series x_t. Following Scafetta and Grigolini (Scafetta & Grigolini, 2002), the signal x_n was interpreted as a jump at time n. It was generated at all walks of time length t:

$$X_{m,t} = \sum_{j=0}^{t-1} x_{j+m}.$$ For a given time t, the ensemble of all the walks of time length t was

considered and distinguished from one another by the initial time m. The range of X was divided in M equal bins, and the probability of finding a walker at that location was estimated by using the fraction of all X that fall in the bin. The results were obtained for M = 500 bins. The entropies were computed using Eqs. (1) and (2). The numerical time series were analyzed searching for a logarithmic dependence of the entropy.

Figure 1 indicates the EMG time series from the right thoracic muscle of the healthy individual and the entropy associated with walks generated from the healthy right thoracic muscle EMG time series as a function of the logarithm of time. At short times, $t < 0.01$ s, the slope is 0.26, 0.32, 0.34 for the Renyi parameter β = 0, 1, 5 respectively. Since the fit was done on only ten data points, there is a large uncertainty for those values. Similar slope values were extracted from the EMG data from all the muscles (both sides of the thoracic and lumbar erector spinae) for both individuals (HEALTHY and LBP subjects). At longer times, for 0.01 s $< t <$ 1 s, the entropies exhibit a plateau. The plateau occurs at an entropy value well below the maximum possible entropy value lnM. Hence, it is not an artifact of the way we estimate the entropy; but it is an intrinsic property of the time series.

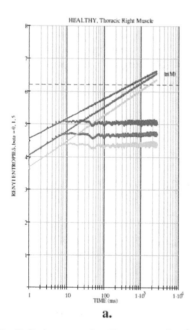
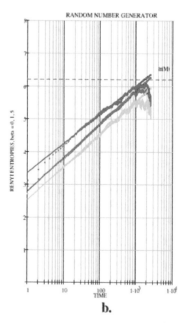

a.   b.

Fig. 1. Entropy vs. ln$t$. Top curve β = 0, middle curve β = 1, bottom curve β = 5. a. Subject without LBP for the right thoracic erector spinae muscle; b. Random number generator.

The entropy plateau corresponds to the Hurst exponent $H \approx 0$. The power spectrum $P(f) \sim f^{\alpha}$ with an exponent $\alpha = 2H +1 \approx 1$ follows $P(f) \sim 1/f$. Self-organization is generally associated with $1/f$ noise, and this is the reason why the entropy plateau can be interpreted as a manifestation of self-organization (Buldyrev et al., 2006). Qualitatively similar dependences were observed in the analysis of the erratic motion of the center of pressure of the human body (Collins & De Luca, 1994; Collins & De Luca, 1995). Though the details are not identical (e.g crossover time and slopes are different), we suspect that this type of crossover from large Hurst exponent random walks at short times to small Hurst exponent random walks at long times characterizes organized complex systems. In Figure 1b, the qualitatively different dependence of entropy on time exhibited by time series was generated with a commercial random number generator. The slopes of S versus $\ln t$ for the random number generator data are 0.38, 0.45, 0.44 for $\beta = 0, 1, 5$ respectively. These values are quite close to the Brownian diffusion value $H = \frac{1}{2}$. There is no plateau in the random number time series.

This comparison between the EMG data on one hand and random data on the other hand supports the idea that the system responsible for the back muscle signal is complex as opposed to noisy. The time evolution of entropy for EMG data also differs qualitatively from the time dependence of the entropy of chaotically advected tracers: the latter does not exhibit a crossover in time to self-organization, but it does exhibit a substantial dependence of the logarithmic amplitude on the Renyi parameter.

The entropy dependence on time constitutes a potential tool for differentiating between subjects with and without LBP. We show in Figure 2 below, side by side, graphs of the relative entropy $S/\ln(M)$ versus $\ln t$ from four erector spinae (right and left thoracic and right and left lumbar) muscles of a healthy male and a LBP male of the same age. In each case, we computed the entropy using $M = 500$ bins.

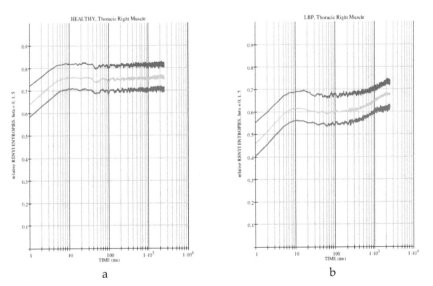

a   b

Fig. 2. Relative Entropy on lumbar right muscle vs. $\ln t$. Top $\beta = 0$, middle $\beta = 1$, bottom $\beta = 5$; a. Subject without LBP; b. Subject with LBP.

The plateau entropy is consistently higher for the healthy individual than for the LBP individual. A previous pilot study in our lab also demonstrated similar results involving ten healthy and ten LBP individuals, who were matched by gender, but not by age (Sung *et al.*, 2007b). The question of whether the plateau entropy constitutes a useful diagnostic tool for LBP needs further investigation with large groups of individuals matched by age, gender, body mass index, etc. It is worth emphasizing that Costa et al. and Chialvo argued based on heart time series that pathology is associated with less variability (lower entropy) as indicated in our study (Chialvo, 2002; Costa *et al.*, 2002).

To better understand the entropy time evolution, we show in Figure 3 the histograms used to determine the entropy for the left thoracic muscle of LBP subjects. In Figure 3a, we see the widening of the probability distribution with time corresponding to the entropy increase at short times $t < 10$ ms. In Figure 3b, the probability distribution is practically stationary corresponding to the entropy plateau at longer times 10 ms $< t <$ 500 ms. In Figure 3c, we show the probability distribution at $t = 1000$ ms, attempting to understand the increase in entropy apparent for $t > 500$ ms. We observe the occurrence of two peaks which may correspond to some sort of phase transition. In order to check this hypothesis, we computed the histogram using 66,000 data points rather than the 6,000 points window used in all other computations.

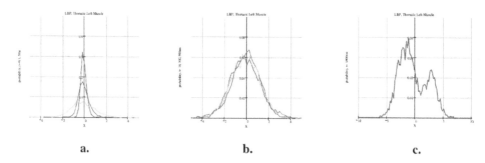

a.   b.   c.

Fig. 3. Probability distributions at short time, intermediate time, and long time for the thoracic left muscle in subjects with LBP at: (a) $t = 0, 1, 5$ms; (b) $t = 10, 100, 500$ms; (c) $t = 1000$ms.

We reduced the original time series to 6,000 entries by averaging over 10 consecutive entries of the original time series. We labeled the resulting time series as x_n, where the index n ('time') runs from 1 to 6,000. Nonlinear time series analysis assumes that the signal is stationary. To test this assumption, we calculated the mean and variance of 100 data points. The results for the subjects with and without LBP are shown in Figures 4A and 4B, respectively. Clearly, the EMG signal is stationary in both cases. Note that the average of the mean (μ) is nonzero, which reflects an offset in the calibration. For the numerical analysis below, we correct the offset by replacing x_n with $x_n - \mu$. For nonlinear systems, signals at different times are correlated as shown in a phase portrait where the signal x_{n+1} at time $n+1$ is plotted vs the signal x_n at time n.

For the subject without LBP (Figure 5A), the phase portrait has a circular shape. This portrait shows that the signals at consecutive times n and $n+1$ are statistically independent of each other. On the other hand, the phase portrait for the subject with LBP has the shape of an ellipse with the long axis directed along the diagonal (Figure 5B). The elliptical shape along the diagonal indicates the presence of correlations. Physicists have developed several

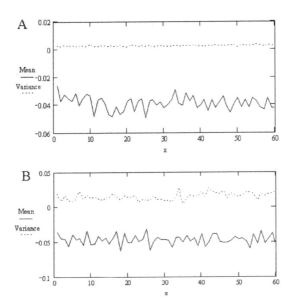

Fig. 4. Mean (solid line) and standard deviation (dashed line) for (A) subjects without and (B) subjects with LBP.

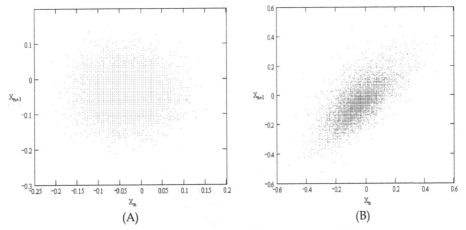

(A)   (B)

Fig. 5. Phase portrait of (A) subjects without and (B) subjects with LBP.

methods to quantify the complexity of time series. One method explores the connection with random walks, or Brownian motion (Denny & Gaines, 2000). To this end, we interpret the signal x_n as a jump at time n. It follows that the sum $X(t)=x_n+x_{n+1}+...+x_{n+t}$ is the displacement between times n and $n+t$. The average is zero $\langle X(t)\rangle=0$. The mean-square displacement is obtained by taking the square and then calculating the average with respect to the initial time n, $\Delta(t) = \langle X2(t)\rangle$. For deterministic motion, $\Delta(t) \sim t2$, while $\Delta(t) \sim t$ is for diffusion. In the general case, we write $\Delta(t) \sim t2h$ so that $0< h < 0.5$ and $0.5 < h< 1$ correspond to subdiffusive (negative correlations) and super-diffusive (positive correlations) behavior, respectively. In Figures 6A and 6B, we show the dependence of $\Delta(t)$ vs t in double-logarithmic plots.

A straight line corresponds to power-law behavior, and the Hurst exponent H (Mandelbrot, 1977) is determined by the slope. For the subject without LBP, we find $H=0.5$, corresponding to diffusive behavior. For the subject with LBP, we have $H=0.2$, which indicates the presence of long-time correlations in the EMG signal, in agreement with the results from the phase portrait. The mean-square follows (fractional) Brownian motion only for short-times. For long-times, $\Delta(t)$ appears to plateau. The determination of the Hurst Exponent is affected by large statistical fluctuations. In order to get a more reliable estimate of the Hurst exponent, an analysis of the entropy of the time series was undertaken.

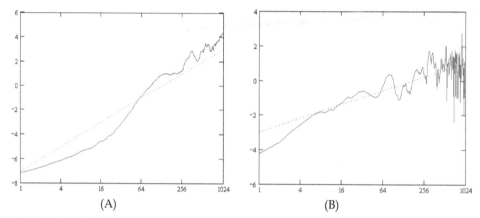

(A)   (B)

Fig. 6. Log-log plot Δvs. t for (A) subjects without and (B) subjects with LBP.

One can characterize the complexity of time series by using the information (Shannon) entropy $S=-\Sigma pj\log pj$, where pj is the probability for outcome number 'j' of a given experiment (Allen et al., 2004; Bezerianos et al., 1995; Bezerianos et al., 2003; Costa et al., 2003). The above equation is the standard formulation of uncertainty as it has the following features: (i) the lowest entropy ($S = 0$) corresponds to one of the outcomes being certain [i.e. probability one] and the others never occurring [i.e. probability zero]; (ii) the largest value for the entropy, $S=\ln(M)$, is achieved when all outcomes are equally likely [all probabilities are equal to each other, $pj = 1/M$]; and (iii) S is additive over partitions of the outcomes. The results reported here were obtained for $M = 1000$ bins. The variation of S with t is expected to be logarithmic: $S(t)\sim H\ln t$, where H is the Hurst exponent introduced before. The entropic analysis of the time series from the subject without LBP and from the subject with LBP shows significant differences in how fast the entropy saturates.

In addition, there is a difference between the slopes of entropy and time function for subjects without and with LBP (Figure 7). The slopes represent estimates for the Hurst exponent H. In agreement with the variance of displacement analysis presented, there was a difference of the Hurst exponent between the subjects without LBP ($H=0.5$; Figure 6, A) and subject with LBP ($H=0.4$; Figure 6, B) were indicated. Note that the value of the exponent H for the LBP subject refers to short-times, while the behavior for long-times is characterized by the value 0.2 quoted before. The difference in the entropy vs time dependence exhibited

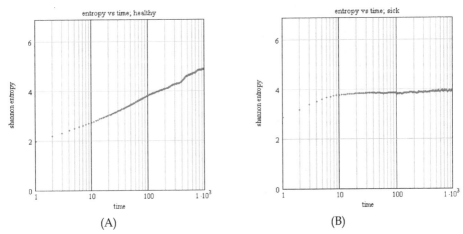

Fig. 7. Shannon entropy versus ln(t) for (A) subjects without and (B) subjects with LBP.

by the healthy and LBP subjects goes beyond the issue of the value of the Hurst exponent. The entropy associated with the LBP subject saturates at very short-times; two orders of magnitude shorter than for the healthy subject. Furthermore, the long time entropy of LBP is lower than for the healthy subject, a result consistent with non-linear analysis of other medical time series (Bezerianos et al., 1995). It is generally observed that injuries result in a decrease in the complexity of biological systems.

In conculsion, nonlinear analysis of time series based on entropy can differentiate between complex biological sources and random sources of the data. While the EMG signal from an erector spinae muscle exhibits an entropy time dependence with a crossover from subdiffusive regime at short times to a self-organization regime (plateau) at longer time scales, time series generated with random number generators do not exhibit the plateau. The Renyi entropy time evolution also differentiates between this complex biological system and deterministic processes (e.g. tracers advection in polymer flows). The presence of the plateau points to the existence of anti-correlations of EMG signals separated in time by at least 0.01 s. Therefore, it is a manifestation of a complex self-organizing system in which individual units interact in a nonlinear fashion such that feedback loops operate over long temporal ranges (Goldberger et al., 2002a).

2.3 Reliability of surface electromyography analysis

The reliability of surface EMG could be different between nonlinear analysis of time series and power spectrum analysis. Our previous study results indicated that the measurement of back muscle fatigability, especially the erector spinae muscle, indicated that the entropy analysis was a more reliable measure than the power spectral analysis (Sung et al., 2008b).

It is well known that the observed EMG signal depends on anatomical factors, such as muscle geometry, subcutaneous fat, gender, and other confounding factors (Lindstrom et al., 1974; Mannion et al., 1997c; Pullman et al., 2000; Roy et al., 1997; Solomonow et al., 1990). As a result, observed quantities from EMG signals show considerable variations even among a group of healthy subjects. A clinical diagnosis of musculoskeletal dysfunction using surface EMG is based on the assumption that dysfunction changes the values of the observed quantities. This underlying assumption is difficult to prove, however, because the EMG signal prior to an injury is generally not available.

One reliable indicator is MF, which is defined by dividing the area under the spectrum into two equal parts. However, use of the MF has led to contradictory results in muscle fatiguing experiments. It still remains to be seen whether a shift in the MF differentiates the various stages of non-acute LBP. The fatigability of back muscles might predispose individuals to LBP. A number of investigators have attempted to classify LBP via changes in the EMG signal during prolonged contraction of the paraspinal muscles (Lariviere *et al.*, 2002a; Lariviere *et al.*, 2002b; Mayer *et al.*, 1989; Peach & McGill, 1998; Roy *et al.*, 1997; Roy *et al.*, 1990). The MF of the back muscles is typically of the order of 100 Hz and is determined by the propagation of the action potential across the electrodes. That is, the MF reflects the behavior of the EMG signal on short-time scales.

Several studies have suggested that surface EMG power spectrum analysis could be used to evaluate patients undergoing rehabilitation in a non-invasive fashion (De Luca, 1984; Mannion *et al.*, 1998; Merletti *et al.*, 1999). The connection between fatigue and EMG spectral parameters is the basis for the use of EMG as an objective and noninvasive method of assessment of back muscle endurance (De Luca, 1984; Mannion *et al.*, 1997a). The original study linking LBP with fatigue was presented by De Luca (De Luca, 1984) who found that subjects with LBP have less endurance, and thus smaller MF slopes, during sustained muscle contractions (Merletti *et al.*, 1999; Roy *et al.*, 1989). However, contradictory results have subsequently been reported and have shown that MF slope is not better than chance in predicting LBP (Humphrey *et al.*, 2005; Lee *et al.*, 2010; Mannion *et al.*, 2001). Thus, a connection between spectral quantities and musculoskeletal pain/dysfunction remains elusive despite considerable efforts.

In recent studies, we applied methods from nonlinear analysis of time series and found that the time-dependent entropy calculated from the EMG signal shows a distinct plateau-like behavior for intermediate times (Kaufman, 2007; Sung *et al.*, 2005; Sung *et al.*, 2007b). The signal from EMG is the instantaneous algebraic summations of action potentials from muscle fibers, and its power spectrum is obtained from a fast Fourier transform of the signal. Recently, several studies in entropy measurements based on nonlinear time series analysis were published without reporting reliability and validity concerns (Goldberger *et al.*, 2002b; Kaufman, 2007; Sung *et al.*, 2007b). Therefore, it would be valuable to confirm the reliability of measurements for characterizing neuromuscular alterations by investigating differences between the power spectrum analysis and nonlinear time series analysis of entropy measures.

It has been found that the degree of randomness is a characteristic property of time series. Entropy is generally used to quantify the complexity. In particular, entropy is used to characterize non-periodic, random phenomena and indicates the rate of information production as it relates to dynamic systems (Richman & Moorman, 2000). Several research groups have compared entropy values for subjects with and without illness/dysfunction (Chialvo, 2002; Costa, 2002; Goldberger *et al.*, 2002a; Stanley *et al.*, 1992; West, 1990). This concept has been used to differentiate healthy subjects from those with heart disease using electrocardiogram time series as well; it is generally found that disease is associated with a lowering of the entropy. In several papers, we applied these ideas to EMG time series for the low back muscles. We found that subjects with LBP have lower entropies than healthy subjects, which is in agreement with the general finding. The traditional approach of EMG is based within the framework of linear systems for which a given input leads to a well-defined periodicity. This connection led to the notion of homeostasis, namely that the normal function of physiologic systems operates in a steady state and that fluctuations are suppressed. However, contradictory results have subsequently been reported without clear understanding of the reliability of entropy measures (Humphrey et al., 2005; Sung et al., 2008b).

Our previous studies indicated that the plateau entropy value was consistently higher for the healthy individual than for the LBP individual. However, the question of whether the plateau entropy constitutes a reliable assessment tool for LBP needs further investigation with large groups of individuals matched by age, gender, body mass index, etc. It is important to understand that Costa et al. and Chialvo argued that pathology/dysfunction is associated with less variability (lower entropy), which was consistent with our findings (Kaufman, 2007; Sung et al., 2005; Sung et al., 2007b).

Nonlinear analysis has proved to be useful in the analysis of a variety of physiologic time series such as human heartbeats (Ivanov et al., 1999) and the shapes of red blood cells under flow stress (Korol & Rasia, 2003). Based on these empirical studies, it has been found that the time series from healthy subjects have higher entropy values than the time series from those with pathology/dysfunction. There are also several other studies indicating that traditional approaches to measuring the complexity of biological signals fail to account for the multiple time scales inherent in such time series. Generally, biological time series are complex data that need to be distilled to useful application to assess a pathology/dysfunction. However, no study has investigated the reliability of entropy measures to assess pathology/dysfunction. In addition, despite much effort, the MF and the MF slope have not shown consistent measurements (De Luca, 1984; Mannion et al., 1998; Merletti et al., 1999; Sung, 2003).

In previous studies, we explored the use of entropy derived from time series as an alternative quantitative measure of EMG signals that can be used in a clinical assessment. We compared the values of the entropy between subjects with LBP and healthy subjects and found that healthy subjects have significantly higher entropies than subjects with LBP (Sung et al., 2007b). However, it is important to examine the between-day variability of entropy, the MF, and the MF slope within the same sample group. In our current study, we compared the values of MF, MF slope, and entropy for two different measurements; and the results indicated the highest correlation for entropy, while the MF slope and MF demonstrated relatively weak correlations.

The results for the right back muscle are illustrated in Figures 8-13 in order to compare values with different measures. The consistent responses of the non-dominant side of the back could be less affected by hand dominance. The histogram of the entropy (Figure 8) demonstrated consistent distributions between pre- and post- measurement entropy values, which are plotted in Figure 9. The points representing the 32 subjects were plotted closely along the diagonal line, indicating that the two measurements reveal a relatively high correlation ($R=0.75$).

The mean and the standard deviations of the MF slope values for two measurements were analyzed, and the correlations ranged from 0.15-0.18, which does not indicate a significant difference between the MF slopes at two different observations. The intra class correlation coefficients (ICCs) ranged from 0.26-0.30, and the standard error of means (SEM) varied between 0.03 and 0.04, which were not significantly different for the distributions for two different times. Figure 10 compared two measurements of the MF slope for the right back muscle, and the number of subjects repeatedly demonstrated less similar results between the two measurements. The Pearson correlation coefficients ranged from 0.15-0.18 and were not statistically different. This result confirms the values of the MF slope of the right back muscle for post-measurement, which was plotted versus the values of pre-measurement in Figure 10 and shows no obvious difference. The points representing the subjects were distributed rather broadly, which was reflected in the low correlation coefficient (R=0.18).

The distribution of MF values from post-measurement shifted towards larger values. The correlations ranged from 0.38-0.47 and were statistically significant. Thus, there was a significant correlation between the distributions of the MF values from the measurements at two different times. The ICCs ranged from 0.54-0.64, and the SEM ranged from 3.10-3.60. The Pearson correlation coefficients ranged from 0.38-0.47 and were statistically significant. In Figure 12, two measurements of the MF for the right back muscle are compared, and the number of subjects repeatedly demonstrated less similar results between two measurements. Figure 12 depicts the histograms of the MF values. The two histograms indicated little difference except for two outliers for post-measurement values. Figure 13 depicts the MF values of the right back muscle, and the linear regression analysis yielded R=0.15. The values of MF for the two measurements were more highly correlated than those for the MF slope, although the correlation (R=0.38) was much lower than that for the entropy (Sung *et al.*, 2005).

Overall, the ICC values of entropy for between-day measurements were higher, and the SEM for entropy was lower than the MF and its slope. Therefore, the results of this study indicated that the entropy analysis could provide reliable measurements for muscle fatigability.

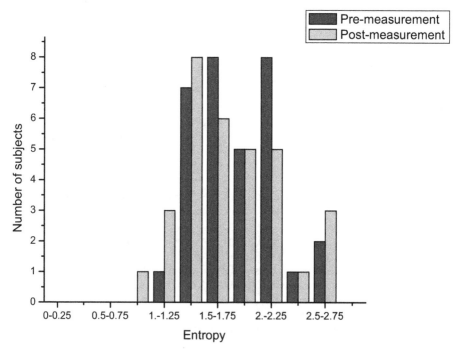

Fig. 8. Histogram of entropy measurements for the right back muscle.

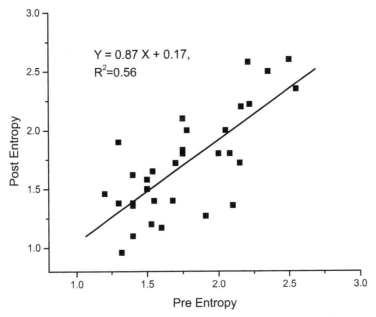

Fig. 9. The entropy values taken at two different measurements for the right erector spinae muscle. The correlation coefficient is $R=0.75$.

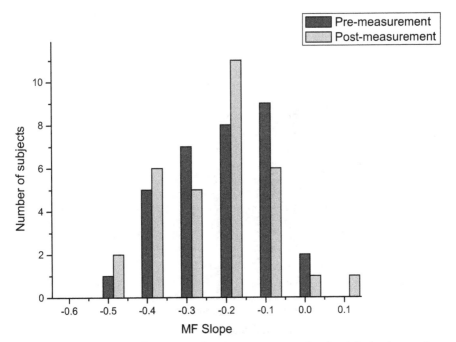

Fig. 10. Histogram of median frequency slope measurements for the right back muscle.

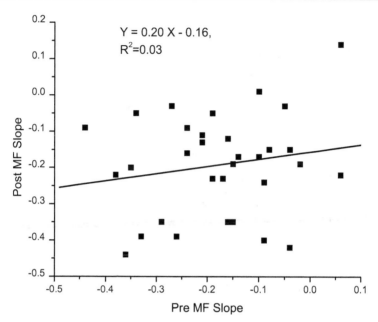

Fig. 11. The median frequency slope taken at two different measurements for the right back muscle. The correlation coefficient is R=0.18.

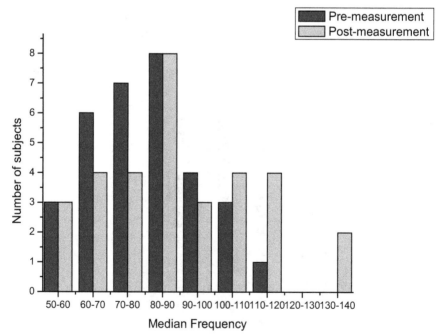

Fig. 12. Histogram of median frequency measurements for the right back muscle.

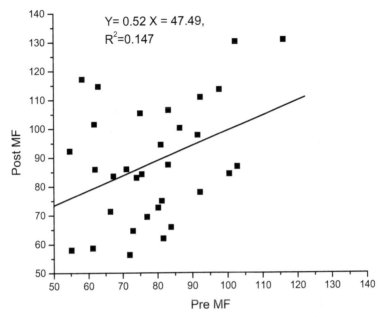

Fig. 13. The median frequency for the right back muscle at two different measurements. The correlation coefficient is $R=0.38$.

Overall, the entropy measurements for back muscles were more reliable than the power spectrum measures based on between-day reliability. Although there were no significant differences for between-day reliability for both entropy and MF slope, the test-retest reliability based on ICC values was higher for the entropy measure. The results of this study indicated that the complexity of time series analysis is a more reliable measure for the adaptability of biological systems than power spectral analysis.

A clinical assessment of LBP is important to objectively identify subjects with genuine pain and to assess the efficacy of therapeutic interventions. The entropy values from two measurements had the highest correlation, and we concluded that entropy is the most reliable measure from the low back muscles. The correlation of the MF slope and MF also demonstrated weak correlations and were statistically insignificant. Although there is a positive correlation between pain level and MF slope in back muscles, it is possible that the statistical use of correlation coefficients based on several validation studies was poor for reliability studies (Meyer, 1994).

In conclusion, it is important to compare the difference between nonlinear time series and power spectrum analysis regarding the irregularity of signals in biological systems. The quantities derived from nonlinear time series analysis of EMG signals will be compared with power spectrum analysis between subjects with and without musculoskeletal dysfunction/pain.

2.4 Sensitivity of surface electromyography analysis

As reported in our previous studies, the complexity of physiologic time series is a sensitive measure for muscle fatigability (Lee *et al.*, 2010). However, it is necessary to determine whether the observed Shannon (information) entropy, as compared with MF, was able to differentiate fatigability of the thoracic and lumbar parts of the erector spinae muscle following the intervention. Previously, our lab investigated tools for evaluating back muscle fatigability after spinal stabilization exercises in participants with chronic LBP (Lee *et al.*, 2010; Sung *et al.*, 2005; Sung *et al.*, 2008a; Sung *et al.*, 2010). The results of our previous study indicated that Shannon entropy might be a valuable tool to measure the differences of outcomes following the exercise intervention. The results indicated that the participants' pain levels decreased significantly after 4 weeks of spinal stabilization exercises. The entropy of the EMG signals also decreased and significantly interacted with pain level. The slope of the MF based on power spectrum analysis also decreased but did not demonstrate any interaction with pain level. Therefore, the entropy of the EMG signals might be a useful tool for measuring LBP.

In addition, the results indicated that the entropy clearly differentiated the two groups. However, the results of power spectrum analysis based on complexity of the EMG signal could be calculated with the entropy of the time series. The results indicated that healthy subjects revealed significantly larger entropy values than the subjects with LBP. These findings consistently demonstrated a connection between physiologic "health" and complexity (Costa *et al.*, 2003; Costa *et al.*, 2005; Li & Huston, 2002). Another important finding indicated that the entropy levels of the EMG signals demonstrated significant interactions between muscles and groups following treatment for muscle endurance. However, the MF did not demonstrate this interaction. The significant interaction effect of the entropy between muscles and groups following treatment during the one-minute back extension test supports the characteristics of the recorded signals that occurs with fatigue (Roy *et al.*, 1989). Exercises for graded activity programs can be used to increase trunk muscle endurance and to decrease pain (Jorgensen & Nicolaisen, 1986; Jorgensen & Nicolaisen, 1987). Undoubtedly, other muscles participated in the load sharing during the testing as well as when subjects performed the intervention exercises. The attachment of the lumbar muscles, rather than the thoracic back muscles, results in an effective lever arm for lumbar stabilization. Therefore, the lumbar muscle is more effective in creating a stabilizing moment over the lumbar vertebral segments during the test (Flicker *et al.*, 1993; MacIntosh & Bogduk, 1986).

Research in biology and medicine has shown that fluctuations in physiological systems may play a significant role (Costa, 2002; Goldberger *et al.*, 2002a; Liu *et al.*, 2002). In fractal physiology, the apparent random, or chaotic, signal is observed on different (time) scales. It is found that the signal looks similar, or self-similar. This means that a single time scale (e.g., the period of oscillation) is replaced by a family of time scales. It follows that the single state of the system is replaced by multiple non-equilibrium states that are correlated with each other. If the signal is completely random with no characteristic time scale, it would be modeled by "white noise" and the power spectrum would be flat with $P(f) \sim f0$. In general, the frequency spectrum is fitted to a power law $P(f) \sim 1/f\alpha$, with $0 < \alpha < 2$. In this case, the power spectrum does not define a MF. Other studies reported that for physiologic systems, a constant "output" requires other variables to fluctuate so that the system can adapt to sudden changes in demand or stimulus (Costa *et al.*, 2005). This extent of fluctuations in physiologic signals can be quantified by entropy calculated from their time series.

Nonlinear analysis is used to characterize "hidden" properties of physiologic time series. Following this approach, we interpreted the EMG signal in terms of a one-dimensional random walk in discrete time. We found that the mean-square displacement increased linearly for short times $t < 20$ ms and is nearly flat for intermediate times 20 ms $< t < 400$ ms. This plateau behavior has been found for other biological systems and implies the existence of correlations in the signal (Costa et al., 2005; Goldberger et al., 2002a). However, these correlations cannot be explained within a linear model, and thus support the use of nonlinear analysis for EMG time series. This may also explain why the MF fluctuates during a sustained contraction, and why the connection between MF slope and LBP has proven elusive despite considerable efforts.

In conclusion, the nonlinear analysis to EMG time series was reviewed for low back muscles. The Shannon entropy is a standard measure of complexity and has been applied in cognitive science research, aging studies, heart failure research, and other fields (Allen et al., 2004; Costa et al., 2003; Costa et al., 2005; Goldberger et al., 2002a; Liu et al., 2002). The time-dependent entropy of the EMG signal exhibits a plateau-like behavior which indicates the presence of long-time correlations in the signal. The plateau value of the entropy was lower for subjects with LBP than for individuals in the control group. This connection might prove to be useful in a clinical assessment of LBP. The existence of long-time correlations in the signal explains the large variability in the MF obtained from the power spectrum. The entropy clearly differentiated the two groups, whereas the MF exhibited significant overlaps between the groups.

3. Conclusion

This chapter covered comprehensive articles comparing the difference between nonlinear time series and power spectrum analysis regarding the irregularity of signals in biological systems. A clinical assessment of pain/dysfunction using EMG should be considered on properties of the signal that change drastically in the presence of pain/dysfunction. A shift in the MF of the spectrum is explained by the change in the velocity of the action potential, and it reflects a quantitative change of the signals. A change in the entropy of the signal also reflects a qualitative change in the physiologic system.

In this chapter, the quantities derived from nonlinear time series analysis of EMG signals was compared with power spectrum analysis between subjects with and without musculoskeletal dysfunction/pain. The fluctuations in physiologic signals can be quantified by entropy calculated from the nonlinear time series. The value of the entropy reflects the adaptability of biological systems; healthy systems are thus expected to have higher values than unhealthy systems. Finally, the distribution of the values of the entropy and power spectrum for a group of subjects with LBP and a group of healthy subjects was discussed.

4. Acknowledgment

This work was supported by Korea University and the Basic Science Research Program through the National Research Foundation of Korea funded by the Ministry of Education, Science and Technology (2010-0003015). This material is also the result of work supported in part by Drs. Miron Kaufman and Ulrich Zurcher of Cleveland State University, Cleveland, Ohio, for their critical analyses of the important intellectual content and interpretation of data. The author declares that no competing interests exist.

5. References

Allen, P. A., Kaufman, M., Smith, A. F. & Propper, R. E. (1998). A molar entropy model of age differences in spatial memory. *Psychol Aging*, Vol. 13, No. 3, Sep, pp. 501-518

Allen, P. A., Murphy, M. D., Kaufman, M., Groth, K. E. & Begovic, A. (2004). Age differences in central (semantic) and peripheral processing: the importance of considering both response times and errors. *J Gerontol B Psychol Sci Soc Sci*, Vol. 59, No. 5, Sep, pp. P210-219

Belair, J., Glass, L., An Der Heiden, U. & Milton, J. (1995a). Dynamical disease: Identification, temporal aspects and treatment strategies of human illness. *Chaos*, Vol. 5, No. 1, Mar, pp. 1-7

Belair, J., Glass, L., Heiden, U. & Milton, J. (1995b). Dynamical Disease: Mathematical Analysis of Human Illness.

Bezerianos, A., Bountis, T., Papaioannou, G. & Polydoropoulos, P. (1995). Nonlinear time series analysis of electrocardiograms. *Chaos*, Vol. 5, No. 1, Mar, pp. 95-101

Bezerianos, A., Tong, S. & Thakor, N. (2003). Time-dependent entropy estimation of EEG rhythm changes following brain ischemia. *Ann Biomed Eng*, Vol. 31, No. 2, Feb, pp. 221-232

Buldyrev, S. V., Ferrante, J. & Zypman, F. R. (2006). Dry friction avalanches: experiment and theory. *Phys Rev E Stat Nonlin Soft Matter Phys*, Vol. 74, No. 6 Pt 2, Dec, pp. 066110, ISSN 1539-3755 (Print) 1539-3755 (Linking)

Chaffin, D. B. (1969). Surface electromyography frequency analysis as a diagnostic tool. *J Occup Med*, Vol. 11, No. 3, Mar, pp. 109-115, ISSN 0096-1736 (Print) 0096-1736 (Linking)

Chialvo, D. R. (2002). Physiology: unhealthy surprises. *Nature*, Vol. 419, No. 6904, Sep 19, pp. 263

Cholewicki, J. & VanVliet, J. J. T. (2002). Relative contribution of trunk muscles to the stability of the lumbar spine during isometric exertions. *Clin Biomech (Bristol, Avon)*, Vol. 17, No. 2, Feb, pp. 99-105

Collins, J. J. & De Luca, C. J. (1994). Random walking during quiet standing. *Physical Review Letters*, Vol. 73, No. 5, Aug 1, pp. 764-767

Collins, J. J. & De Luca, C. J. (1995). Upright, correlated random walks: A statistical-biomechanics approach to the human postural control system. *Chaos*, Vol. 5, No. 1, Mar, pp. 57-63

Costa, M., Goldberger, A. L. & Peng, C. K. (2002). Multiscale entropy to distinguish physiologic and synthetic RR time series. *Comput Cardiol*, Vol. 29, pp. 137-140

Costa, M., Goldberger, A. L. & Peng, C. K. (2003). Multiscale entropy analysis: A new measure of complexity loss in heart failure. *J Electrocardiol*, Vol. 36 Suppl, pp. 39-40

Costa, M., Goldberger, A. L. & Peng, C. K. (2005). Multiscale entropy analysis of biological signals. *Phys Rev E Stat Nonlin Soft Matter Phys*, Vol. 71, No. 2 Pt 1, Feb, pp. 021906

Costa, M. G., A.J. Peng, C.K. (2002). Multiscale entropy analysis of complex physiologic time series. *Phys Rev Lett*, Vol. 89, No. (6)

Cybulski, O., Babin, V. & Holyst, R. (2004). Minimization of the Renyi entropy production in the stationary states of the Brownian process with matched death and birth rates. *Phys Rev E Stat Nonlin Soft Matter Phys*, Vol. 69, No. 1 Pt 2, Jan, pp. 016110, ISSN 1539-3755 (Print) 1539-3755 (Linking)

De Luca, C. J. (1984). Myoelectrical manifestations of localized muscular fatigue in humans. *Crit Rev Biomed Eng*, Vol. *11*, No. 4, pp. 251-279

Denny, M. & Gaines, S. (2000). Chance in Biology- Using Probability to Explore Nature.

Flicker, P. L., Fleckenstein, J. L., Ferry, K., Payne, J., Ward, C., Mayer, T., Parkey, R. W. & Peshock, R. M. (1993). Lumbar muscle usage in chronic low back pain. Magnetic resonance image evaluation. *Spine*, Vol. *18*, No. 5, pp. 582-586.

Furey, C. A. (1963). Clinical Indications for Electromyography. *J Med Soc N J*, Vol. *60*, Nov, pp. 514-517, ISSN 0025-7524 (Print) 0025-7524 (Linking)

Gage, J. S. (1992). The concept of meaning and the mathematical theory of communication. *MD Comput*, Vol. *9*, No. 3, May-Jun, pp. 146-148, ISSN 0724-6811 (Print) 0724-6811 (Linking)

Glass, L. (2001). Synchronization and rhythmic processes in physiology. *Nature*, Vol. *410*, No. 6825, Mar 8, pp. 277-284

Goldberger, A. L., Amaral, L. A., Hausdorff, J. M., Ivanov, P., Peng, C. K. & Stanley, H. E. (2002a). Fractal dynamics in physiology: alterations with disease and aging. *Proc Natl Acad Sci U S A*, Vol. *99 Suppl 1*, Feb 19, pp. 2466-2472

Goldberger, A. L., Peng, C. K. & Lipsitz, L. A. (2002b). What is physiologic complexity and how does it change with aging and disease? *Neurobiol Aging*, Vol. *23*, No. 1, Jan-Feb, pp. 23-26

Herzog, W., Nigg, B. M., Robinson, R. O. & Read, L. J. (1987). Quantifying the effects of spinal manipulations on gait, using patients with low back pain: a pilot study. *J Manipulative Physiol Ther*, Vol. *10*, No. 6, Dec, pp. 295-299, ISSN 0161-4754 (Print) 0161-4754 (Linking)

Hobbie, R. K. (1997). Intermediate Physics for Medicine and Biology.

Hoffmann, W. (1968). [Significance of clinical electromyography in childhood. 3. Electromyographic findings in movement disorders of central nervous origin]. *Padiatr Grenzgeb*, Vol. *7*, No. 1, pp. 13-25, ISSN 0030-932X (Print) 0030-932X (Linking)

Humphrey, A. R., Nargol, A. V., Jones, A. P., Ratcliffe, A. A. & Greenough, C. G. (2005). The value of electromyography of the lumbar paraspinal muscles in discriminating between chronic-low-back-pain sufferers and normal subjects. *Eur Spine J*, Vol. *14*, No. 2, Mar, pp. 175-184

Ivanov, P. C., Amaral, L. A., Goldberger, A. L., Havlin, S., Rosenblum, M. G., Struzik, Z. R. & Stanley, H. E. (1999). Multifractality in human heartbeat dynamics. *Nature*, Vol. *399*, No. 6735, Jun 3, pp. 461-465

Jorgensen, K. & Nicolaisen, T. (1986). Two methods for determining trunk extensor endurance. A comparative study. *Eur J Appl Physiol Occup Physiol*, Vol. *55*, No. 6, pp. 639-644

Jorgensen, K. & Nicolaisen, T. (1987). Trunk extensor endurance: determination and relation to low-back trouble. *Ergonomics*, Vol. *30*, No. 2, pp. 259-267.

Kantz, H. S., T. (2003). Nonlinear Time Series Analysis. Vol. *2nd Ed., Cambridge UP, Cambridge,*

Kaufman, A. (1985). Nonlinear Dynamics: Statistical Physics and Chaos in Fusion Plasmas. *Science*, Vol. *228*, No. 4698, Apr 26, pp. 485-486

Kaufman, M., Zurcher, U., Sung P. (2007). Entropy of Electromyography Time Series. *Physica A Statistical Mechanics and its Applications*, Vol. *386*, No. 2, 2007, pp. 698-707

Knowlton, G. C., Bennett, R. L. & Mc, C. R. (1951). Electromyography of fatigue. *Arch Phys Med Rehabil*, Vol. 32, No. 10, Oct, pp. 648-652, ISSN 0003-9993 (Print) 0003-9993 (Linking)

Koppell, N. (2000). We Got Rhythm: Dynamical Systems of the Nervous System. Vol. 47, pp. 6-16

Korol, A. M. & Rasia, R. (2003). Signatures of deterministic chaos in dyslipidemic erythrocytes under shear stress. *Chaos*, Vol. 13, No. 1, Mar, pp. 87-93

Lariviere, C., Arsenault, A. B., Gravel, D., Gagnon, D. & Loisel, P. (2002a). Evaluation of measurement strategies to increase the reliability of EMG indices to assess back muscle fatigue and recovery. *J Electromyogr Kinesiol*, Vol. 12, No. 2, Apr, pp. 91-102

Lariviere, C., Arsenault, A. B., Gravel, D., Gagnon, D., Loisel, P. & Vadeboncoeur, R. (2002b). Electromyographic assessment of back muscle weakness and muscle composition: reliability and validity issues. *Arch Phys Med Rehabil*, Vol. 83, No. 9, Sep, pp. 1206-1214

Lee, T. R., Kim, Y. H. & Sung, P. S. (2010). Spectral and entropy changes for back muscle fatigability following spinal stabilization exercises. *Journal of Rehabilitation Research & Development*, Vol. 47, No. 2, pp. 133-142, ISSN 1938-1352 (Electronic) 0748-7711 (Linking)

Li, J. S. & Huston, J. P. (2002). Non-linear dynamics of operant behavior: a new approach via the extended return map. *Rev Neurosci*, Vol. 13, No. 1, pp. 31-57

Lindstrom, L., Magnusson, R. & Petersen, I. (1974). Muscle load influence on myo-electric signal characteristics. *Scand J Rehabil Med*, Vol. 0, No. Suppl, pp. 127-148.

Liu, J. Z., Dai, T. H., Sahgal, V., Brown, R. W. & Yue, G. H. (2002). Nonlinear cortical modulation of muscle fatigue: a functional MRI study. *Brain Res*, Vol. 957, No. 2, Dec 13, pp. 320-329

MacIntosh, J. E. & Bogduk, N. (1986). The biomechanics of the lumbar multifidus. *Clinical Biomechanics*, Vol. 1, pp. 205-213

Mandelbrot, B. (1977). The Fractale Geometry of Nature.

Mandelbrot, B. (1983). Fractal Geometry of Nature.

Mannion, A. F., Connolly, B., Wood, K. & Dolan, P. (1997a). The use of surface EMG power spectral analysis in the evaluation of back muscle function. *J Rehabil Res Dev*, Vol. 34, No. 4, Oct, pp. 427-439

Mannion, A. F., Connolly, B., Wood, K. & Dolan, P. (1997b). The use of surface EMG power spectral analysis in the evaluation of back muscle function. *Journal of Rehabilitation Research & Development*, Vol. 34, No. 4, pp. 427-439

Mannion, A. F. & Dolan, P. (1994). Electromyographic median frequency changes during isometric contraction of the back extensors to fatigue. *Spine*, Vol. 19, No. 11, Jun 1, pp. 1223-1229

Mannion, A. F., Dumas, G. A., Cooper, R. G., Espinosa, F. J., Faris, M. W. & Stevenson, J. M. (1997c). Muscle fibre size and type distribution in thoracic and lumbar regions of erector spinae in healthy subjects without low back pain: normal values and sex differences. *J Anat*, Vol. 190 (Pt 4), May, pp. 505-513

Mannion, A. F., Dumas, G. A., Stevenson, J. M. & Cooper, R. G. (1998). The influence of muscle fiber size and type distribution on electromyographic measures of back muscle fatigability. *Spine*, Vol. 23, No. 5, Mar 1, pp. 576-584

Mannion, A. F., Muntener, M., Taimela, S. & Dvorak, J. (2001). Comparison of three active therapies for chronic low back pain: results of a randomized clinical trial with one-year follow-up. *Rheumatology (Oxford)*, Vol. 40, No. 7, Jul, pp. 772-778

Mayer, T. G., Kondraske, G., Mooney, V., Carmichael, T. W. & Butsch, R. (1989). Lumbar myoelectric spectral analysis for endurance assessment. A comparison of normals with deconditioned patients. *Spine*, Vol. 14, No. 9, pp. 986-991.

Merletti, R., Roy, S. H., Kupa, E., Roatta, S. & Granata, A. (1999). Modeling of surface myoelectric signals--Part II: Model-based signal interpretation. *IEEE Trans Biomed Eng*, Vol. 46, No. 7, Jul, pp. 821-829

Meyer, J. J. (1994). The validity of thoracolumbar paraspinal scanning EMG as a diagnostic test: an examination of the current literature. *J Manipulative Physiol Ther*, Vol. 17, No. 8, Oct, pp. 539-551

Nigg, B. M., Herzog, W. & Read, L. J. (1988). Effect of viscoelastic shoe insoles on vertical impact forces in heel-toe running. *Am J Sports Med*, Vol. 16, No. 1, Jan-Feb, pp. 70-76, ISSN 0363-5465 (Print) 0363-5465 (Linking)

Panjabi, M. M. (1992). The stabilizing system of the spine. Part II. Neutral zone and instability hypothesis. *Journal of Spinal Disorders*, Vol. 5, No. 4, pp. 390-396; discussion 397

Peach, J. P. & McGill, S. M. (1998). Classification of low back pain with the use of spectral electromyogram parameters. *Spine*, Vol. 23, No. 10, May 15, pp. 1117-1123

Pincus, S. M. (2001). Assessing serial irregularity and its implications for health. *Ann N Y Acad Sci*, Vol. 954, Dec, pp. 245-267

Pullman, S. L., Goodin, D. S., Marquinez, A. I., Tabbal, S. & Rubin, M. (2000). Clinical utility of surface EMG: report of the therapeutics and technology assessment subcommittee of the American Academy of Neurology. *Neurology*, Vol. 55, No. 2, Jul 25, pp. 171-177

Rack, M. H. & Ross, H. F. (1975). Electromyography of human biceps during imposed sinusoidal movement of the elbow joint. *J Physiol*, Vol. 244, No. 1, Jan, pp. 44P-45P, ISSN 0022-3751 (Print) 0022-3751 (Linking)

Richman, J. S. & Moorman, J. R. (2000). Physiological time-series analysis using approximate entropy and sample entropy. *Am J Physiol Heart Circ Physiol*, Vol. 278, No. 6, Jun, pp. H2039-2049

Roy, S. H., De Luca, C. J. & Casavant, D. A. (1989). Lumbar muscle fatigue and chronic lower back pain. *Spine*, Vol. 14, No. 9, pp. 992-1001

Roy, S. H., De Luca, C. J., Emley, M., Oddsson, L. I., Buijs, R. J., Levins, J. A., Newcombe, D. S. & Jabre, J. F. (1997). Classification of back muscle impairment based on the surface electromyographic signal. *Journal of Rehabilitation Research & Development*, Vol. 34, No. 4, pp. 405-414

Roy, S. H., De Luca, C. J., Snyder-Mackler, L., Emley, M. S., Crenshaw, R. L. & Lyons, J. P. (1990). Fatigue, recovery, and low back pain in varsity rowers. *Med Sci Sports Exerc*, Vol. 22, No. 4, Aug, pp. 463-469

Scafetta, N. & Grigolini, P. (2002). Scaling detection in time series: diffusion entropy analysis. *Phys Rev E Stat Nonlin Soft Matter Phys*, Vol. 66, No. 3 Pt 2A, Sep, pp. 036130, ISSN 1539-3755 (Print) 1539-3755 (Linking)

Scafetta, N. & West, B. J. (2003). Solar flare intermittency and the earth's temperature anomalies. *Phys Rev Lett*, Vol. 90, No. 24, Jun 20, pp. 248701

Scafetta, N. & West, B. J. (2004). Multiscaling comparative analysis of time series and a discussion on "earthquake conversations" in California. *Phys Rev Lett*, Vol. *92*, No. 13, Apr 2, pp. 138501

Shannon, C. E. (1997). The mathematical theory of communication. 1963. *MD Comput*, Vol. *14*, No. 4, Jul-Aug, pp. 306-317, ISSN 0724-6811 (Print) 0724-6811 (Linking)

Solomonow, M., Baten, C., Smit, J., Baratta, R., Hermens, H., D'Ambrosia, R. & Shoji, H. (1990). Electromyogram power spectra frequencies associated with motor unit recruitment strategies. *J Appl Physiol*, Vol. *68*, No. 3, Mar, pp. 1177-1185

Sprott, J. (2003). Chaos and Time-Series Analysis.

Stanley, H. E., Buldyrev, S. V., Goldberger, A. L., Hausdorff, J. M., Havlin, S., Mietus, J., Peng, C. K., Sciortino, F. & Simons, M. (1992). Fractal landscapes in biological systems: long-range correlations in DNA and interbeat heart intervals. *Physica A*, Vol. *191*, No. 1-4, Dec 15, pp. 1-12

Strogatz, S. H. (2001). Exploring complex networks. *Nature*, Vol. *410*, No. 6825, Mar 8, pp. 268-276

Sung, P. S. (2003). Multifidi muscles median frequency before and after spinal stabilization exercises. *Arch Phys Med Rehabil*, Vol. *84*, No. 9, Sep, pp. 1313-1318

Sung, P. S., Zurcher, U. & Kaufman, M. (2005). Nonlinear analysis of electromyography time series as a diagnostic tool for low back pain. *Med Sci Monit*, Vol. *11*, No. 1, Jan, pp. CS1-5, ISSN 1234-1010 (Print) 1234-1010 (Linking)

Sung, P. S., Zurcher, U. & Kaufman, M. (2007a). Comparison of spectral and entropic measures for surface electromyography time series: a pilot study. *Journal of Rehabilitation Research & Development*, Vol. *44*, No. 4, pp. 599-609, ISSN 1938-1352 (Electronic) 0748-7711 (Linking)

Sung, P. S., Zurcher, U. & Kaufman, M. (2007b). Comparison of spectral and entropic measures for surface electromyography time series: A pilot study. *J Rehabil Res Dev*, Vol. *44*, No. 4, pp. 599-610

Sung, P. S., Zurcher, U. & Kaufman, M. (2008a). Gender differences in spectral and entropic measures of erector spinae muscle fatigue. *Journal of Rehabilitation Research & Development*, Vol. *45*, No. 9, pp. 1431-1439, ISSN 1938-1352 (Electronic) 1938-1352 (Linking)

Sung, P. S., Zurcher, U. & Kaufman, M. (2008b). Reliability difference between spectral and entropic measures of erector spinae muscle fatigability. *J Electromyogr Kinesiol*, Dec 31

Sung, P. S., Zurcher, U. & Kaufman, M. (2010). Reliability difference between spectral and entropic measures of erector spinae muscle fatigability. *J Electromyogr Kinesiol*, Vol. *20*, No. 1, Feb, pp. 25-30, ISSN 1873-5711 (Electronic) 1050-6411 (Linking)

Vinga, S. & Almeida, J. S. (2004). Renyi continuous entropy of DNA sequences. *J Theor Biol*, Vol. *231*, No. 3, Dec 7, pp. 377-388, ISSN 0022-5193 (Print) 0022-5193 (Linking)

West, B. (1990). Fractal Physiology & Chaos in Medicine.

Wilder, D. G., Aleksiev, A. R., Magnusson, M. L., Pope, M. H., Spratt, K. F. & Goel, V. K. (1996). Muscular response to sudden load. A tool to evaluate fatigue and rehabilitation. *Spine*, Vol. *21*, No. 22, pp. 2628-2639.

7

Nonlinear Analysis for Evaluation of Age-Related Muscle Performance Using Surface Electromyography

Hiroki Takada[1], Yasuyuki Matsuura[1],
Tomoki Shiozawa[2] and Masaru Miyao[3]
[1]University of Fukui, Fukui
[2]Aoyama Gakuin University, Shibuya, Tokyo
[3]Graduate School of Information Science, Nagoya University, Nagoya
Japan

1. Introduction

Several electromyographic methods are currently used, but needle electromyography (nEMG) and surface electromyography (sEMG) are most often applied. To physiologically evaluate electromyographic wave patterns for the detection of abnormalities, the wave patterns obtained with nEMG or sEMG have been macroscopically examined, and subjectively judged by physicians.

- nEMG findings are used for the evaluation of whether a disorder is neurogenic or myogenic, and if it is both neurogenic and myogenic, they provide important information about whether it is acute, subacute, or chronic (KIMURA, 1989). However, the probe is a needle electrode, which is percutaneously inserted into muscular tissues.

- sEMG findings are used for various evaluations, such as the classification of trembling for the diagnosis of involuntary motion, the diagnosis or differential diagnosis of dystonia and spasm, and the identification of involuntary constrictor muscles (KIZUKA et al., 2006).

- sEMG is further used for the determination of the electric potential through a nerve conduction examination (evoked EMG). In evoked EMG, the electrostimulation of peripheral nerves is percutaneously performed (KIMURA, 1989).

The examination methods described, except for method B), are invasive and cause severe pain in patients. Generally, "smoothing" and "integration" refer to two ways of quantifying EMG energy over time; smoothing refers to continuously averaging out the peaks and valleys of a changing electrical signal. On the other hand, integration refers to measuring the area under a curve over a period of time. These methods are used to examine the relative degree of muscular contraction, and are also employed to provide a parameter for the evaluation of muscular training conditions (Aukee, 2002). However, the results obtained are affected by the location of the measuring electrodes and the shape and size of the probes. That is, EMG findings are macroscopically and subjectively evaluated, as described above, and no algorithm for the quantification of the degree of muscular abnormalities or recovery has been established. In this study, we apply and discuss the measurement parameters that have been developed for evaluating the average rectified sEMG (ARS) data obtained from perineal muscles during biofeedback training (BFT) for the treatment of dysuria (Tries & Eisman, 1995) (Fig. 1), and we evaluated the effects of this training (SHIOZAWA et al., 2007). Kegel (1948; 1951) was the first to use BFT for the treatment of urinary incontinence (UI), and it was observed that if the pelvic floor muscles are hypotonic, bladder suspension surgery is less effective for treating stress-related incontinence. In order to improve the contractability of the pubococcygeus portion of the levator ani muscle, Kegel invented the pressure perineometer (KEGEL, 1951). In the U.S.A., at least 13 million community-living adults and more than 50% of all residents in nursing facilities suffer from UI (FANTL et al., 1996). The direct medical expenditure incurred for the care of these people is estimated to be >$15 billion annually, in addition to the $35.2 billion incurred annually for nursing home residents (PEEK et al., 1995). There is a consensus that in most cases, behavioral treatment modalities, including biofeedback, should be used before invasive modalities such as surgery.

A biofeedback instrument has three tasks (PEEK et al., 1995): i) To monitor (in some way) a physiological process of interest, ii) To measure (objectify) what is monitored, and iii) To present what is monitored or measured as meaningful information. The contributions of many previous researchers and practitioners can be cited as the forerunners of biofeedback.

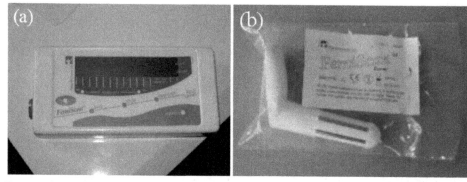

Fig. 1. A biofeedback system (FemiScan Co. Ltd., Finland). The main body (a), and a disposable electrode that can be inserted into perineal muscles (b).

Edmund Jacobsen commenced research at Harvard in 1908, and throughout the 1920s and 1930s worked to develop progressive muscle relaxation as an effective behavioral technique for the alleviation of neurotic tensions and many functional medical disorders (JACOBSEN, 1938). He used crude electromyographic equipment to monitor the levels of muscle tension in his patients during the course of treatment. The classification of and historical perspectives on biofeedback applications can be found in Gaarder and Montgomery (GAARDER and MONTGOMERY, 1981), Gatchel and Price (GATCHEL and PRICE, 1979), and Basmajian (BASMAJIAN, 1989).

Recently, the rapid atrophy of the muscles used for bending at the hip joint during walking (flexor muscles around the hip joint) with age has drawn attention. The flexor muscles around the hip joint consist of the femoral rectus and abdominal muscles. It has been indicated that a lack of these muscles is responsible for the falling of the elderly. In this study, we examined the ARS of the femoral rectus muscles performed during the BFT of the dominant leg, using the measurement parameters mentioned above, and evaluated changes with age.

2. Sensor output signal evaluation system

The sensor output signal evaluation (SOSE) system was developed in 2006 (Shiozawa et al., 2006a). The SOSE system can evaluate the exponential curve-fitting in BFT.

2.1 Participants
The subjects consisted of 31 healthy adults aged 20-73 years (mean, 44.3±19.9 years). All of the subjects were Japanese and lived in Nagoya and its environs. The following were the exclusion criteria for the subjects: subjects working in a night shift, subjects with a dependence on alcohol, subjects who consumed alcohol and caffeine-containing beverages after waking up and within two hours of eating a meal, subjects who may have had a previous history of bone, joint, or nerve problems, and special strength training exercises were not usually done. The subjects were not prescribed drugs for any disease.

2.2 Design
The subject sat back on a four-legged stool, and electromyographic electrodes were applied at an interval of several centimeters to the center of the femoral rectus muscles in the dominant left or right leg (Fig.2). The subjects were instructed to kick a fixed belt by moving the bottom of the lower leg forward (kicking motion).

2.2.1 Biofeedback training
Temporal data were obtained using sEMG, and they are expressed here as $\{y(t)\}$. Generally, sEMG data are recorded by a computer at 2 kHz. Here, the integral calculation was performed every 0.1 s using the following equation:

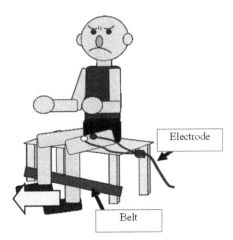

Fig. 2. Biofeedback training instruction signal. The BFT instruction signal produced by superimposing the ARS on the target instruction signal.

$$x(t) = \sum_{k=0}^{199} \left| y(t + 0.0005k) \right|, \tag{1}$$

and the ARS $\{x(t)\}$ was calculated in real time and outputted. The subject was told to observe the outputted wave patterns and the rectangular waves $f(t)$ of a 10-s cycle superimposed on the same display (Fig. 3), and then perform intermittent continuous contractions of the femoral rectus muscles corresponding to the patterns (BFT).

The subjects performed BFT for 2 min. We ensured that the body sway was not affected by environmental conditions; using an air conditioner, we adjusted the *temperature* to 25 °C in the exercise room, which was large, quiet, and *bright*. All subjects were tested from 10 am to 5 pm in an exercise *room*. All subjects gave consent in writing after a sufficient explanation of this study.

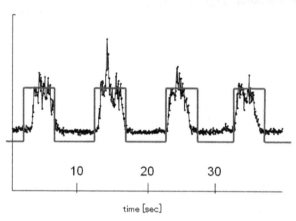

time [sec]

Fig. 3. Biofeedback training instruction signal. BFT instruction signal produced by super-imposing the ARS on the target instruction signal.

2.2.2 Materials
A special electromyographic transformation box (AP-U027, TEAC Co.) was connected to a commercially available portable and versatile amplifier and recorder (Polymate AP1532, TEAC Co.), and electromyographic electrodes (bipolar) with preamplifiers were used.

2.2.3 Procedure
First, the electromyographic wave patterns obtained over 5 seconds at the maximum effort of the kicking motion (maximum voluntary contraction (MVC) (CARLO and DELUCA, 1997) were integrated in real time using a computer, and the ARS data on the display were shown to the subject. Next, the threshold line at 75% of the mean ARS (mV) during the muscular contraction period was shown to the subject, who was requested to perform muscular training aiming at the threshold line for 1 min 20 s. In other words, BFT was performed at 75% of the MVC. During BFT, data were recorded in a notebook computer (AP Monitor, NoruPro) at a sampling rate of 2 kHz. The low frequency cut-off filters were used at 16 Hz, and an alternating current-eliminating filter was also used.

2.3 Algorithm in the SOSE system

The initial 20 s of the sEMG data recorded over a total of 1 min 20 s were excluded, because the subjects may have required this time to adjust to the training. The sEMG data of the 6-cycle rectangular waves that occurred over the remaining minutes of training (target value) $f(t)$ and the ARS were analyzed in accordance with the Double-Wayland algorithm (TAKADA et al., 2006a) and our own mathematical algorithms of the sensor output signal evaluation system. Fig. 4 shows a revision of the flow chart in SHIOZAWA et al. (2006a). Taking a mean of the ARS (MARS) as a threshold H for determining continuous muscular contractions, the time sequences above the threshold H were regarded as continuous muscular contractions. Based on whether differences such as $x(t) - x(t - 0.1)$ and $(x(t + 0.1) - x(t))(x(t) - x(t - 0.1))$ were positive or negative, a maximal series for the continuous muscular contractions was extracted as shown in Fig. 5.

a. The value of the MARS during the muscular relaxation period (x^a) and the measurement parameters in the other terms (SHIOZAWA et al., 2006b; SHIOZAWA et al., 2006c; TAKADA et al., 2006b) indicating the shape of the ARS were determined every cycle, and the ARS values obtained from the femoral rectus muscles were evaluated.
b. Maximum amplitude (x^b): This maximum value was examined and recorded.
c. Duration of continuous muscular contraction (x^c): The duration between the first and last maximal values in a cycle exceeding the MARS sEMG was measured (Fig. 5).
d. The time constant of the exponential decay curve fit to the maximal points during the muscular contraction period in the BFT (x^d): All maximal values between the first and last maximal values exceeding the MARS in a cycle were extracted as $\{x_m(t)\}$ and fit to the exponential decay curve $\hat{x}_m(t) = C\exp[-x^d t]$. On a semi-log graph, the time constant (x^d) was estimated using the mean least square method, which minimized the sum of the squared residuals;

$$L = \sum_t \{\log \hat{x}_m(t) - \log x_m(t)\}^2 . \tag{2}$$

In order to estimate the time constant (x^d), the following simultaneous equation should be solved.

$$\frac{\partial L}{\partial \log C} = 0, \frac{\partial L}{\partial x^d} = 0 \tag{3}$$

The numerical sequences of the 4 measurement parameters were determined at a repetition number of 6. The relationship between the age (z) of the subjects who had undergone sEMG and the value $x^i(z)$ $(i = a,b,c,d)$ estimated in the 5th cycle was statistically examined to evaluate correlations between each measurement parameter and age (Appendix).

2.4 Practical study of the SOSE system

The numerical sequences of each of the measurement parameters at a repetition number of 6 were obtained by sEMG performed during BFT. The relationship between the age (z) of the subjects who had undergone sEMG and the value $x^i(z)$ $(i = a,b,c,d)$ was examined in 5th cycle. Fig. 6 shows the $x^i(z)$ of all 50 subjects. The linear regression analysis using the least-square method, demonstrated that the coefficients by which age (z) was multiplied were 0.071, -0.268, -0.006, and -0.010 for (a), (b), (c), and (d), respectively, and the parameters,

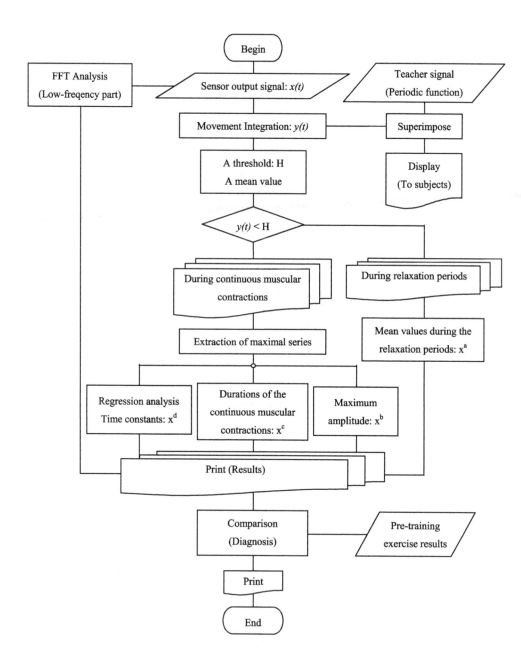

Fig. 4. A part of the flow chart of our mathematical algorithm of the sensor output signal evaluation system.

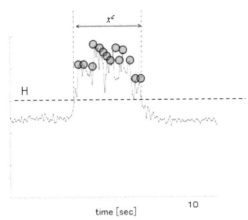

Fig. 5. A series of maximal values of the ARS during the muscular contraction periods in the BFT were extracted by our mathematical algorithm of the sensor output signal evaluation system.

except for (a), decreased with age. Since the linear regression coefficients varied with the measurement parameters, correlations between these parameters and age could not be judged using only the coefficients by which age (z) was multiplied. When using the t-test to evaluate the null hypothesis ($\hat{b} = 0$) for the regression coefficient ($\hat{b}$), the test values (A.3) were 1.105, 0.238, 1.621, and 3.245 for (a), (b), (c), and (d), respectively, and the only parameter exceeding $t_{48}(0.975)$ was the time constant of the exponential decay curve fit to the maximal points of the muscular contraction period in the BFT (x^d).

We examined correlations between the parameters of the ARS and age. Regression equations (A.1) for each parameter (i = a,b,c,d) were determined, and the null hypothesis ($\hat{b} = 0$) for the regression coefficient ($\hat{b}$) was examined using the t-test. Since the test value (A.3) was larger than the two-sided 5% point, t_{48} (0.975), in the t distribution with a latitude of 48, the null hypothesis was rejected in the case of i = d. Therefore, the time constant of the exponential decay curve fit to the maximal points during the continuous muscular contraction period (x^d) is significantly dependant on age (p<0.05).

2.5 Problem
The analysis of sEMG data is generally performed by the fast Fourier transformation (FFT), which is a linear analytical method. A Fourier series expansion of the function $f(t)$, showing target levels (instruction signals) for BFT, is possible, and the following expansion equation (MATSUMOTO and MIYAHARA, 1990) is useful for evaluating the differences between the ARS and the rectangular waves:

$$f(t) = 1 + \sum_{k=1}^{\infty} \frac{2}{k\pi} \{1 + (-1)^{k+1}\} \sin\frac{2\pi k}{T} t \ . \tag{4}$$

Higher-order terms (high-frequency components) are included in this expansion equation, but the coefficients are small due to the presence of the order in the denominator. Accordingly, the high-frequency power was considered to be theoretically irrelevant for the

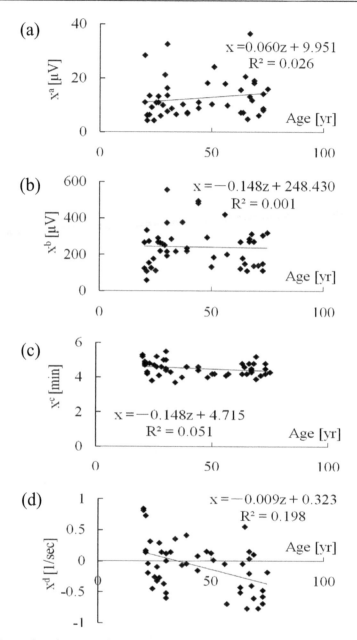

Fig. 6. Relationships between the measurement parameters of the ARS and age and their linear regressions. R^2 shows the coefficient of determination. MARS during the muscular relaxation period, x^a (a). Maximum amplitude, x^b (b). Duration of continuous muscular contraction, x^c (c). Time constant of the exponential curve fit to the maximal points of the continuous muscular contraction period, x^d (d).

evaluation shown in Eq. (4). Since muscular conditions always vary, signals should be regarded as non-steady (BEYER, 1987). Since a spectral estimation by the Fourier analysis is based on the assumption that the signals to be analyzed are steady and linear, this linear analysis of sEMG data is inappropriate.

Myopotentials are induced by changes in the firing patterns of nerve impulses. Several muscle fibers controlled by a motor nerve are collectively called a motor unit (MU), and several MUs can be excited by nerve impulses, causing an MU action potential. The MU action potential measured on the skin's surface is a superficial myopotential, and it is observed at a site spatially distant from the local region where the MU action potential waves are generated. In sEMG, a very large number of MU action potential waves are superimposed, and the activity states of whole muscles are observed by this method (YOSHIDA et al., 2004). Therefore, sEMG signals should be considered nonlinear, or more generally, sEMG shows a time series produced by stochastic processes. Recently, it has been recognized that sEMG data can be examined by nonlinear analytical methods, such as the recurrence plot and the Wayland algorithm (YOSHIDA et al., 2004; TAKADA et al, 2006c). However, the measurement parameters used in the present study, such as the time constant of the exponential decay curve fit to the maximal points of the continuous muscular contraction period (x^d), are used as a linear analytical method for sEMG. In the next section, we discuss the reason why we have succeeded in findings a linear index showing a correlation with age.

3. Solution & recommendations

The complexity of the bio-signal or the degree of visible determinism generating those signals can be measured by our Double-Wayland algorithm (TAKADA et al, 2006a), which is introduced in this section.

3.1 Double-Wayland algorithm

The translation error is a statistical index that measures the smoothness of flow in an attractor generating a time series. In addition, randomness can be evaluated by the Double-Wayland algorithm by comparing the translation errors in the temporal differences of the time series (differenced time series) with the results of the Wayland algorithm in each embedding space (Wayland et al., 1993).

An attractor is reconstructed from a time series. The attractor is constructed by means of embedding the time series data proposed by Takens (1981) in the phase space. Embedding is a method that draws an orbit in phase space supposing a vector whose elements are the values for when the time elapses from t to Δt, $2\Delta t$, ..., $(N-1)\Delta t$ as a point in N dimensional phase space (embedding space). N and Δt are referred to as the embedding dimension and the sampling time, respectively. The delay coordinates $\{x(t)\}$ can reconstruct a continuous trajectory without crossing into an embedding space that has a high dimension. If we only resample the time series at every delay time τ when the auto-correlation coefficient $\rho(\tau)$ is regarded as zero, components of the delay coordinate $x(t) = (x(t), x(t+\tau),..., x(t+(N-1)\tau))$ cannot linearly correlate with each other. In this study, the auto-correlation function $\rho(t)$ was estimated from the time series data (Matsumoto et al., 2002) and regarded as zero when $\rho(t)$ decreased below $1/e \cong 0.37$ for the first time ($t \geq 0$).

The Wayland algorithm assumes that the difference vectors $v(t) = x(t+\tau) - x(t)$ in the embedding space characterize the nonlinear variations of the trajectories and estimate the translation error in an m-dimensional embedding space (m = 1, 2, ..., 10). Here, τ was estimated at 73-76 times the sampling time. A linear correlation between adjacent vectors $\mathbf{x}(t)$ and $\mathbf{x}(t+\tau)$ is eliminated by resampling the time series with respect to each embedding delay τ.

i. A series of delay coordinate vectors $\{\mathbf{x}(t)\}$ is embedded in each space.

ii. M onset periods t_0 are randomly selected.

iii. The values of

$$E_{\text{trans}}(t_0) = \frac{1}{K+1}\sum_{i=0}^{K}\frac{\left|\mathbf{v}(t_i)-\overline{\mathbf{v}}\right|}{\left|\overline{\mathbf{v}}\right|} \tag{5}$$

are standardized by the average of the difference vectors at $K+1$ points $\{\mathbf{x}(t_i)\}_{i=0}{}^K$.

$$\overline{\mathbf{v}} = \frac{1}{K+1}\sum_{i=0}^{K}\mathbf{v}(t_i) \tag{6}$$

is obtained at every onset period, where the K points nearest to $\mathbf{x}(t_0)$ are selected as $\{\mathbf{x}(t_i)\}_{i=0}{}^K$.

iv. The median of the M values of Eq. (5) is extracted.

v. Q medians are obtained by repeating the above steps. The translation error E_{trans} is estimated by the expectation value of these Q medians.

The Double-Wayland algorithm includes the following additional steps.

vi. Translation errors, E_{trans}', are derived from temporal differences in the time series data (differenced time series) $\{\mathbf{x}(t+\tau) - \mathbf{x}(t)\}$ by the Wayland algorithm outlined above.

vii. If a differential equation system that included stochastic factors was the generator of the time series, the flow would not be smooth. In such a case, a significantly higher number of translation errors might be estimated in the last step than in step (v).

In this study, we set the conditions of the coefficients M, K, and Q to be 51, 3, and 10, respectively (Wayland et al., 1993).

If a time series is produced from a chaos process, the translation vectors point in almost the same direction unless the time implementation τ is too large, since deterministic aspects remain in time development. The minimum translation error would be estimated in such an embedding space that has no false intersection along the orbit and best reflects the degree of freedom. Hereby, the optimum embedding dimension to capture the chaos process can be obtained.

The differenced time series produced in the stochastic process often reconstitutes an indifferentiable orbit in embedding space. This indicates that the translation error estimated from the differenced time series exceeds the translation error estimated from the time series data. Accordingly, we weighed the translation error estimated from the time series data against the error estimated from the differenced time series in m dimensional phase space.

In general, the threshold of the translation error for classifying the time series data as deterministic or stochastic is 0.5, which is half of the translation error resulting from a random walk (MATSUMOTO et al., 2002). The abovementioned E_{trans} is compared with the translation error (E_{trans}') estimated from the differenced time series.

3.2 Non-linear analysis of the sEMG in the BFT

Using the Double-Wayland algorithm, translation errors were estimated from the sEMG measured during a continuous muscle contraction period and during BFT. We compared the translation errors E_{trans} and E_{trans}' in each embedding space (Figs.7). Intermittent muscle the differenced sEMG's of the younger subjects. E_{trans}' would be less than E_{trans} if the degree of determinism involved in the generator were reduced. The form of a rectangular wave as a teacher signal might reduce the nonlinearity involved in the generator of sEMG for the young. Moreover, we employed the method of surrogate data to ascertain the cause of the correlation between age and a linear index for the ARS. According to the Fourier shuffle algorithm, 20 surrogate sequences were generated from each ARS during the 3 s continuous muscle contraction period and the 3 s of BFT shown in Fig. 7. Using the Wayland algorithm, translation errors were estimated from the surrogate sequences. The embedding delay was estimated as 0.064 ± 0.003 s and 0.290 ± 0.135 s from the surrogate data of the ARS during the continuous muscle contraction period and BFT, respectively. A significant difference was observed between the translation errors, E_{trans}, estimated during the continuous muscle contraction period and the BFT ($p < 0.01$). The E_{trans} calculated during the continuous muscle contraction period was greater than that taken after this period. BFT could enhance the linearity in the generator of sEMG.

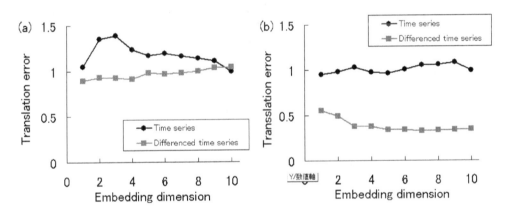

Fig. 7. Results of the calculations involved in sEMG using the Double-Wayland algorithm. Translation errors, E_{trans} and E_{trans}', were estimated from sEMG data measured during a continuous muscle contraction period for 3 s (a) and during 3 s of BFT (b) (TAKADA et al., 2010).

3.3 Stability of the sEMG in the BFT

Since there were differences in not only the unit of measurement but also the numerical order between the parameters, they were normalized using the intermediate values $\bar{x}^i$ for each cycle, and the reproducibility (stability) of the measurements was evaluated using the standard deviation $\sigma[x^i / \bar{x}^i]$. The normalized value is 1 when the measurement is equal to the intermediate value. When the reproducibility (stability) of repeated measurements is high, the deviations from this value are small, and the standard deviation is close to 0.

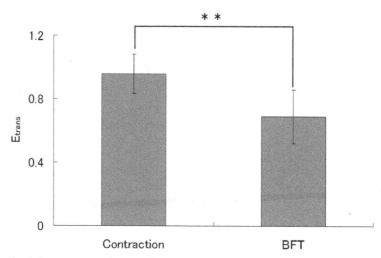

Fig. 8. Result of the surrogate data analysis. In 10 dimensional embedding space, translation errors were estimated from the surrogate data of the ARS during the continuous muscle contraction period and the BFT.

The intermediate values of the parameters and the standard deviations (σ) of normalized measurements were determined for each subject, and the medians of σ in the age groups are compared in Table 1. The duration of continuous muscular contraction (x^c) alone showed $\sigma < 0.1$ for any age group.

Age group	N	Mean during relaxation	Maximal amplitude	Duration of continuous muscular contraction	Time constant
≤25	8	0.24	0.13	0.06	1.51
≤45	9	0.21	0.14	0.08	0.55
≤65	6	0.33	0.14	0.08	1.84
65 <	8	0.07	0.06	0.06	0.89

N expresses the number of subjects in each age group.

Table 1. Standard deviations of normalized indices $x/\overline{x}$ [8]

4. Future research directions

The decline in translation errors, E_{trans}', was not always seen in the middle-aged and the elderly. Poor muscular control might enhance the instability of the temporal variations involved in the ARS, which should be maintained as a constant during a muscular contraction in BFT. The relationship between age and the decline in the translation errors, E_{trans}', should be investigated in future work.

We will employ a time series analysis, such as a surrogate method, to ascertain the cause of the correlation between age and a linear index of ARS.

5. Conclusion

Recently, there has been an increasing focus on the rapid reduction of the muscles that are required for bending the hip joint during walking with age. Atrophy of the flexor muscles has been implicated in falling in the elderly. In this study, we examined the ARS of the femoral rectus muscles during BFT of the dominant leg. To this end, we developed parameters for the measurement of the shapes in the ARS, and evaluated the changes in these parameters as the muscles age. A statistical analysis indicated that it was necessary to include the time constant of the exponential decay curve fit to the maximal points during prolonged muscular contraction to evaluate changes with age using the ARS during BFT. A reduction in the function of muscular control due to aging can be detected by performing sEMG during BFT using this time constant. Using our Double-Wayland algorithm, we have also confirmed the stationarity of the ARS during the muscle contraction period.

6. Appendix

The relationship between each of the above measurement parameters and age was examined. $x^i_j(z_j)$ of subject j ($j = 1, 2, \cdots, 50$) was plotted, and a linear regression analysis of these 50 points was performed by the least-square method (MATSUMOTO and MIYAHARA, 1990). The regression equation of each measurement parameter was determined.

$$x^i = \hat{a} + \hat{b}\, z \tag{A.1}$$

$$\text{s.t.} \quad \hat{a} = \frac{1}{50}\left(\sum_{j=1}^{50} x^i_j - \hat{b} \sum_{j=1}^{50} z_j \right), \tag{A.2.1}$$

$$\hat{b} = \frac{1}{S_{zz}} \sum_{j=1}^{50} x^i_j \left(z_j - \frac{1}{50} \sum_{j=1}^{50} z_j \right). \quad (i = \text{a, b, c, d}) \tag{A.2.2}$$

Here, S_{zz} denotes a variance of age. The dependence of each measurement parameter on age was statistically evaluated by a two-sided t-test with the null hypothesis that the regression coefficient $\hat{b} = 0$.

$$\left| \hat{b} - 0 \right| / \sqrt{S_E / 48 S_{zz}} \tag{A.3}$$

If the above value is larger than $t_{48}(1-\alpha/2)$, the null hypothesis is rejected, and the measurement parameter is considered to be correlated with age (SHIMIZU and TAKADA, 2001). Here, S_E denotes the residual sum of squares by the least-square method, and $t_{48}(1-\alpha/2)$ represents the t distribution at a probability of $1-\alpha/2$ and a latitude of 48. In this study, since the significance level (α) was defined as 0.05, $t_{48}(1-\alpha/2)$ was approximately 2.010.

7. Acknowledgment

This work was supported in part by a ground-based study proposal for the fiscal year of 2005-2007 (17659189) and the Hori Information Science Promotion Foundation.

8. References

Aukee, P., Penttinen, J., Immonen, P. & Airaksinen, O. (2002) Intravaginal surface EMG probe design test for urinary incontinence patients. *Acupunt. Electro-Ther. Res. Int. J.*, Vol.27, 2002, pp.37–44, 0360-1293.

Basmajian, S. (1989) *An anthology of visual poetry and collage*, Sober Minute Press, 0921280009, Toronto.

Beyer, W.H. (eds.) (June 30,1987) *CRC Standard Mathematical Tables and Formulae* (28th ed.), CRC Press, ISBN 0849306280,Boca Raton, FL.

Bosco, C. & Komi, P. V. (1980) Influence of aging on the mechanical behaviour of leg extensor muscles. *European Journal of Applied Physiology*, Vol.45, Dec 1980, pp.209-219, 1439-6319.

Carlo, J. & Deluca, C.J. (1997) The use of surface electromyography in biomechanics. *Journal of Applied Biomechanics*, Vol.13, July 1993, pp.135–163, 1065-8483.

Chang, T., Schiff, S.J., Sauer, T., Gossard, J.P. & Burke, R.E. (1994) Stochastic Versus Deteriministic Variability in Simple Neuronal circuits: I. Monosynaptic Spinal Cord Reflexes, *Biophysical Journal*, Vol.67, No.2, Aug 1994, pp.671-683, 0006-3495.

Chang, T., Sauer, T. & Schiff, S.J. (1995) Tests for nonlinearity in short stationary time series, *Chaos*, Vol.5, No.1, Mar 1995, pp.118-126, 1054-1500.

Fantl, J.A., Newman, D.K., Colling, J., Delancey, J., Keeys, C.,Loughery, R., Mcdowell, J., Norton, P., Ouslander, J., Schnelle, J., Staskin, D., Tries, J., Urich, V., Vitousek, S.H., Weiss, B.D., & Whitmore, K. (Mar 1996) *Urinary Incontinence in Adults : Acute and Chronic Management.* Clinical practice guideline. Rockville, MD: Agency for Health Care Policy and Research, Public Health Service, US Department of Health and Human Services.

Gaarder, K.R. & Montgomery, P.S. (Jun, 1981) *Clinical Biofeedback-Procedural Manual for Behavioral Medicine*, Williams & Wilkins, 0683034014, London.

Gatchel, R. J. & Price, K. P. An introduction and historical overview, In: Gatchel, R.J. and Price, K.P.(eds.), Mar 1979. *Critical Applications of Biofeedback: Appraisal and Status*, Pergamon Press, 0080229786, New York.

Hanayama, K. (2001) Evaluation of muscle fatigue with muscle fiber conduction velocity, Clinical Electroencephalography, Vol.43, No.3, pp.144-147, 0009-9155.

Jacobsen, E.(Dec, 1938) *Progressive relaxation*, University of Chicago Press, 0226390586, Chicago.

Kegel, A.H. (1948) Progressive resistance exercise in the functional restoration of the perineal muscles. *American Journal of Obstetrics and Gynecology*, Vol.56, Aug 1948, pp.238-248, 0002-9378.

Kegel, A.H.(1951) Physiologic therapy for urinary stress incontinence. *Journal of the American Medical Association*, Vol.146, 1951, pp.915-917, 0098-7484.

Kiryu, T. (1997) Monitoring local muscle fatigue using surface electromyography. *Journal of the Society of Biomechanisms*, Vol.21, No.2, Feb 1997,pp.75-80, 0285-0885.

Kimura, J. (Jun 15, 1989) *Electrodiagnosis in Diseases of Nerve and Muscles: Principles and Practice* (2nd), Oxford University Press, pp.209-304, 0803653425, Philadelphia.

Kizuka, T., Masuda, T., Kiryu, T. & Sadoyama, T. (Mar 2006) *Practical usage of surface electromyography*, Tokyo Denki University Press, pp.65-92, 4501325100, Tokyo.

Matsumoto, H. & Miyahara, Y. (Jun 1999) *Introduction to mathematical statistics*, Gakujutsu Tosho, pp.106-108, 4873611741, Tokyo.

Matsumoto, T., Tokunaga, R., Miyano, T. & Tokuda, I. (Nov 2002) *Chaos and time series,* Baihukan, pp.49–64, 4563014974, Tokyo.

Peek, C. J. (Jan 1, 1995) A primer of biofeedback instrumentation, In: *Biofeedback a Practitionaer's Guide,* Schwartz, M.S., pp.597-629, Guilford Press, 0898628067, New York.

Shimizu, Y. & Takada, H. (2001) Verification of air temperature variation with form of potential, *Forma,* Vol.16, No.4, 2001, pp.339-356, 0911-6036.

Shiozawa, T., Takada, H. & Miyao, M. (2006a) Sensor output signal evaluation system, Japan Patent P2006-111387.

Shiozawa, T., Takada, H., Miyao, M. & Kawasaki, H.(2006b) Propositions of evaluating indices of muscle performancs detected by using surface electromyography and evaluation of stability of the indices, *Proceedings of the 21th Symposium on Biological and Physiological Engineering 2006,* Kagoshima(Japan), Nov 2006.

Shiozawa, T., Takada, H., Miyao, M., Takada, M., Kawasaki, H. & Watanabe, Y. (2006c) Evaluation of muscle performances detected by using surface electromyography, *Japanese Journal of Ergonomics,* Vol.42, Jun 2006, pp.S440-S441. 0549-4974.

Shiozawa, T., Takada, H. & Miyao, M. (2007) Sensor output signal evaluation system, PCT Patent Publication No. WO 2007/129452.

Takada, H., Morimoto, T., Tsunashima, H., Yamazaki, T., Hoshina, H. & Miyao, M. (2006a) Applications of Double-Wayland Algorithm to Detect Anomalous Signals, *Forma,* Vol.21, No.2, 2006, pp.159-167, 0911-6036.

Takada, H., Shiozawa, T., Miyao, M., Takada, M. & Kawasaki, H. (2006b) Mathematical analysis of skeletal muscle electromyogram and the aging, *Japanese Journal of Ergonomics,* Vol.42, Jun 2006, pp.S444-S445. 0549-4974.

Takada, H., Shiozawa, T., Miyao, M., Nakayama, M. & Kawasaki, H.(2006c) Theoretical consideration to set the amplitude of teacher signal in the biofeedback training, *Proceedings of the 21th Symposium on Biological and Physiological Engineering 2006,* Kagoshima(Japan), Nov 2006.

Takada, H., Shiozawa, T., Takada, M., Miyao, M. & Kawasaki, H.(2007) Propositions of evaluaing indices of muscle performances detected by using surface electromyography and the aging, *Bulletin of Gifu University of Medical Science,* Vol.1, Mar 2007, pp.91-95, 1881-9168.

Takada, H., Shiozawa, T., Miyao, M. Matsuura, Y. & Takada, M. (Oct 6, 2010) Consideration of indices to evaluate age-related muscle performance by using surface electromyography. In: *Advances in computational biology,* Arabnia, H. R., pp.585-591, Springer, 9781441959126, New York

Takens, F. (1981) Detecting strange attractors in turbulence, *Lecture Notes in Mathematics,* Vol.898, 1981, pp.366-381, 0075-8434.

Theiler, J., Eubank, S., Longtin, A., Galdrikian, B. & Farmer, J.D. Testing for nonlinearity in time series: The method of surrogate data, Physica D, 58, pp.77-94, 1992, 0167-2789.

Tries, J. & Eisman, E. (Jan 1, 1995) Urinary incontinence — evaluation and biofeedback treatment. In: *Biofeedback a Practitionaer's Guide,* Schwartz, M. S., pp.597-629, Guilford Press, 0898628067, New York.

Wayland, R., Bromley, D., Pickett, D. & Passamante, A. (1993) Recognizing determinism in a time series, *Phys. Rev. Lett.,* Vol.70, No.5, Feb 1993, pp.580–582, 0031-9007.

Yoshida, H., Ujiie, H., Ishimura, K. & Wada, M. (2004) The estimation of muscle fatigue using chaos analysis, *Journal of the Society of Biomechanisms*, Vol.28, No.4, 2004, pp.201-212, 0285-0885.

Young, A. (1997) Ageing and physiological functions. *Philos Trans R Soc Lond B*, Vol.352, Dec 1997, pp.1837–1843, 0264-3839.

8

The Usefulness of Wavelet Transform to Reduce Noise in the SEMG Signal

Angkoon Phinyomark, Pornchai Phukpattaranont and Chusak Limsakul
Department of Electrical Engineering, Prince of Songkla University, Songkhla,
Thailand

1. Introduction

This chapter presents a usefulness of wavelet transform (WT) algorithm in pre-processing stage of surface electromyography (sEMG) signal analysis particularly in application of noise reduction. The successful pre-processing stage based on wavelet decomposition and denoising algorithm is proposed in this chapter together with the principle, theory, up-to-date literature review and experimental results of the wavelet denoising algorithms. Main application of this algorithm is sEMG control systems, notably prosthetic devices or computers.

SEMG signal is one of the useful electrophysiological signals. It is measured by surface electrodes that are placed on the skin superimposed on the muscle. Rich useful information has occurred in the muscles subjacent to the skin as a mixture of the whole motor unit action potentials (MUAPs). Such information is also useful in a wide class of clinical and engineering researches which may lead to providing the diagnosis tools of neuromuscular and neurological problems and to providing the control systems of assistive robots and rehabilitation devices (Merletti & Parker, 2004). Generally, in order to use the sEMG as a diagnosis signal or a control signal, a feature is often extracted before performing classification stage due to a lot of information obtained from raw sEMG data and a low computational complexity required in the embedded devices (Boostani & Moradi, 2003). However, the sEMG signals that originate in a wide class of human muscles and activities are definitely contaminated by different types of noise (De Luca, 2002; Reaz et al., 2006). This becomes a main problem to extract certain features and thus the reach to high accurate classification. In the last decade, many research works have been interested in developing better algorithms and improving the existing methods to reduce noises and to estimate the useful sEMG information (De Luca et al., 2010; Mewett et al., 2004; Phinyomark et al., 2011).

Generally, noises contaminated in the sEMG signal can be categorized into four major types: ambient noise, motion artifact, inherent instability of the sEMG signal, and inherence in electronic components in the detection and recording equipment (De Luca, 2002). The first three types have specific frequency band and do not fall in the energy band of the sEMG signal. For instance, power-line interference has the frequency component at 50 Hz (or 60 Hz), and motion artifact and instability in nature of sEMG signal have most of their energy in the frequency range of 0 to 20 Hz. Usage of conventional filters, i.e. band-pass filter and band-stop filter, can reduce noises in these types (De Luca et al., 2010). However, the last noise type is a central concern in analysis of the sEMG signal. It is an inherent noise that is generated by electronic equipment. The frequency components of this noise are random in nature and range in the usable energy of sEMG frequency band from 0 to several thousand Hz. It causes difficulty in elimination using the conventional filters. Moreover, using high-quality electronic components, intelligent circuit design and construction techniques, noises can be only reduced but it cannot be entirely eliminated (De Luca, 2002). Hence, it may cause a problem in extracting the robust features (Phinyomark et al., 2008; Zardoshti-Kermani, 1995).

Wavelet transform and adaptive filter are used in advanced filtering methods that are commonly used as a powerful tool to remove random noise in non-stationary signals. Nonetheless, the drawback of adaptive filter is the complexity of devising an automatic procedure. Its performance depends on a reference input signal which is difficult to apply in the real-world applications. On the other hand, wavelet transform method does not require any reference signals. The pre-processing stage based on wavelet denoising algorithm for sEMG upper- and lower- limb movement recognitions have been a huge success over the past few years (Hussain et al., 2007, 2009; Khezri & Jahed, 2008; Phinyomark et al., 2010a, 2011; Ren et al., 2006). To achieve the best performance in wavelet denoising algorithm, five wavelet parameters must be addressed. Hence, in this chapter, we have evaluated all wavelet denoising parameters for improving the classification performance of sEMG control systems. As a result, the improvement of classification accuracy of the sEMG recognition system has been presented and a robustness of the system has also been improved.

The rest of this chapter is as follows: Section 2 presents various types of electrical noises in sEMG signals and discusses how to simulate these artificial noises. In Section 3, principle and theory of wavelet transform algorithm in both general and denoising viewpoints are described. Extensive review and careful survey of up-to-date wavelet denoising methods in numerous biomedical signals and applications are summarized in Section 4 and recent trend of wavelet denoising algorithms in the sEMG signal analysis is discussed in Section 5. In Section 6, the experimental results of using wavelet denoising algorithms with real sEMG signals are presented and discussed. Lastly, conclusion and future trends of using wavelet transform to reduce noise in the sEMG signal are proposed in Section 7.

2. Electrical noises in the SEMG signal

2.1 Different types of the noises

Noises contaminated in the sEMG signal can be categorized into four main types: ambient noise, motion artifact, sEMG signal inherent instability, and inherence in electronic components in the detection and recording equipments (De Luca, 2002; Kale & Dudul, 2009; Reaz et al., 2006). More details about source and characteristics of each noise type are explained in the following discussion:

1. Ambient noise: This kind of noise originates from electromagnetic radiation sources such as electrical-power wires, light bulbs, fluorescent lamps, radio and television transmission, computers, etc. Essentially any electromagnetic device or device that is plugged into the A/C power supply generates and may contribute ambient noises. Moreover, our body surfaces are persistently flooded with electric-magnetic radiation and it is practically impossible to avoid exposure to it on the surface of the earth. The dominant frequency of the ambient noise arises from the 50 Hz (or 60 Hz) radiation from power sources. Generally, the main concern noise in this type is also called "Power-line noise or 50 Hz interference". The amplitude of the ambient noise is one to

three orders of magnitude greater than the sEMG signal. Therefore, in analysis of the sEMG signal in various research works have implemented a notch filter (band-stop filter) at this frequency (Mewett et al., 2004). Theoretically, this type of filter would only remove the unwanted power-line frequency; however, practical implementations also remove portions of the adjacent frequency components. Because the dominant energy of the sEMG signal is located in the 50-100 Hz range, the use of notch filter is not advisable (De Luca, 2002). One of our previous studies (Phinyomark et al., 2009a), the effect of this kind of noises with the sEMG feature extraction was investigated. The robust features for this kind of noise, notably Willison amplitude, have been found in order to avoid the implementing a notch-filter.

2. Motion artifact: This kind of noise causes irregularities in the signal. When motion artifact is putted into the data, the sEMG information may be skewed. There are two main sources of motion artifact: 1) the interface between the detection surface of electrode and skin 2) the movement of the cable connecting electrode to the amplifier. The dominant energy of the electrode motion artifact has been concerned in the frequency range from 0 to 20 Hz. The second type of noise source, cable motion artifact typically has a frequency range of 1 to 50 Hz. However, both of these sources can be essentially reduced by proper design of the electronics circuitry and set-up. Moreover, some research works suggest implementing a high-pass filter into the measurement instrumentation with a corner frequency of 10 Hz (Clancy et al., 2002) or 20 Hz (De Luca et al., 2010).

3. SEMG signal inherent instability: Amplitude of the sEMG signal is quasi-random in nature. This kind of noise is affected by the random in nature of the firing rate of the motor units which, in most conditions, fire in the frequency components between 0 and 20 Hz. Because of the unstable nature of these components of the sEMG signal, it is advisable to consider them as unwanted noise and remove them from the sEMG signal. Nevertheless, it can be removed using a high-pass filter with a cut-off frequency of 20 Hz which has already been implemented in the removing of motion artifact.

4. Inherence in electronic components in the detection and recording equipments: All electronics equipments generate electrical noise. This noise has the frequency components that range from 0 Hz to several thousand Hz. The problem is that this kind of noise cannot be eliminated. It can only be reduced by using high-quality electronic components, intelligent circuit design and construction techniques. Therefore, this kind of noise is becoming a major problem in analysis of the sEMG signal. Our previous studies, we have paid more interest in reducing the effect of noise in this group (Phinyomark et al., 2008, 2009b, 2009c, 2009d, 2009e, 2009f, 2009g, 2009h, 2010a, 2010b, 2010c, 2011).

Note that during the recording of the sEMG signal, the subject is generally instructed to relax. However, regardless of relaxation, muscles always show a basic level of electrical activity. It has been suggested that this residual sEMG activity may establish a significant part of the total noise level (Huigen et al., 2002). All of these noises also mentioned to the background noise.

2.2 Simulation of noises in SEMG signal analysis

From the above explanation, we can notice that first three types of noises have the specific frequency band and do not fall in the dominant energy band of the sEMG signal. Thus usage of the conventional filters such as band-pass filter, high-pass filter and notch filter can eliminate noises in this group (De Luca et al., 2010). However, noise of the last type is a main concern in analysis of the sEMG signal. It ranges in the usable energy of sEMG frequency band from 0 to several thousand Hz; therefore, it causes difficulty in elimination using the conventional filters. Moreover, using high-quality electronic components, intelligent circuit design and construction techniques, noise in this group can be only reduced but it cannot be entirely eliminated (De Luca, 2002; Kale & Dudul, 2009; Reaz et al., 2006).

To prepare the noisy sEMG signals, random noise is considered to be used as a representative noise, an agent of the fourth noise type. Usually, white Gaussian noise (WGN) is used as a representative random noise in the sEMG signal analysis (Boostani & Moradi, 2003; Kale & Dudul, 2009; Laterza & Olmo, 1997; Law et al., 2011; Wellig & Moschytz, 1998; Zardoshti-Kermani et al., 1995). This noise is also called artificial random noise or simulated random noise. The WGN is a random signal with a flat power spectral density and a normal amplitude distribution. To more clearly understand, the flat power spectral density means that the signal contains equal power within a fixed bandwidth at any center frequency and the normal amplitude distribution means that the signal contains random values that tend to cluster around a single mean value. Usually the WGN is set to a zero mean and a unit standard deviation (Kale & Dudul, 2009; Phinyomark et al., 2009c, 2010a, 2011). In order to evaluate performance of the denoising algorithms, different levels of the WGN are used in the preparation of noisy environment. Zardoshti-Kermani et al. (1995) estimated the WGN with root-mean-square (RMS) amplitude on each muscle position varying from 0% to 50% of the overall average RMS amplitude of the whole muscle activities. The estimated signal-to-noise ratios (SNRs) were varied from 1:3 to 7:1 which depended on level of muscle contraction. Subsequently, Andrade et al. (2006) and Law et al. (2011) estimated the WGN with amplitude ranging from 20% to 100% and from 2% to 40% of the absolute maximum amplitude, respectively. On the other hand, Boostani and Moradi (2003) estimated the WGN with one tenth of the peak-to-peak amplitude range of the sEMG signal. In our previous studies, noisy sEMG signals were simulated by adding synthetic WGNs which resulted in different SNRs. The SNRs ranged from 20 dB (low noise level) to 0 dB (high noise level) with the increasing step of 5 dB SNR (Phinyomark et al., 2009c, 2010a, 2011). In addition, some research studies have used our criterion for simulated noisy EMG environments; for instance, Huang et al. (2010) designed a robust EMG sensing interface for pattern classification by using the simulated WGN in range of 20-0 dB SNRs.

Other three important types of noises that normally are used and considered in the simulated noisy EMG environment are power-line noise, movement artifact, and baseline noise. Firstly, power-line interference is used to evaluate ability of both denoising algorithms and robust sEMG features (Boostani & Moradi, 2003; Phinyomark et al., 2009a). This kind of noise is easy to simulate because its frequency component appears at only one frequency point, 50 or 60 Hz. Secondly, movement artifact can be estimated by the volunteer movement which can be monitored by using an accelerometer sensor (De Luca et al., 2010). The accelerometers were attached in the proximity of the sEMG sensors, such as on the top or the distal. When the subjects move their muscles and a movement at the electrode-skin interface is occurred, the g value from the accelerometer can be shown that event (De Luca et al., 2010). Thirdly, noise that is considered in analysis of the sEMG signal is baseline noise. However, this kind of noise can be problematic only when the sEMG signal is very low SNR (Clancy et al., 2002) such as in the assessment of antagonist muscle co-activation or in the classification of low-level muscle contraction (Baratta et al., 1998; Law et al., 2011).

3. Principle and theory of wavelet transform in denoising viewpoint

3.1 Wavelet decomposition

Wavelet transform (WT) is a time-scale representation technique, which expresses a signal into a two-dimensional function of time and scale (pseudo-frequency). The WT uses the correlation with translation and dilation of a wavelet function to yield this transformation. It represents a signal as a sum of wavelets with different locations and scales that allows to use long time intervals for low-frequency information and to use shorter regions for high-frequency information. The WT can be categorized into two main types: continuous wavelet transform (CWT) and discrete wavelet transform (DWT). Calculating wavelet coefficients at every possible scale as implemented in CWT is a fair amount work and it generates an awful lot of data. Usually in denoising viewpoint, the researchers obtain such an analysis from DWT. The definition of DWT is given by:

$$C(a,b) = \sum_{n \in Z} x(n) g_{j,k}(n) \tag{1}$$

where $C(a,b)$ are dyadic wavelet coefficients, a is dilation or scale ($a=2^{-j}$), b is translation ($b=k \times 2^{-j}$), $x(n)$ is the input signal, and $g_{j,k}(n)$ is discrete wavelet ($g_{j,k}(n)=2^{j/2} \times g(2^{j}n-k)$ where $j \in N$ and $k \in Z$). When the input signal is decomposed to a certain level using the DWT, a set of wavelet coefficients is correlated to the high-frequency components (low-scale) while the other wavelet coefficients are correlated to low-frequency components (high-scale). In details, as shown in Fig. 1, in the first step, the original signal (S) is passed through two complementary filters, a low-pass filter and a high-pass filter, and emerges as two signals, approximations and details. The first-level approximation coefficient array (cA1) is obtained from a low-pass filter which includes down-sampling and the first-level detail coefficient array (cD1) is passed through a high-pass filter with down-sampling. The low-pass and high-pass filtering processes are similar to convolving the signal with a scaling function and a wavelet function, respectively. For many signals, generally, the low-frequency content (cA) is the most important part and the high-frequency content (cD), on the other hand, impacts flavor or nuance (noises). Hence, the second-level approximation coefficient array (cA2) and the second-level detail coefficient array (cD2) are obtained by inputting the cA1 into the filters. This is similar to dilating the original scaling function and wavelet function prior to convolving with the cA1. The process is repeated until the desired final level approximation and detail coefficient arrays are obtained. As shown in Fig. 1, it has 3 decomposition levels. When the decomposition is taken as a whole, the denoising process can be employed. If any modification process is not required, the reconstruction process will be instantaneously done. The reconstructed signal (S'), final level approximation and all level details, are true components of the original signal. This is called the perfect reconstruction. The reconstruction process is performed by up-sampling each coefficient array prior to refiltering.

The DWT provides a great advantage over the Fourier analysis and the short-time Fourier transform (STFT) analysis. Although the traditional Fourier analysis performs greatly for the stationary signals, it has a serious drawback if the interesting signals contain non-stationary or transitory characteristics. The STFT and the DWT, on the other hand, map a signal into a two-dimensional function of time and frequency by using a windowing technique. Both of them thus perform greatly for the non-stationary signals. The DWT shares some similarities to the STFT as we described above, except that the fixed window size in the STFT is no more flexible for many signals.

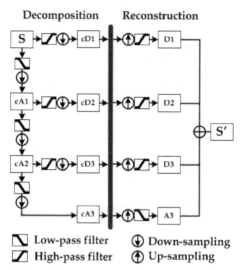

Fig. 1. Wavelet decomposition and reconstruction process.

3.2 Wavelet denoising

The undesired wavelet coefficients containing random noise can be discarded before performing the reconstruction process. The cleaner signal will be obtained from that process. To grab this outcome, thresholding is used in wavelet domain to remove or to shrink some coefficients of DWT detail sub-signals of the measured signal. Usually, the denoising method that applies thresholding in wavelet domain has been proposed by Donoho (1995). The Donoho's method for noise reduction works well for a wide class of one-dimensional and two-dimensional signals. The basic idea of wavelet-based denoising procedure is illustrated in Fig. 2. It consists of three main steps: decomposition, modification of detail coefficients and reconstruction. The first and the last main steps are the general DWT procedure as we described in the Section 3.1. The middle main step is added into the general DWT procedure that involves three parameters: threshold selection rule, threshold rescaling method and thresholding function. In other words, two main points must be addressed: how to choose the threshold value and how to perform the thresholding. In addition, two parameters in decomposition step must be evaluated that are wavelet function and decomposition level.

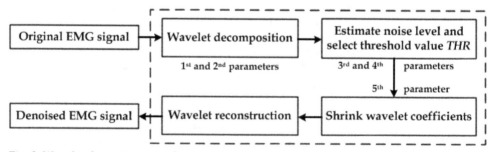

Fig. 2. Wavelet denoising procedure.

In details, the first step in producing a wavelet denoising is to choose a wavelet function (first parameter) to be used in signal decomposition. Different types of wavelet are available which each type has different sub-types. The second step, the selection of a suitable decomposition level (second parameter) must be selected with a candidate wavelet function. The third step, the threshold value *THR* (third parameter) to be applied in the wavelet domain is calculated by the product of the standard deviation of the noise energy σ and the small factor that depends on the length N of the data sample (Donoho and Johnstone, 1994). There are many modified versions of threshold selection rule. In order to rescale the threshold value *THR* obtained from the third step; the estimation of the noise energy σ (fourth parameter) is specified in this step. The fifth step, after threshold *THR* is smoothed, the thresholding is based on a threshold value *THR* which is used to compare with all the detailed coefficients. Ordinarily, two types of thresholding functions (fifth parameter) are often used: hard thresholding and soft thresholding (Donoho and Johnstone, 1994). The choice of threshold values and thresholding functions plays an important role in the global performance of a wavelet processor for noise reduction. Wavelet-based denoising algorithm is based on the underlying model. It is basically of the following form:

$$s(n) = x(n) + \sigma e(n) , \qquad (2)$$

where $s(n)$ is the measured or noisy signal, $x(n)$ is the original or clean signal and $e(n)$ is a Gaussian white noise $N(0,1)$, σ is the strength of the noise, and time n is equally spaced.

4. Review and theory of modified wavelet denoising methods

From the last section, the application of wavelet-based denoising algorithm requires the selection of five processing parameters named "wavelet denoising parameters", including: (1) the type of wavelet basis function, (2) the decomposition level, (3) threshold selection rule (4) threshold rescaling method, and (5) thresholding function. Throughout the extensive review and careful survey of up-to-date wavelet denoising methods in a wide class of biomedical signals and applications, theory and definition of all methods are summarized in the following.

4.1 Wavelet basis functions

Wavelet function or mother wavelet can be categorised into two main types: orthogonal and biorthogonal wavelets. Orthogonal wavelet is entirely defined by the scaling filter (a low-pass finite impulse response (FIR) filter). For analysis with this wavelet, the high-pass filters are calculated as the quadrature mirror filter of the low-pass filters and reconstruction filters are defined as the time reverse of the decomposition filters. In biorthogonal wavelet, decomposition and reconstruction filters are defined as the separate filters. Commonly, there are 6 wavelet families: Daubechies wavelets (10 sub-types), Symlets wavelets (7 sub-types), Coiflet wavelets (5 sub-types), BiorSplines wavelets (15 sub-types), ReverseBior wavelets (15 sub-types) and Discrete Meyer wavelet. All of wavelet functions are presented in Table I. It is important for choosing the right wavelet function (Kania et al., 2007; Tan et al., 2007). The right filter determines perfect reconstruction and performs better analysis.

Wavelet family	Wavelet subtypes
Daubechies	db1 or haar, db2, db3, db4, db5, db6, db7, db8, db9, db10
Symlets	sym2, sym3, sym4, sym5, sym6, sym7, sym8
Coiflet	coif1, coif2, coif3, coif4, coif5
BiorSplines	bior1.1, bior1.3, bior1.5, bior2.2, bior2.4, bior2.6, bior2.8, bior3.1, bior3.3, bior3.5, bior3.7, bior3.9, bior4.4, bior5.5, bior6.8
ReverseBior	rbio1.1, rbio1.3, rbio1.5, rbio2.2, rbio2.4, rbio2.6, rbio2.8, rbio3.1, rbio3.3, rbio3.5, rbio3.7, rbio3.9, rbio4.4, rbio5.5, rbio6.8
Discrete Meyer	dmey

Table 1. List of 53 wavelet functions from 6 wavelet families.

4.2 Decomposition levels

Next step is the selection of the number of decomposition level of the signal. The decomposition level can be varied from 1 (the first level of decomposition) to $J=\log_2 N$ (the maximum depth of decomposition) where N is the length in samples of time-domain signal.

4.3 Threshold selection rules

Threshold selection rule refers to "how to choose the threshold value". Generally, most of research works have used universal threshold selection rule proposed by Donoho. It has been shown that its denoising capability is better than other classical methods such as SURE method, Hybrid method, and minimax method (Phinyomark et al., 2009f). The definition and description of four mainly threshold selection rules are summarized in Table 2. Hence, in our studies, we have interested in numerous modified versions of universal rule (rule 1 in Table 2). Six modified universal rules have been proposed as described in the following. In this chapter, we provide the specific name to each rule as follows.

Thresholding rule	Description
Rule 1: Universal	It uses a fixed form threshold (Donoho & Johnstone, 1994) which can be defined as $THR_{UNI} = \sigma\sqrt{2\log(N)}$, where N is the length in samples of time-domain signal and σ is standard deviation of noise. The parameter σ can be estimated using median parameter which can be calculated as $\sigma = \text{median}\left(\left|cD_j\right|\right)\big/0.6745$ where cD_j is the detail wavelet coefficients at scale level j and 0.6475 is a normalization factor.
Rule 2: SURE	Threshold is selected using the rule of Stein's Unbiased Estimate of Risk (SURE). It gets an estimate of the risk for a particular threshold THR, where risk is defined by SURE (Stein, 1981). Minimizing the risk in THR gives a selection of the threshold.
Rule 3: Hybrid	This rule attempts to overcome limitation of SURE. It is a mixture of the universal and the SURE rules. The exact conditions of this algorithm are described in Donoho and Johnstone (1995).
Rule 4: Minimax	This method was also proposed in Stein (1981) work. It used a fixed threshold chosen to yield minimax performance for mean square error against an ideal procedure.

Table 2. Four main threshold selection rules.

1) Length Modified Universal rule (LMU): It was modified by Donoho to be used with soft-thresholding function (Donoho, 1995). It is defined as

$$THR_{LMU} = \frac{\sigma\sqrt{2\log(N)}}{\sqrt{N}}.$$

(3)

2) Scale Modified Universal rule (SMU): It was modified by Donoho to be used with level dependent method (Donoho, 1992). It can be expressed as

$$THR_{SMU} = \sigma\sqrt{2\log(N)} \cdot 2^{\frac{j-J}{2}},$$

(4)

where j is scale level from 1 to J and J is the maximum level.
3) Global Scale Modified Universal rule (GSMU): It was modified by Zhong and Cherkassky (2000) to be used in denoising of image. It is given by

$$THR_{GSMU} = \sigma\sqrt{2\log(N)} \cdot 2^{\frac{-J}{2}}.$$

(5)

4) Scale Length Modified Universal rule (SLMU): It was modified by Donoho (1992). It is a combination between LMU and SMU rules. It is shown as

$$THR_{SLMU} = \frac{2\sigma\sqrt{2\log(N)}}{\sqrt{N} \cdot 2^{\frac{J-j}{2}}}.$$

(6)

5) Log Scale Modified Universal rule (LSMU): It was modified by Song and Zhao (2001). It takes the different thresholds at different scales. It can be defined as

$$THR_{LSMU} = \frac{\sigma\sqrt{2\log(N)}}{\log(j+1)}.$$

(7)

6) Log Variable Modified Universal rule (LVMU): It was modified by Zhang and Luo (2006). It uses the constant d to adapt the value of threshold THR. Experiment of Zhang and Luo (2006) showed that the constant d is associated to the wavelet function and the SNR. It should be ranging between 0 and 3. In our study, we used $d = 3$. The equation can be defined as

$$THR_{LVMU} = \frac{\sigma\sqrt{2\log(N)}}{\log[e + (j-1)^d]}.$$

(8)

4.4 Threshold rescaling methods

All threshold selection rules can be smoothing their thresholds by using rescaling methods. In threshold rescaling, three categories can be identified: global (GL), first-level (FL) and level dependent (LD) (Elena et al., 2006; Johnstone & Silverman, 1997). In the first one, standard deviation of noise (σ) can be adapted to three categories (GL, FL and LD). While the second one, length of wavelet coefficients (N) can be adapted to only GL and LD thresholding. To identify the threshold rescaling methods, GL defines σ as the estimated standard deviation of all wavelet coefficients and N as the length of the total wavelet coefficients. FL defines σ_1 as the estimated standard deviation of the first-level detail coefficients (cD_1). LD defines σ_j as the estimated standard deviation for every possible decomposition levels and N_j as the length of the wavelet coefficients at decomposition level j.

4.5 Thresholding functions

After threshold values are determined, shrinking can be done using wavelet thresholding functions. In this chapter, after extensive review of the available literatures, fifteen wavelet thresholding functions were described in the following.

1) Hard function (HAD): It is the simplest function. All wavelet's detail coefficients whose absolute values are lower than threshold are set to be zero and other wavelet's detail coefficients are kept (Donoho & Johnstone, 1994). It is defined as

$$cD_j = \begin{cases} cD_j, & if\ |cD_j| > THR_j \\ 0, & otherwise \end{cases} . \tag{9}$$

2) Soft function (SOF): It is an expanded version of HAD (Donoho & Johnstone, 1994). It can be done by first zeroing all wavelet's detail coefficients whose absolute values are lower than threshold same as HAD. Then, non-zero coefficients are shrunk towards zero. SOF function is determined by

$$cD_j = \begin{cases} \text{sgn}(cD_j)(|cD_j| - THR_j), & if\ |cD_j| > THR_j \\ 0, & otherwise \end{cases} , \tag{10}$$

where $\text{sgn}(x)$ is a sign function that extracts the sign of a real number x.

3) Mid function (MID): It is an extension of SOF (Percival & Walden, 2000), small wavelet's coefficients are zeroed, and then large wavelet's coefficients are not affected. However, intermediate wavelet's coefficients are reduced. MID function can be expressed as

$$cD_j = \begin{cases} cD_j, & |cD_j| > 2THR_j \\ 2\,\text{sgn}(cD_j)(|cD_j| - THR_j), & THR_j < |cD_j| \le 2THR_j \\ 0, & otherwise \end{cases} . \tag{11}$$

4) Hyperbolic function (HYP): It is attempted to address the limitation of SOF. It is described in Vidakovic (1999) work and its equation is defined same as modulus squared function (Guoxiang & Ruizhen, 2001) that is given by

$$cD_j = \begin{cases} \text{sgn}(cD_j)\sqrt{(cD_j^2 - THR^2)}, & if\ |cD_j| > THR \\ 0, & otherwise \end{cases} . \tag{12}$$

5) Modified hyperbolic function (MHP): It combines the advantage of HAD and SOF functions. It resembles the variance pattern of HAD and the removing of bias problem of SOF. It is modified by Poornachandra et al. (2005) and is shown as

$$cD_j = \begin{cases} (k \cdot cD_j)\left[1 + (\dfrac{cD_j^2}{6})\right], & if \ |cD_j| > THR_j \\ 0, & otherwise \end{cases} \qquad (13)$$

where k is the scaling function and, in our studies, we used 1 for the constant k.

6) Non-negative Garrote function (NNG): It combines Donoho and Johnstone's thresholding function with Breiman's NNG. The equation is modified by Gao (1998) as

$$cD_j = \begin{cases} cD_j - \dfrac{THR_j^2}{cD_j}, & if \ |cD_j| > THR_j \\ 0, & otherwise \end{cases} \qquad (14)$$

7) Compromising of HAD and SOF function (CHS): It estimates wavelet's coefficients by weighted average of HAD and SOF (Guoxiang & Ruizhen, 2001). For $0<a<1$, when a is 0, it changed into HAD and when a is 1, it changed into SOF. In our study, we used 0.5 for the constant a. It can be expressed as

$$cD_j = \begin{cases} sgn(cD_j)(|cD_j| - \alpha THR_j), & if \ |cD_j| > THR_j \\ 0, & otherwise \end{cases} \qquad (15)$$

8) Weighted Averaging function (WAV): It estimates coefficients by weighted average of HYP and HAD (Zhang & Luo, 2006). It is given by

$$cD_j = \begin{cases} (1-\alpha)sgn(cD_j)\sqrt{(cD_j^2 - THR_j^2)} + \alpha(cD_j), & if \ |cD_j| > THR_j \\ 0, & otherwise \end{cases} \qquad (16)$$

where $0<a<1$. If a is 0, Eq. (16) will change to HYP and Eq. (16) will change to HAD, if a is 1. We used 0.5 for the constant a.

9) Adaptive Denoising function (ADP): It is modified based on SOF (Tianshu et al., 2002). It is given by

$$cD_j = cD_j - THR_j + \dfrac{2THR_j}{1 + e^{2.1cD_j/THR_j}} \qquad (17)$$

10) Improved function (IMP): It is attempted to address the deficiency of HAD and SOF (Su & Zhao, 2005). It can be defined as

$$cD_j = \begin{cases} sgn(cD_j)(|cD_j| - \beta^{(THR_j - |cD_j|)} \cdot THR_j), & if \ |cD_j| > THR_j \\ 0, & otherwise \end{cases} \qquad (18)$$

where $\beta \in \Re^+$ and $\beta > 1$. In our study, we used 15 from the suggestion of Su and Zhao work (2005).

11) Custom function (CUT): Idea of this function is similar to that of NNG function, in the sense that CUT and NNG are continuous and can adapt to the signal characteristics. Denote $0 < \gamma < THR_j$ and $0 < a < 1$. In our studies, we used the same threshold as in Yoon and Vaidyanathan (2004) work with $a = 1$ and $\gamma = THR_j/2$. The equation can be expressed as

$$cD_j = \begin{cases} cD_j + \mathrm{sgn}(cD_j)(1-\alpha)THR_j \, , & if \, |cD_j| \ge THR_j \\ 0 \, , & if \, |cD_j| \le \gamma \, , \\ \alpha \cdot THR_j \left(\dfrac{|cD_j|-\gamma}{THR_j - \gamma} \right)^2 \left\{ (\alpha - 3)\left(\dfrac{|cD_j|-\gamma}{THR_j - \gamma} \right) + 4 - \alpha \right\}, & otherwise \end{cases} \quad (19)$$

12) Firm function (FIM): It remedies the drawbacks of HAD and SOF functions. Gao and Bruce (1997) generalize a general FIM function using double threshold values. The THR_2 is defined by universal rule but THR_1 is scoped to range between 0 and THR_2. According to the previous experiments, Gao and Bruce (1997) suggested that when THR_1 equals $2/3THR_2$, the denoised results would be better. FIM can be expressed as follows

$$cD_j = \begin{cases} 0, & if \, |cD_j| \le THR_1 \\ \mathrm{sgn}(cD_j)\left[\dfrac{THR_2 \left(|cD_j| - THR_1 \right)}{(THR_2 - THR_1)} \right], & if \, THR_1 < |cD_j| < THR_2 \, . \\ cD_j, & if \, |cD_j| > THR_2 \end{cases} \quad (20)$$

13) Modified firm function (MFM): It is a modified version of general FIM function. A higher order polynomial is used to replace the linear function in the interval $[THR_1, THR_2]$. This modification enables to get a differentiable thresholding function. The expression (Gao & Bruce, 1997) can be defined as

$$cD_j = \begin{cases} 0, & if \, |cD_j| \le THR_1 \\ \mathrm{sgn}(cD_j)\left(r_2 - r_1 |cD_j| \right)\left(|cD_j| - THR_1 \right)^2, & if \, THR_1 < |cD_j| < THR_2 \, , \\ cD_j, & if \, |cD_j| > THR_2 \end{cases} \quad (21)$$

where $r_1 = \dfrac{(THR_1 + THR_2)}{(THR_2 - THR_1)^3}$ and $r_2 = \dfrac{2THR_2^2}{(THR_2 - THR_1)^3}$.

14) Qian function (QIN): It is a compromise shrinkage between HAD and SOF by constant parameter Q. Where Q is 1, it is equivalent to SOF and it is equivalent to HAD, when Q is ∞. QIN with $Q = 2$ is suggested from the experiments in (Qian, 2001). It is given by

$$cD_j = \begin{cases} cD_j \dfrac{\|cD_j\|^Q - THR^Q}{\|cD_j\|^Q}, & if \, |cD_j| > THR \\ 0, & otherwise \end{cases} \quad (22)$$

15) Yasser function (YAS): YAS shrinks the wavelet's detail coefficients which are lower than threshold value instead of set to be zero. Moreover, it has a constant parameter γ in

order to apply a nonlinear function to the threshold value. When γ is 3, the good results in speech signal are obtained (Ghanbari & Karami-Mollaei, 2006), which can be expressed as

$$cD_j = \begin{cases} cD_j, & if \ |cD_j| > THR \\ \mathrm{sgn}(cD_j)\dfrac{|cD_j|^{\gamma}}{THR^{\gamma-1}}, & otherwise \end{cases} . \tag{23}$$

5. Review of wavelet denoising in SEMG signal analysis

Selection of suitable wavelet denoising parameters is critical for the success of sEMG signal filtration in wavelet domain, because there is currently no known method to calculate the combination of the above wavelet denoising parameters that gives the best results. Therefore, many works have tried to find the optimal wavelet denoising parameters which lead to maximum filtration performance. All research studies about wavelet denoising parameters in analysis of the sEMG signals have been discussed in this section (Guo et al., 2004a, 2004b, 2005; Hussain et al., 2007, 2009; Jiang & Kuo, 2007; Khezri & Jahed, 2008; Li et al., 2010; Liu & Luo, 2008; Luo et al., 2007; Moshou et al., 2000; Ren et al., 2006; Yang & Luo, 2004; Zhang & Luo, 2006; Zhang et al., 2010) as summarized in Table 3.

In details, the sEMG signal analysis based on WT has been firstly proposed in 2000 by Moshou et al. (2000). Wavelet-based denoising is used to separate coordinated muscle activity of the shoulder of a driver related to certain movements that appear during driving a car. The denoised signals show clearly the real muscle activity bursts that mean the small activity peaks covered by the screen of noises are now observable. In Moshou et al. (2000) work, the simplest thresholding function, HAD, is used with a decomposition using db5 at 5 decomposition levels. Afterwards, Guo et al. (2004a, 2004b, 2005) compared four classical threshold selection rules: Universal, SURE, Hybrid and Minimax, and two classical thresholding functions: HAD and SOF, with real sEMG signal acquired from normal walking on the flat. They used the sym5 at 3 decomposition levels in their application. Evaluation criterion of both Moshou et al. (2000) and Guo et al. (2004a, 2004b, 2005) works is based on the observation of the sEMG waveforms between noisy sEMG signal and denoised sEMG signal. Jiang and Kuo (2007) compare the similar wavelet denoising parameters as Guo et al. (2004a, 2004b, 2005), but the acquired sEMG signals are changed from the normal walking activity to the mouse clicking activity; in addition, the simulated signals at 16-dB SNR have also been deployed. In Jiang and Kuo (2007) work a new evaluating function is proposed which is called signal-to-noise estimator (SNE). They prove that this evaluating function works well for the simulated signals but it does not work for the real sEMG signals. Subsequently, Jiang and Kuo concluded that the denoised sEMG signal is insensitive to the selection of wavelet denoising parameters. Furthermore, the db2 at 6 decomposition levels is used in their work due to the suggestion of previous study (Wellig & Moschytz, 1998). Zhang and Luo (2006) pay attention to apply wavelet denoising technique with control of the upper-limb prostheses. Some classical threshold selection rules and thresholding functions are employed (Liu & Luo, 2008; Luo et al., 2007; Yang & Luo, 2004). In addition, in one of their works, Zhang and Luo (2006) propose the new modified threshold selection rule and thresholding function. The sym8 at 4 decomposition levels is performed in denoising and extracting procedures. However, the results in Zhang, Luo and Liu works (Liu & Luo, 2008; Luo et al., 2007; Yang & Luo, 2004; Zhang & Luo, 2006) are also only observed from the figures as same as employed in Moshou et al. (2000) and Guo et al. (2004a, 2004b, 2005) works.

Reference	Application	Wavelet denoising parameters				
		1	2	3	4	5
Moshou et al. (2000)	Identifying car driver fatigue and movement	db5	5	-	-	HAD, SOF
Guo et al. (2004a, 2004b, 2005)	Lower limb prosthesis control	sym5	3	Universal, SURE, Hybrid, Minimax	-	HAD, SOF
Jiang & Kuo (2007)	MUAP detection	db2	6	Universal, SURE, Hybrid, Minimax	-	HAD, SOF
Zhang & Luo (2006)	Upper limb prosthesis control	sym8	4	LVMU	-	HAD, SOF, WAV
Yang & Luo (2004)	Upper limb prosthesis control	sym8	4	Hybrid	-	SOF
Khezri & Jahed (2008)	Upper limb prosthesis control	Daubechies Symlets Coiflet Biorthogonal	6	Hybrid Bayes Shrink	-	SOF
Hussain et al. (2007)	Detecting muscle fatigue	db2, db6, db8, dmey	4	-	-	HAD
Hussain et al. (2009)	Determining muscle contraction (walking speed)	db2, db4, db5, db6, db8, sym4, sym5, dmey	4	Universal	-	HAD
Li et al. (2010)	Upper limb prosthesis control	-	4	-	-	SOF
Zhang et al. (2010)	-	sym2	5	Minimax	-	SOF

Table 3. Applications of wavelet denoising algorithms with the sEMG signal. Note that wavelet denoising parameters: (1) the type of wavelet basis function, (2) the decomposition level, (3) threshold selection rule (4) threshold rescaling method, and (5) thresholding function.

Later, Khezri and Jahed (2008) proposed a usefulness of classical threshold selection rule, called Hybrid, to estimate the denoised upper-limb sEMG signals. It improved the accuracy of the sEMG classification compared with the one without denoising pre-processing stage and Bayes Shrink threshold selection rule. Following that, in one of our works (Phinyomark et al., 2009f), we compared Hybrid with three other classical threshold selection rules. The results showed that Universal yields better denoising performance than the others including Hybrid. Moreover, Hussain et al. (2007, 2009) suggested that pre-processing stage using the

Universal threshold selection rule and HAD thresholding function was able to improve the classification of the lower- and upper- limb activities, respectively. All of these introduced literatures work well for the surface EMG signal. On the other hand, for the intramuscular EMG signal, Ren et al. (2006) developed a technique for extracting and classifying motor unit action potentials (MUAPs) for needle EMG signal decomposition. In that technique, noise reduction based on threshold estimation calculated in the WT was proposed. The needle EMG signal is decomposed by the WT at ninth level with the db5. HAD thresholding is implemented with the semi-automatic threshold estimator, which is defined as $THR = \sigma \cdot \lambda$ where λ is set to be between 8 and 15 by the user in accordance with the SNR and σ is the noise energy estimated from the minimum value of the second moment feature in time domain. However, this threshold estimator is not suitable for surface EMG signal because in the MUAP detection, useful MUAP components have most of their energy in low-frequency components. Therefore, threshold obtained by this estimator has a large value (most high frequency components could be set to zeros). On the contrary, some high frequency components are still important for surface EMG signal, thus proposed technique in Ren et al. work (2006) is not included in our study. However, even though the results from most of previous works are not presented using the quantitative results, the improving ability in those applications based on wavelet denoising algorithm has been definitely established (Hussain et al., 2009; Khezri & Jahed, 2008; Ren et al., 2006; Zhang et al., 2010). In order to more clearly understand the effectiveness of wavelet denoising algorithm over conventional filters, discussion and illustration have been presented in review of Zhang et al. (2010).

6. Experimental results with real sEMG signals

The sEMG data that are used to demonstrate and evaluate the wavelet denoising parameters in our study were recorded from two forearm muscles and six upper-limb movements. Two forearm muscles are flexor carpi radialis muscle and extensor carpi radialis longus muscle and six upper-limb movements are hand open, hand close, wrist extension, wrist flexion, pronation, and supination. The sEMG signals were recorded by two pairs of surface electrodes (3M red dot 25 mm. foam solid gel). Each electrode was separated from the other by 20 mm. A band-pass filter of 10-450 Hz bandwidth and an amplifier with 60 dB gain were used. Sampling rate was set at 1000 samples per second using a 16 bit A/D converter board (IN BNC-2110, National Instruments Corporation). The sample size of each EMG data is 256 ms for the real-time constraint that the response time should be less than 300 ms (Englehart et al., 2001).

To evaluate the ability of wavelet denoising algorithm, two criteria are usually used based on: (1) the difference between signal values implied by a wavelet denoising method and the original signal values; and (2) the difference between classification accuracy obtained from the denoised signal and classification accuracy obtained from the raw signal (Phinyomark et al., 2010b). However, most studies have focused to evaluate the quality of wavelet denoising method based on the first criterion. In this chapter, we have evaluated the ability of wavelet denoising methods with only the first criterion; however, the relationship between the first criterion and the second criterion has been discussed.

The first criterion is error measure. One of the most popular methods is mean square error (MSE) that is also employed in our study. However, there are a lot of error measures; for instances, mean absolute error (MAE), mean absolute percentage error (MAPE), mean error (ME), mean percentage error (MPE), root mean square error (RMSE), percentage root-mean-square difference (PRD), signal-to-noise ratio output (SNR$_{out}$), and improved signal-to-noise ratio (ISNR). Due to the similarity of these measured indices, normally only one of these indices is selected to use in evaluating study. Definition of the MSE can be expressed as

$$MSE = \frac{\sum_{i=1}^{N}(f_i - fe_i)^2}{N},$$ (24)

where f_i represents the estimated sEMG signal from the original signal and fe_i is estimated sEMG signal from the noisy signal. The performance of wavelet denoising method is better when these indices including MSE are smaller. It means that useful information in the sEMG signal is remained and undesirable parts of the sEMG signal are removed. To guarantee the best wavelet denoising method achieved and optimized for estimating of useful sEMG signals, more than one times of additional noises should be done and in each time the level of noises shoud be varied from low noise level to high noise level; for example, 20-0 dB SNRs. The effect of different noise levels could be observed through this procedure. Example of the original sEMG signal and the sEMG signal with the WGN at 5 dB SNR are shown in Fig. 3. The SNR can be calculated by

$$SNR = 10\log\frac{P_{clean}}{P_{noise}},$$ (25)

where P_{clean} is power of the original sEMG signal and P_{noise} is power of the WGN.

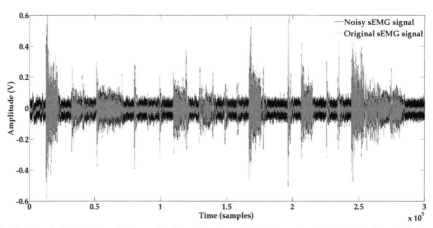

Fig. 3. Original sEMG signal (gray line) and noisy sEMG signal at 5 dB SNR (black line) with random and repeatable six upper-limb movements.

6.1 Wavelet basis functions
Firstly, the selection of an optimal wavelet function was done. The MSE calculated from 53 wavelet functions (in Table 1) were employed. The results are respectively shown in Fig. 4(a) and Fig. 4(b) at two levels of noises, low and high noise levels. The figure is plotted in log-lin type of a semi-log graph, defined by a logarithmic scale on the y axis, and a linear scale on the x axis. From the figure, the results of wavelet functions in high and low levels of

noises have the similar trend. As SNR increases, the MSE of each wavelet function also increases. The smallest MSE is db1, bior1.1 and rbio1.1. Their MSEs are 0.00407, 0.01242, 0.04090, 0.12739 and 0.41242 at SNR value of 20, 15, 10, 5 and 0 dB, respectively. It produces the best denoising wavelets. The db2, db7, sym2, bior5.5 and rbio2.2 provide marginally better performance than the rest candidates. Furthermore, the various orders of Daubechies (db1-db10), Symlets (sym2-sym8), BiorSplines (bior1.1-bior1.5, bior4.4, bior5.5, and bio6.8), Coiflet (coif1-coif2), and ReverseBior (rbio1.1-rbio3.9, rbio6.8) can be used to reduce noises. The most terrible wavelet function is bior3.1. Its MSE is as much as seven of the minimum MSE. The third order of decomposition of BiorSplines (Bior3.3, bior3.5, bior3.7, and bior3.9) and Discrete Meyer (dmey) are worse performance. Its MSE is as much as two of the minimum MSE. Moreover, in high noise, the second order of decomposition of BiorSplines (bior2.2-bior2.8) and the fifth order of decomposition of ReverseBior (rbio5.5) are not good. Therefore, these functions are not recommended to use for denoising sEMG signal.

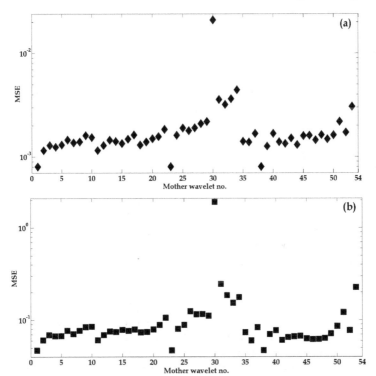

Fig. 4. MSE calculated from all wavelet functions (mother wavelet no. refer to the wavelets in Table I, i.e. #1-Daubechies order 1, #2-Daubechies order 2, ..., #11-Symlets order 2, ...,#18-Coiflet order 1, ..., #53-Discrete Meyer) (a) at 20 dB SNR (b) at 0 dB SNR. Note that decomposition level is 4, threshold selection rule is Universal, threshold rescaling method is GL for N parameter and LD for σ parameter, and thresholding function is SOF.

If we consider only optimal wavelets for denoising, we can conclude that db1, bior1.1 and rbio1.1 are the best ones. However, the ability of these functions in classification viewpoint is poor. Hence, for real-world application, these wavelet functions are not recommended.

The db2, db7, sym2, bior5.5 and rbio2.2 are prospective to have good performance in both denoising and classification performance. At this point we recommend wavelet functions in this group to be used in future works. Note that we are not reported the classification results in this work because the suitable wavelet functions depend on the classifier types (such as neural network, fuzzy logic, neuro-fuzzy classifier, probabilistic classifier, etc.). One of the useful results in classification viewpoint is presented in Englehart (1998) work. In Englehart study, wavelet coefficients are extracted from upper-limb sEMG signals and are subjected to dimensionality reduction method. As a result, classification errors are reported. Within the Daubechies, Coiflet and Symlet families, the best performance is db18, coif4 and sym8, respectively. Interesting trend is the improvement of classification performance that it tends to increase with the order of wavelet function. Hence, if balance between class separability and robustness is considered, the db7, sym5 and coif4 are some compromise wavelets.

6.2 Decomposition levels
Secondly, the selection of an optimal decomposition level was done. Fig. 5(a) and Fig. 5(b) present the effects of decomposition levels for five wavelet functions. When decomposition levels are more than seven, the MSE rapidly increases. Therefore, in Fig. 5(a) and Fig. 5(b), only first eight levels are shown. We found that the third and the fourth levels are better than other levels for low level of noises (20-10 dB SNRs). On the other hand, the fourth and the fifth levels are better than the others for high level of noises (10-0 dB SNRs). The effect of wavelet function with an optimal wavelet function is a little bit. The decomposition level 4 is suggested to be used as a compromise level between high and low level of noises.

6.3 Threshold selection rules
Thirdly, the selection of an optimal threshold selection rule was done. For the classical threshold selection rules, Universal rule is better than other classical methods as can be observed in Fig. 6. Hence, modified versions of Universal threshold selection rule are proposed and also evaluated. The MSE of LSMU rule is the lowest, followed closely by LVNU, SMU and Universal rules. GSMU rule have slightly larger error, and LMU and SLMU rules have a large error. However, in classification viewpoint, GSMU rule is the best threshold selection rule (Phinyomark et al., 2009f).

6.4 Threshold rescaling methods
Fourthly, the selection of an optimal threshold rescaling method was done. From our previous study (Phinyomark et al., 2009f), the optimal rescaling method is dependent on type of threshold selection rules. However, the general trend can be observed. For the threshold rescaling of N parameter, the GL is better than the LD. For the threshold rescaling of σ parameter, the suitable rescaling method is dependent on the level of noises. At very high noise, the LD is better than the FL. On the other hand, at medium to low noise, the FL is better than the LD.

6.5 Thresholding functions
Fifthly, the selection of an optimal thresholding function was done. In Fig. 7, the MSEs of 15 thresholding functions and no denoising case with only WT are presented. At medium and high levels of noises, SNR is lower than 10 dB, all functions are better than WT except MFM. However, at low level of noises, 15 dB SNR, CUT, FIM and MFM are worse than WT. In addition, HAD, MHP, CUT and MFM are worse than WT at very low noise, 20 dB SNR.

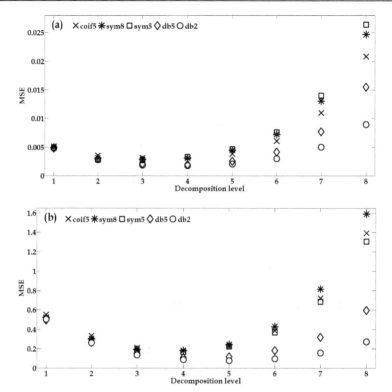

Fig. 5. MSE of five wavelet functions with eight decomposition levels (a) at 20 dB SNR (b) at 0 dB SNR. Note that threshold selection rule is Universal, threshold rescaling method is GL for N parameter and LD for σ parameter, and thresholding function is SOF.

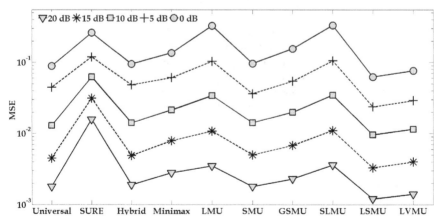

Fig. 6. MSE of four classical and six modified threshold selection rules at 20-0 dB SNR. Note that wavelet function is db2, decomposition level is 4, threshold rescaling method is GL for N parameter and LD for σ parameter, and thresholding function is SOF.

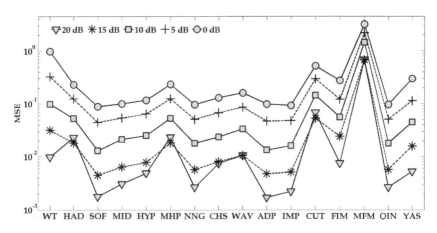

Fig. 7. MSE of WT and fifteen modified universal thresholding rules at 20-0 dB SNR. Note that wavelet function is db2, decomposition level is 4, threshold selection rule is Universal, and threshold rescaling method is GL for N parameter and LD for σ parameter.

As SNR increases, the MSE of each function as well increases. From the experimental results, the MSE of ADP is lowest, followed closely by SOF and IMP. It means that ADP is the best thresholding function in denoising viewpoint. MSE of WT is seven times the MSE of ADP at low noise and is three times the MSE of ADP at high noise. Moreover, in classification viewpoint, ADP is also the best thresholding function (Phinyomark et al., 2010b); whereas, the classification performance of SOF is not good.

7. Conclusion and future trends

Noises contaminated in the sEMG signals are an unavoidable problem during recording data; whereas noises are a main problem in analysis of the sEMG signal both in clinical and engineering applications. Random noises that have their frequency components fall in the energy band of the sEMG signal are the major problem. Conventional filters do not effectively remove random noises but wavelet denoising algorithm is not problematical in this way. Hence, numerous wavelet denoising methods have been proposed during the last decade. Suggestion of five wavelet denoising parameters in a compromise between two viewpoints, denoising and classification, is presented in the following:

- wavelet function: db2, db7, sym2, sym5, coif 4, bior5.5 and rbio2.2;
- decomposition level: 4;
- threshold selection rule: GSMU;
- threshold rescaling methods: LD for N parameter and FL or LD for σ parameter; and
- thresholding function: ADP.

Recommendation above can be useful to apply for many sEMG applications. However, for analysis of intramuscular EMG signal, re-evaluation of wavelet denoising parameters should be done because the purpose in interpretation is different (Ren et al., 2006). However, the pre-processing stage based on wavelet denoising algorithm is recommended to be implemented in analysis of sEMG signal, especially in multifunction myoelectric control system.

8. Acknowledgment

This work was supported in part by the Thailand Research Fund (TRF) through the Royal Golden Jubilee Ph.D. Program (Grant No. PHD/0110/2550), and in part by NECTEC-PSU Center of Excellence for Rehabilitation Engineering, Faculty of Engineering, Prince of Songkla University through Contact No. EMG540014S.

9. References

Andrade, A. O.; Nasuto, S.; Kyberd, P.; Sweeney-Reed, C. M. & Van Kanijn, F. R. (2006). EMG Signal Filtering based on Empirical Mode Decomposition. *Biomedical Signal Processing and Control*, Vol.1, No.1, (January 2006), pp. 44-55, ISSN 1746-8094

Baratta, R. V.; Solomonow, M.; Zhou, B. H. & Zhu, M. (1998). Methods to Reduce the Variability of EMG Power Spectrum Estimates. *Journal of Electromyography and Kinesiology*, Vol.8, No.5, (1991), pp. 279–285, ISSN 1050-6411

Boostani, R. & Moradi, M. H. (2003). Evaluation of the Forearm EMG Signal Features for the Control of a Prosthetic Hand. *Physiological Measurement*. Vol.24, No.2, (February 1980), pp. 309-319, ISSN 0967-3334

Clancy, E. A.; Morin, E. L. & Merletti, R. (2002). Sampling, Noise-reduction and Amplitude Estimation Issues in Surface Electromyography. *Journal of Electromyography and Kinesiology*, Vol.12, No.1, (1991), pp. 1–16, ISSN 1050-6411

De Luca, C. J. (2002). Surface Electromyography: Detection and Recording, In: *DelSys Incorporated*, 10.05.2011, Available from http://www.delsys.com/Attachments_pdf /WP_SEMGintro.pdf

De Luca, C. J.; Gilmore, L. D.; Kuznetsov, M. & Roy, S. H. (2010). Filtering the Surface EMG Signal: Movement Artifact and Baseline Noise Contamination. *Journal of Biomechanics*, Vol.43, No.8, (January 1968), pp. 1573-1579, ISSN 0021-9290

Donoho, D. L. (1992). Wavelet Analysis and WVD: A Ten Minute Tour, In: *Progress in Wavelet Analysis and Applications*, Meyer, Y. & Roques, S., pp. 109–128, Frontières Ed.

Donoho, D. L. (1995). De-noising by Soft-thresholding. *IEEE Transactions on Information Theory*, Vol.41, No.3, (1955), pp. 613-627, ISSN 0018-9448

Donoho, D. L. & Johnstone, I. M. (1994). Ideal Spatial Adaptation by Wavelet Shrinkage. *Biometrika*, Vol.81, No.3, (October 1901), pp. 425-455, ISSN 0006-3444

Donoho, D. L. & Johnstone, I. M. (1995). Adapting to Unknown Smoothness via Wavelet Shrinkage. *Journal of the American Statistical Association*, Vol.90, No.432, (March 1888), pp. 1200-1224, ISSN 0162-1459

Elena, M. M. ; Quero, J. M. & Borrego, I. (2006). An Optimal Technique for ECG Noise Reduction in Real Time Applications. *Proceedings of CinC 2006 Computers in Cardiology*, pp. 225-228, ISBN 978-1-4244-2532-7, Valencia, Spain, September 17-20, 2006

Englehart, K. (1998). *Representation and Classification of the Transient Myoelectric Signal*. Ph.D. Thesis, University of New Brunswick, Fredericton, N.B., Canada.

Englehart, K.; Hudgins, B. & Parker, P. A. (2001). A Wavelet-Based Continuous Classification Scheme for Multifunction Myoelectric Control. *IEEE Transactions on Biomedical Engineering*, Vol.48, No.3, (1953), pp. 302-311, ISSN 0018-9294

Gao, H. Y. (1998). Wavelet Shrinkage Denoising Using the Non-negative Garrote. *Journal of Computational and Graphical Statistics*, Vol.7, No.4, (1992), pp. 469-488, ISSN 1061-8600

Gao, H. Y. & Bruce, A. G. (1997). WaveShrink with Firm Shrinkage. *Statistica Sinica*, Vol.7, No.4, (January 1991), pp. 855-874, ISSN 1017-0405

Ghanbari, Y. & Karami-Mollaei, M. R. (2006). A New Approach for Speech Enhancement based on the Adaptive Thresholding of the Wavelet Packets. *Speech Communication*, Vol.48, No.8, (May 1982), pp. 927–940, ISSN 0167-6393

Guo, X. ; Yang, P. ; Li, Y. & Yan, W. L. (2004a) The SEMG Analysis for the Lower Limb Prosthesis Using Wavelet Transform. *Proceedings of IEMBS 2004 26th Annual International Conference of the IEEE Engineering in Medicine and Biology Society*, pp. 341-344, ISBN 0-7803-8439-3, San Francisco, CA, USA, September 1-5, 2004

Guo, X.; Yang, P.; Li, L. F. & Yan, W. L. (2004b) Study and Analysis of Surface EMG for the Lower Limb Prosthesis. *Proceedings of ICMLC 2004 3rd International Conference on Machine Learning and Cybernetics*, pp. 3736-3740, ISBN 0-7803-8403-2, Shanghai, China, August 26-29, 2004

Guo, X.; Yang, P.; Liu, H. C. & Yan, W. L. (2005). Research and Analysis on the Effect of Joint Angle on EMG in Thigh Muscles. *Proceedings of CNIC 2005 1st International Conference on Neural Interface and Control Proceedings*, pp. 139-142, ISBN 0-7803-8902-6, Wuhan, China, May 26-28, 2005

Huang, H.; Zhang, F.; Sun, Y. L. & He, H. (2010). Design of a Robust EMG Sensing Interface for Pattern Classification. *Journal of Neural Engineering*, Vol.7, No.5, (March 2004), pp. 056005-1-056005-10, ISSN 1741-2560

Huigen, E.; Peper, A. & Grimbergen, C. A. (2002). Investigation into the Origin of the Noise of Surface Electrodes. *Medical and Biological Engineering and Computing*, Vol.40, No.3, (January 1963), pp. 332-338, ISSN 0140-0118

Hussain, M.S.; Reaz, M. B. I.; Ibrahimy, M. I.; Ismail, A. F. & Yasin, F. M. (2007). Wavelet based Noise Removal from EMG Signals. *Informacije MIDEM*, Vol.37, No.2, (1971), pp. 94-97, ISSN 0352-9045

Hussain, M. S. ; Reaz, M. B. I. ; Yasin, F. M. & Ibrahimy, M. I. (2009). Electromyography Signal Analysis Using Wavelet Transform and Higher Order Statistics to Determine Muscle Contraction. *Expert Systems*, Vol.26, No.1, (July 1984), pp. 35-48, ISSN 0266-4720

Jiang, C. F. & Kuo, S. L. (2007). A Comparative Study of Wavelet Denoising of Surface Electromyographic Signals. *Proceedings of EMBS 2007 29th Annual International Conference of the IEEE Engineering in Medicine and Biology Society*, pp. 1868-1871, ISBN 978-1-4244-0787-3, Cite Internationale, Lyon, France, August 22-26, 2007

Johnstone, I. M. & Silverman, B. W. (1997). Wavelet Threshold Estimators for Data with Correlated Noise. *Journal of the Royal Statistical Society: Series B (Statistical Methodology)*, Vol.59, No.2, (1934), pp. 319-351, ISSN 1369-7412

Kale, S. N. & Dudul, S. V. (2009). Intelligent Noise Removal from EMG Signal Using Focused Time-Lagged Recurrent Neural Network. *Applied Computational Intelligence and Soft Computing*, Vol.2009, Article ID 129761, (2008), 12 pages, ISSN 1687-9724

Kania, M.; Fereniec, M. & Maniewski, R. (2007). Wavelet Denoising for Multi-lead High Resolution ECG Signals. *Measurement Science Review*, Vol.7, No.4, (2001), pp. 30-33, ISSN 1335-8871

Khezri, M. & Jahed, M. (2008). Surface Electromyogram Signal Estimation based on Wavelet Thresholding Technique. *Proceedings of EMBS 2008 30th Annual International Conference of the IEEE Engineering in Medicine and Biology Society*, pp. 4752-4755, ISBN 978-1-4244-1814-5, Vancouver, British Columbia, Canada, August 20-25, 2008

Laterza, F. & Olmo G. (1997). Analysis of EMG Signals by Means of the Matched Wavelet Transform. *Electronics Letters*, Vol.33, No.5, (March 1965), pp. 357-359, ISSN 0013-5194

Law, L. F.; Krishnan, C. & Avin, K. (2011). Modeling Nonlinear Errors in Surface Electromyography due to Baseline Noise: A New Methodology. *Journal of Biomechanics*, Vol.44, No.1, (January 1968), pp. 202-205, ISSN 0021-9290

Li, Y. ; Tian, Y. & Chen, W. (2010). Multi-pattern Recognition of sEMG based on Improved BP Neural Network Algorithm. *Proceedings of CCC 2010 29th Chinese Control Conference*, pp. 2867-2872, ISBN 978-1-4244-6263-6, Beijing, China, July 29-31, 2010

Liu, Z. & Luo, Z. (2008). EMG De-noising by Multi-scale Product Coefficient Hard Thresholding. *Journal of Huazhong University of Science and Technology (Natural Science Edition)*, Vol.36, No.1, (1972), pp. 134-136, ISSN 1671-4512

Luo, Z. Z. ; Zhang, Q. J. & Jiang, J. P. (2007). Improving Method for Surface Electromyography Denoising based on Wavelet Transform. *Journal of Zhejiang University (Engineering Science)*, Vol.41, No.2, (1956), pp. 213-216, ISSN 1008-973X

Merletti, R. & Parker, P. (2004). *ELECTROMYOGRAPHY Physiology, Engineering, and Noninvasive Applications*, John Wiley & Sons, ISBN 0-471-67580-6, USA

Mewett, D. T. ; Reynolds, K. J. & Nazeran, H. (2004). Reducing Power Line Interference in Digitised Electromyogram Recordings by Spectrum Interpolation. *Medical and Biological Engineering and Computing*, Vol.42, No.4, (January 1963), pp. 524-531, ISSN 0140-0118

Moshou, D.; Hostens, I.; Papaioannou, G. & Ramon, H. (2000). Wavelets and Self-organising Maps in Electromyogram (EMG) Analysis. *Proceedings of ESIT 2000 European Symposium on Intelligent Techniques*, pp. 186-191, Aachen, Germany, September 14-15, 2000

Percival, D. B. & Walden, A. T. (2000). *Wavelet Methods for Time Series Analysis*, Cambridge University Press, ISBN 0-521-64068-7, USA

Phinyomark, A. ; Limsakul, C. & Phukpattaranont, P. (2008). EMG Feature Extraction for Tolerance of White Gaussian Noise. *Proceedings of I-SEEC 2008 International Workshop and Symposium Science Technology*, pp. 178-183, Nong Khai, Thailand, December 15-16, 2008

Phinyomark, A. ; Limsakul, C. & Phukpattaranont, P. (2009a). EMG Feature Extraction for Tolerance of 50 Hz Interference. *Proceedings of ICET 2009 4th PSU-UNS International Conference on Engineering Technologies*, pp. 289-293, ISBN 978-86-7892-227-5, Novi Sad, Serbia, April 28-30, 2009

Phinyomark, A. ; Limsakul, C. & Phukpattaranont, P. (2009b). A Novel EMG Feature Extraction for Tolerance of Interference. *Proceedings of ANSCSE 13 13th International*

Annual Symposium on Computational Science and Engineering, pp. 407-413, Bangkok, Thailand, March 25-27, 2009

Phinyomark, A. ; Limsakul, C. & Phukpattaranont, P. (2009c). A Novel Feature Extraction for Robust EMG Pattern Recognition. *Journal of Computing*, Vol.1, No.1, (December 2009), pp. 71-80, ISSN 2151-9617

Phinyomark, A. ; Limsakul, C. & Phukpattaranont, P. (2009d). Evaluation of Wavelet Function Based on Robust EMG Feature Extraction. *Proceedings of PEC 7 7th PSU-Engineering Conference*, pp. 277-281, Hat Yai, Thailand, May 21-22, 2009

Phinyomark, A. ; Limsakul, C. & Phukpattaranont, P. (2009e). Evaluation of Mother Wavelet Based on Robust EMG Feature Extraction Using Wavelet Packet Transform. *Proceedings of ANSCSE 13 13th International Annual Symposium on Computational Science and Engineering*, pp. 333-339, Bangkok, Thailand, March 25-27, 2009

Phinyomark, A. ; Limsakul, C. & Phukpattaranont, P. (2009f). A Comparative Study of Wavelet Denoising for Multifunction Myoelectric Control. *Proceedings of ICCAE 2009 International Conference on Computer and Automation Engineering*, pp. 21-25, ISBN 978-1-4244-3564-7, Bangkok, Thailand, March 8-10, 2009

Phinyomark, A. ; Limsakul, C. & Phukpattaranont, P. (2009g). An Optimal Wavelet Function Based on Wavelet Denoising for Multifunction Myoelectric Control. *Proceedings of ECTI-CON 2009 6th International Conference on Electrical Engineering/Electronics, Computer, Telecommunications and Information Technology*, pp. 1098-1101, ISBN 978-1-4244-3388-9, Pattaya, Thailand, May 6-9, 2009

Phinyomark, A. ; Limsakul, C. & Phukpattaranont, P. (2009h). EMG Denoising Estimation Based on Adaptive Wavelet Thresholding for Multifunction Myoelectric Control. *Proceedings of CITISIA 2009 3rd IEEE Conference on Innovative Technologies in Intelligent Systems and Industrial Applications*, pp. 171-176, ISBN 978-1-4244-2886-1, Monash University, Sunway Campus, Malaysia, July 25-26, 2009

Phinyomark, A. ; Limsakul, C. & Phukpattaranont, P. (2010a). Optimal Wavelet Functions in Wavelet Denoising for Multifunction Myoelectric Control. *ECTI Transactions on Electrical Eng., Electronics, and Communications*, Vol. 8, No.1, (2003), pp. 43-52, ISSN 1685-9545

Phinyomark, A. ; Limsakul, C. & Phukpattaranont, P. (2010b). EMG Signal Estimation Based on Adaptive Wavelet Shrinkage for Multifunction Myoelectric Control. *Proceedings of ECTI-CON 2010 7th International Conference on Electrical Engineering/Electronics, Computer, Telecommunications and Information Technology*, pp. 351-355, ISBN 978-1-4244-5607-9, Chiang Mai, Thailand, May 19-21, 2010

Phinyomark, A. ; Phukpattaranont, P. & Limsakul, C. (2010c). EMG Signal Denoising via Adaptive Wavelet Shrinkage for Multifunction Upper-limb Prosthesis. *Proceedings of BMEiCON 2010 3rd Biomedical Engineering International Conference*, pp. 35-41, Kyoto, Japan, August 27-28, 2010

Phinyomark, A. ; Phukpattaranont, P. & Limsakul, C. (2011). Wavelet-based Denoising Algorithm for Robust EMG Pattern Recognition. *Fluctuation and Noise Letters*, Vol.10, No.2, (March 2001), pp. 157-167, ISSN 0219-4775

Poornachandra, S.; Kumaravel, N.; Saravanan, T. K. & Somaskandan, R. (2005). WaveShrink Using Modified Hyper-shrinkage Function. *Proceedings of IEEE-EMBS 2005 27th Annual International Conference of the Engineering in Medicine and Biology Society*, pp. 30-32, ISBN 0-7803-8741-4, Shanghai, China, January 17-18, 2006

Qian, J. (2001). Denoising by Wavelet Transform, In: *Department of Electrical Engineering, Rice University*, 11.05.2011, Available from: http://www.daimi.au.dk/~pmn/spf02/CDROM/pr1/Litteratur/Denoising%20by%20wavelet%20transform.pdf

Reaz, M. B. I.; Hussain, M. S. & Mohd-Yasin, F. (2006). Techniques of EMG Signal Analysis: Detection, Processing, Classification and Applications. *Biological Procedures Online*, Vol.8, No.1, (May 1998), pp. 11-35, ISSN 1480-9222

Ren, X.; Hu, X.; Wang, Z. & Yan, Z. (2006). MUAP Extraction and Classification based on Wavelet Transform and ICA for EMG Decomposition. *Medical and Biological Engineering and Computing*, Vol.44, No.5, (1963), pp. 371-382, ISSN 0140-0118

Song, G. & Zhao, R. (2001). Three Novel Models of Threshold Estimator for Wavelet Coefficients. *Proceedings of WAA 2001 2nd International Conference on Wavelet Analysis and Its Applications*, pp. 145-150, ISBN 3-540-43034-2, Hong Kong, China, December 18-20, 2001

Su, L. & Zhao, G. (2005). De-noising of ECG Signal Using Translation-invariant Wavelet De-noising Method with Improved Thresholding. *Proceedings of IEEE-EMBS 2005 27th Annual International Conference of the Engineering in Medicine and Biology Society*, pp. 5946-5949, ISBN 0-7803-8741-4, Shanghai, China, January 17-18, 2006

Tan, H. G. R.; Tan, A. C.; Khong, P. Y. & Mok, V. H. (2007). Best Wavelet Function identification System for ECG Signal Denoise Applications. *Proceedings of ICIAS 2007 International Conference on Intelligent and Advanced Systems*, pp. 631-634, ISBN 978-1-4244-1355-3, Kuala Lumpur, Malaysia, November 25-28, 2007

Tianshu, Q.; Shuxun, W.; Haihua, C. & Yisong, D. (2002). Adaptive Denoising based on Wavelet Thresholding Method. *Proceedings of ICOSP 2002 6th International Conference on Signal Processing*, pp. 120-123, ISBN 0-7803-7488-6, Beijing, China, August 26-30, 2002

Vidakovic, B. (1999). *Statistical Modeling by Wavelets*, John Wiley & Sons, ISBN 978-0-471-29365-1, USA

Wellig, P. & Moschytz, G. S. (1998). Analysis of Wavelet Features for Myoelectric Signal. *Proceedings of ICECS 1998 IEEE International Conference on Classification. Electronics, Circuits and Systems*, pp. 109-112, ISBN 0-7803-5008-1, Lisboa, Portugal, September 7-10, 1998

Yang, Q. Y. & Luo, Z. Z. (2004). Surface Electromyography Disposal based on the Method of Wavelet De-noising and Power Spectrum. *Proceedings of ICIMA 2004 IEEE International Conference on Intelligent Mechatronics and Automation*, pp. 896-900, ISBN 0-7803-8748-1, Chengdu, China, August 26-31, 2004

Yoon, B. J. & Vaidyanathan, P. P. (2004). Wavelet-based Denoising by Customized Thresholding. *Proceedings of ICASSP 2004 IEEE International Conference on Acoustics, Speech, and Signal Processing*, pp. ii-925-ii-928, ISBN 0-7803-8484-9, Montreal, Canada, May 17-21, 2004

Zardoshti-Kermani, M.; Wheeler, B. C.; Badie, K. & Hashemi, R. M. (1995). EMG Feature Evaluation for Movement Control of Upper Extremity Prostheses. *IEEE Transactions on Rehabilitation Engineering*, Vol.3, No.4, (March 1993), pp. 324-333, ISSN 1063-6528

Zhang, Q. J. & Luo, Z. Z. (2006). Wavelet De-noising of Electromyography. *Proceedings of ICMA 2006 IEEE International Conference on Mechatronics and Automation*, pp. 1553-1558, ISBN 1-4244-0465-7, Luoyang, China, June 25-28, 2006

Zhang, X.; Wang, Y. & Han, R. P. S. (2010). Wavelet Transform Theory and its Application in EMG Signal Processing. *Proceedings of FSKD 2010 7th International Conference on Fuzzy Systems and Knowledge Discovery*, pp. 2234-2238, ISBN 978-1-4244-5931-5, Qingdao, China, August 10-12, 2010

Zhong, S. & Cherkassky, V. (2000). Image Denoising Using Wavelet Thresholding and Model Selection. *Proceedings of ICIP 2000 International Conference on Image Processing*, pp. 262-265, ISBN 0-7803-6297-7, Vancouver, BC, Canada, September 10-13, 2000

sEMG Techniques to Detect and Predict Localised Muscle Fatigue

M. R. Al-Mulla[1], F. Sepulveda[2] and M. Colley[2]

[1]*Kuwait University*
[2]*Essex University*
[1]*Kuwait*
[2]*UK*

1. Introduction

Recent advances in physiological studies have demonstrated the importance of muscle fatigue detection and prediction in various aspects of our lives, including sports, rehabilitation and ergonomics. Automating muscle fatigue detection/prediction in wearable technology has the potential to aid in many applications. However, current research has made little progress towards automating muscle fatigue detection/prediction in computational models. The work presented in this chapter supports the idea that an automated muscle fatigue detection/prediction system can be used to aid sporting performance and to avoid injury. In support of this view, a wearable system that operates based on the detection and classification of three different stages of muscle fatigue (Non-Fatigue, Transition-to-Fatigue and Fatigue) has been developed. Current research focuses on only two muscle fatigue stages (Non-Fatigue and Fatigue); with this limitation in mind, data was analysed with the aim to develop features that best extract muscle fatigue content, using both statistical models and evolutionary computations tools to help find the number of muscle fatigue stages. This enabled the development of an automated muscle fatigue detection system, which provides true prediction capabilities. In doing so, a third stage of fatigue was identified, the so-called Transition-to-Fatigue stage, which occurs before the onset of fatigue. By identifying this transitional fatigue stage, it is possible to predict when fatigue will occur, which provides the foundation of the automated system. To demonstrate the applicability of the Transition-to-Fatigue class, the classification performance of the two class (Non-Fatigue and Fatigue) and three class approaches (Non-Fatigue, Transition-to-Fatigue and Fatigue) were compared. This chapter will include various studies that identify the most suitable methods to apply in the real-time autonomous system. The first section of studies developed various statistical features that best distinguished between the different classes of fatigue, resulting in new combined feature extraction methods called 1D spectro and 1D spectro_std. The second section used evolutionary computation, evolving features and creating pseudo-wavelets improving current state of the art. The various features evolved in this work all produced high classification accuracy from surface electromyography (sEMG) signals emanating from the biceps brachii during both isometric and non-isometric contractions. In the third section, a method to predict the time to fatigue was established using artificial neural network classification based on the three classes of fatigue. This technique was also implemented in the final study that developed a working prototype of the wearable autonomous system. One of the developed feature extraction methods, 1D spectro, was selected for implementation into the wearable autonomous system. This chapter presents preliminary empirical evidence demonstrating that the developed features and methods for fatigue detection/prediction improve the current state of the art. In this chapter, a definition of muscle fatigue is set, then, an overview of the detection of muscle fatigue will be given, followed by a discussion of specific approaches for extracting sEMG features which are related to muscle fatigue. The chapter then concludes with a summary of challenges for the future of this new and exciting technology.

1.1 Muscle fatigue definition

The term 'muscle fatigue' was first introduced by Bills (1943), who categorised it into three groups: subjective fatigue, which is influenced by psychological factors such as a lack of motivation; objective fatigue, which indicates a decline in productivity; and finally, physiological fatigue, which manifests itself by changes in physiological processes. Chaffin (1973) introduced the term 'localised muscle fatigue' as an example of physiological fatigue, which refers to the inability of a given muscle to maintain a desired force and is associated with localised pain.

Studies on localised muscle fatigue have focused mainly on the decline in the force of a muscle contraction during a sustained activity (Barry & Enoka, 2007), which results in a definition of fatigue as the inability of a muscle to continue exerting force or power. Barry & Enoka argue that this definition indicates that fatigue occurs quickly after the onset of a sustained period of exercise, although the subject may be able to sustain the activity. However, the muscle impairment will eventually lead to total fatigue, where it is impossible for the subject to continue performing the task (Bigland-Ritchie & Woods, 1984).

Muscle fatigue is a physiological phenomenon that can only be measured precisely by invasive means, which is clearly unsuitable for most applications, such as in sport science, human-computer interaction, ergonomics and occupational therapy. Therefore, non-invasive techniques have been developed to detect signals that are related to muscle fatigue. Generally, non-invasive clinical studies of muscle fatigue acquire such signals using two main techniques: mechanomyography (MMG) and/or electromyography (EMG). Historically, EMG has been chosen as the most suitable clinical research tool. MMG, on the other hand, is considered to be a mechanical equivalent of surface electromyography (sEMG), that works by recording the low-frequency oscillations that are produced by the muscle fibres when the muscle contracts and expands (Gordon & Holbourn, 1948). Nevertheless, there are other established techniques that are used to detect localised muscle fatigue, such as near infrared spectroscopy (NIRS) and ultrasound, and methods for assessing muscle fatigue, such as the Moore-Garg strain index and the CR Borg scale (Borg, 1970).

It has been known for at least 40 years that the sEMG signal carries information related to muscle fatigue (Edwards, 1981; Lindstrom et al., 1977), making it a suitable method for non-invasive muscle fatigue detection. Furthermore, the sEMG signal provides useful information when measuring and analysing localised muscle fatigue (Hagberg, 1981; Jorgensen et al., 1988; Petrofsky et al., 1982). Myoelectric manifestations of muscle fatigue can be seen in changes in signal frequency and amplitude and in the muscle conduction velocity (CV), while the mechanical factors related to muscle fatigue are manifested in a loss in the force exerted by the muscle (Asghari Oskœi et al., 2008). The myoelectric manifestations are perceived as an objective means by which to analyse muscle fatigue, since they disregard subjective motivators and, compared to mechanical factors, they provide early indicators of fatigue. In addition, sEMG is a very portable, easy to use and fairly inexpensive method.

1.2 How can muscle fatigue be detected ?

There are several techniques for signal detection which are often used in conjunction with each other for the study of muscle fatigue and it may be difficult to determine which to use in a particular application. Most modern research uses one or more of the methods described here in conjunction, such as an accelerometer with sEMG electrodes. Usually, the aim of combining sensors with sEMG or other sensors is validation, labelling or improving the signal to noise ratio.

To date, no consensus has been reached upon the ideal sensor technology to use for MMG recordings (Courteville et al., 1998; Gregori et al., 2003; Watakabe et al., 1998). The literature suggests that accelerometers are more appropriate than condenser microphones due to the effects of background noise. Also, accelerometers are inexpensive and reliable devices whereas condenser microphones are more expensive and have a much larger frequency range (20-2000 Hz) than that needed for accurately recording muscle vibrations (13-35 Hz) (Armstrong, 2010).

Compared to sEMG data collection, accelerometers are physically bulkier, more susceptible to noise from sudden movement and are significantly more expensive than sEMG electrodes. Limitations of NIRS are related to inconsistencies regarding muscle oxygenation during isometric exercise, making it a less reliable method. NIRS sensors are also very sensitive to movement, which makes NIRS an unsuitable candidate technique in sports and other movement-rich scenarios. It is possible to use the goniometer sensor to measure the development of fatigue in a realistic scenario. However, currently available goniometer sensors are expensive, have a short lifetime and must be handled with care. Electronic force gauges are also applicable in measuring fatigue but suffer from fragile construction, high cost and subject encumbrance in most scenarios. The Moore-Garg strain index and the modified Borg Scale can be used for fatigue detection in terms of translating facial/body cues using video processing, but these techniques suffer from privacy issues and can be highly subjective. In addition the Moore-Garg and Borg methods require a second person to measure the subjects' fatigue stages.

1.3 EMG signal pre-processing

Signal filtering is an important process that attenuates unwanted or erroneous electrical signals picked up by sensors and thus allows the experimenter to focus on a narrow energy band of interest. In general, filters attenuate signals within certain frequency ranges (the so-called stopband), thus limiting the frequency spectrum of the recorded signal to that of the so-called passband (De Luca, 1997). Filters can be categorised into four main types: low-pass, high-pass, bandpass and bandstop. Modern technologies have enabled the measurement of EMG signals of low noise and high signal fidelity (i.e., high signal to noise ratio). Filters can also be characterised by the width of their transition zone (De Luca, 1997), with more complex filter designs needed to produce tighter transition ranges. In general, the more complex the filter, the higher is its so-called 'order', i.e., a first order filter is a very simple order filter. The full effective bandwidth of the EMG signal can be measured using differential amplification. Bandpass refers to the range of frequencies from the low frequency to the high frequency limit of a signal. Typical bandpass frequency ranges are from between 10 and 20 Hz (high pass filtering) to between 500 and 1000 Hz (low-pass filtering). Movement artifacts, which are normally comprised of low frequency components (typically < 10 Hz), are removed by high-pass filtering, and signal aliasing is avoided by removing high frequency signal components through the use of low-pass filtering (Gerdle et al., 1999). Merletti (1999) states that the sEMG signals should be between the range of 5-500 Hz due to negligible contribution of the signals power density function outside of this range. Invasive EMG, on the other hand, should have a low-pass cut-off at no less than 1.5 kHz.

EMG signals are filtered by several classical filter types, including the Butterworth filter, Fourier series, the Chebyshev filter, the Elliptic filter and the Thompson or Bessel Filter, and filter equations are frequently recursive, such as in the Butterworth filter (De Luca, 1997). The purpose of the Butterworth filter is to produce a flat as possible frequency response in the passband, resulting in steep rolloffs in higher order filters, making it an ideal filter for conditioning the EMG signal (De Luca, 1997). Additionally its maximum passband gain, the cutoff frequency and the filter order are all clearly specified. In the past, sharp notch filtering was commonly used to remove power-line (A/C) noise components (i.e., either 50 or 60 Hz). However, since there are large signal contributions at these frequencies in EMG experiments, notch filtering results in a loss of information in this setting, and is thus usually avoided (Day, 2010).

Prior to the use of computers in signal processing, signals were mostly filtered by analogue means. Analogue filters usually employ electronic circuits, making use of three fundamental components: resistors, capacitors and inductors, which are arranged in circuits designed to meet particular needs (De Luca, 1997). The performance of an analogue filter is heavily dependent on the quality of the circuit design and the physical components that are used in building the circuit.Hence, digital filtering is often considered to be superior to analogue filtering (Hong & Bartlett, 2008). In the context of this thesis, the versatility of digital filtering makes it particularly suitable for the filtering of sEMG signals, where they are mostly used to remove noise, i.e., a band-pass filter, which combines low and high-pass filters, is used to cut off frequencies from 10-500 Hz. Signals can also be filtered through the application of a low-pass filter, so that slow changes in the signal amplitude are displayed and the signal is thus smoothed. According to Basmajian & De Luca (1985), the RMS signal voltage is the most suited approach to quantify the EMG signal, which is the mathematical equivalent to the standard deviation of the EMG signal.

1.4 Application of EMG in muscle fatigue research

EMG is an easy to use technique and has therefore been used in a vast range of research on muscle physiology. Generally, localised muscle fatigue occurs after a prolonged, relatively strong muscle activity, when a muscle or a group of muscles are fatigued. Due to the variability of inter-person muscle characteristics, there is no simple function of muscle load and timing that defines a precise muscle fatigue threshold. Changes in the EMG signals caused by fatigue are either measured in the time or frequency domain. Integrated EMG (IEMG) usually uses the time domain, and an increase in the signal period, amplitude and power reflect a higher muscle fibre recruitment for a fixed external force. The changes in EMG signal in the frequency domain relate to mean power frequency and median power frequency, which varies due to a shift towards lower frequencies, a small increase in low-frequency signal power, a relative decrease in high-frequency signal power, a decrease in low-frequency spectrum slope and an increase in high-frequency spectrum slope (Eberstein & Beattie, 1985; Gross et al., 1980; Petrofsky et al., 1982; Sato, 1982; Viitasalo & Komi, 1977). There are several reasons for these changes in the EMG signal, such as signal synchronisation, modulation of the recruitment firing rate, grouping and slowing of the CV (De Luca, 1979; Hermens et al., 1986; Viitasalo & Komi, 1977).

Although sEMG has been applied in many studies of localised muscle fatigue, it is not without its limitations, in particular, in studies of dynamic muscle contractions. The use of sEMG requires proper knowledge of the mechanisms of signal generation and propagation. Although signal acquisition *per se* is easy, inaccurate conclusions are easily drawn when inappropriate experimental methods are used (Merletti et al., 2003).

Most research concentrates on isometric contractions to establish typical sEMG readings when conducted in controlled settings. Changes in sEMG amplitude and centre frequency have been studied by Petrofsky et al. (1982), who found a decrease in the centre frequency of the spectrogram for all muscle groups. Research has also shown that a development in muscle fatigue correlates with changes in sEMG signal amplitude and MDF (Hagberg, 1981). Muscle fatigue causes MU recruitment, and the MU firing rate increases as a function of the elapsed time. These changes are not reflected in the EMG changes which occur during fatiguing isometric contraction of the arm flexors at 20-30% MVC (Maton & Gamet, 1989). However, it was recently found that the changes due to fatigue in the sEMG signal (increased amplitude and decreased frequency) suggest that the recruitment of MU firing rates correlates with sEMG amplitude (Calder et al., 2008).

Although CV strongly influences the power spectrum density (PSD) and has the highest inter-person repeatability, it has been argued that fatigue also compresses the frequency content of the sEMG signal in a proportional manner (Linssen et al., 1993). The PSD time-dependency can also be analysed, and is usually estimated from the instantaneous sEMG parameters, although there are shortcomings in the identification of changes in the short-period sEMG signals. A time-varying autoregressive (AR) model was proposed by Zhang et al. (2010), which produced a more stable and accurate instantaneous parameter estimation. Minning et al. (2007) studied differences in the rate of fatigue in the shoulder muscles during voluntary isometric contractions. They discovered day-to-day inconsistencies in the rate of fatigue in the middle deltoid muscle, which also fatigued more rapidly than other muscle groups. However, for the other muscles they found a consistent relationship between trial, day and muscle type. In a study on the relationship between short-time Fourier transform (STFT) and continuous wavelet transforms to analyse EMG signals from the back and hip muscles during fatiguing isometric contractions, it was found that the two methods reveal similar information regarding EMG spectral variables (Coorevits et al., 2008).

Although the success of sEMG is likely to be more prevalent in isometric muscle contractions, more recently EMG has been applied to the study of dynamic contractions (Singh et al., 2007). The analysis of the sEMG spectrum during cycling activities reveals a strong correlation between the onset of fatigue and the reduction of the MDF in dynamic contractions (Singh et al., 2007), and sEMG has been validated using biochemical analysis, indicating that the low-frequency band is a reliable indicator of muscle fatigue in dynamic contractions (Soo et al., 2009). By analysing the quantitative and qualitative changes in EMG patterns, such as IEMG and the frequency of the mean power, it has been argued that in dynamic contractions fatigue is related to qualitative changes in the pattern of MU recruitment, which occurs at a faster rate when the muscle has a higher degree of fast twitch muscles fibres. For the quantitative changes, only a small reduction in the amplitude of the IEMG signal was related to a high percentage of slow twitch muscle fibres (Komi & Tesch, 1979). Masuda et al. (1999) studied changes in sEMG patterns during static and dynamic fatiguing contractions by looking at the muscle fibre CV, MDF and mean amplitude in the vastus lateralis muscle. The muscle fibre CV appeared to be influenced by the metabolic state in the muscle, as it decreased significantly in isometric contractions, while it remained constant during dynamic contractions. This suggests that changes in the MDF cannot be explained wholly by shifts in the muscle fibre CV. Farina (2006) proposed a technique for detection and processing of muscle CV during dynamic contractions, and showed that a decline in CV reflects muscle fatigue. Another method for estimating muscle fatigue during dynamic contraction is to use a source separation technique related to independent component analysis to test whether the firing of MUs becomes more synchronised at the onset of localised muscle fatigue. As argued by Naik et al. (2009), it is widely accepted that lower-frequency sEMG signals indicate muscle fatigue due to MU synchronisation; however, there is little experimental evidence of this theory. Naik et al. concluded that during cycling movements, a global matrix is an applicable measurement for estimating localised muscle fatigue.

Several studies have identified the state of peripheral fatigue (Dimitrov et al., 2006; Gonzalez-Izal, Malanda, Navarro-Amezqueta, Gorostiaga, Mallor, Ibanez & Izquierdo, 2010). In a recent study, Gonzalez-Izal, Malanda, Navarro-Amezqueta, Gorostiaga, Mallor, Ibanez & Izquierdo (2010) compared several EMG parameters to assess peripheral fatigue during dynamic contractions. In that study, new spectral indices (FInsmX) developed by Dimitrov et al. (2006) were based on discrete wavelet transforms (DWT) and were compared to spectral parameters, such as mean average voltage, median spectral frequency and ratios between different scales obtained by DWT. Results showed the newly proposed spectral indices to be the best for assessing peripheral fatigue, both in correlation with the power output changes and in their regression. These new spectral indices have also been shown to be a useful tool in detecting changes in muscle power output in fatiguing dynamic contractions, and they can be used as predictors of changes in muscle power output (Gonzalez-Izal, Rodriguez-Carreno, Malanda, Mallor-Gimenez, Navarro-Amezqueta, Gorostiaga & Izquierdo, 2010).

Detecting muscle fatigue in an automated system requires a real-time measurement of changes in localised muscle fatigue. Stulen & De Luca (1982) developed a muscle fatigue monitor, which was a non-invasive device measuring localised muscle fatigue by spectral compression calculating median frequencies and two other parameters of the spectrum. This study used the MDF, which the author states is a more reliable analysis feature than other traditional parameters, e.g. mean or mode frequencies. Kramer et al. (1987) proposed a robust and relatively reliable parameter of fatigue that could be calculated off-line from computed, real-time sEMG data obtained from a simple analogue device. Wavelet coefficients can be used in non-stationary and time-varying signal processing, hence they have been applied in the assessment of localised muscle fatigue for both static and dynamic contractions using sEMG signals. The amplitude of approximation coefficients coincide with muscle fatigue development. Moshou et al. (2005) proposed a method for automating the detection of muscle fatigue by using NNs, where a two-dimensional self-organising map visualises the approximation of wavelet coefficients, enabling the visualisation of the onset of fatigue over time, and thus separating the EMG signal from fresh and fatigued muscles. Tepavac & Schwirtlich (1997) developed a technique which utilises the processed sEMG signal as an activation signal that changes the pattern to control a functional electrical stimulation (FES) system. Their technique is able to notify the user that a rapid drop in the muscle force is approaching, providing the capability of a simple on-off fatigue detection in FES applications. In the development of this technique the authors used seven different sEMG parameters, however the best relationship was established between the MDF and force changes, which were the parameters used to determine the prediction of the onset of fatigue and detection of fatigue. This is an interesting technique although it is not performed in autonomous, real-time system.

1.5 sEMG signal analysis and feature characterisation

Feature extraction is used in pattern recognition, being a form of dimensionality reduction (Samet, 2006). This method is used for transforming input data to a certain set of features which will extract the relevant information from that data. sEMG signals can be analysed to detect muscle fatigue by examining the changes in EMG measurements. Studies on sEMG show that an increase in EMG signal amplitude or shifts in the spectrogram are indicators of muscle fatigue in static contractions (Chaffin, 1973; De Luca, 1997; Duchene & Goubel, 1993; Kadefors et al., 1968; Lindstrom et al., 1977; Marras, 1990). Hagberg (1981) established that significant changes in the sEMG signal indicate muscle fatigue. Studies on muscle fatigue during isometric contraction have established typical sEMG readings when conducted in controlled settings. Changes in sEMG amplitude and centre frequency were studied by Petrofsky et al. (1982), who found a decrease in the centre frequency of the spectrogram for all muscle groups. It has also been shown that a development in muscle fatigue correlates with changes in amplitude and MDF (Hagberg, 1981). A variety of parameters have been used to investigate sEMG signals to determine muscle fatigue; however it is common to study the signal in terms of its frequency at a certain time, in both the time and time-frequency domains. Table 1 categorized the papers according to the feature extraction methods used by authors.

Feature extraction method	Refrence ID
RMS	(Basmajian & De Luca, 1985; Kumar & Mital, 1996)
STFT	(Merletti & Parker, 2004)
Total Band Power	(Welch, 1967)
New spectral parameter FI 1 to FI 5	(Dimitrov et al., 2006)
PSD	(Ortengren et al., 1975)
MDF	(Kumar & Mital, 1996)
IMDF	(Asghari Oskœi et al., 2008; Roy et al., 1998)
Cohen class transformations	(Cohen, 1995; Raez et al., 2006; Ricamato et al., 1992)
Gabor Transform	(Gabor, 1946)
Wavelet analysis	(Kumar et al., 2003; Laterza & Olmo, 1997)
Autogression analysis	(Graupe & Cline, 1975; Kim et al., 2005; Tohru, 1992)
Entropy	(Jaynes, 1957; Sung et al., 2008)
Recurrence Quantification Analysis	(Filligoi et al., 2010; Morana et al., 2009)
HOS	(Hussain et al., 2008; Kanosue et al., 1979)
Composite Features	(Boostani & Moradi, 2003; Hudgins et al., 1993; Phinyomark et al., 2009)

Table 1. Signal analysis and feature characteristics

1.5.1 Time domain and frequency domain analysis

A signal is acquired, and in some circumstances, analysed, in the time domain where the signal amplitude/voltage is represented as a function of time. However, for many analysis techniques, it is the frequency of the signal that is of greater value, and consequently the signal should be analysed in the frequency-domain, whereby the signal undergoes a Fourier transform so that it is represented as a function of frequency, rather than time.

Both the average rectified value, which measures the average of the absolute signal value, and the RMS, which is a measure of the signal power (Kumar & Mital, 1996), are used in the analysis of the raw EMG signal in the time domain. The RMS of the EMG signal calculates the square root of the average power of the raw EMG signal over a specific time period (Basmajian & De Luca, 1985). De Luca's group acknowledged both the average rectified value and RMS as appropriate analysis methods, however, several authors prefer the RMS (De Luca, 1997;

Merletti et al., 2003), since it can be used to obtain a moving average (Basmajian & De Luca, 1985). The moving average approach is used for processing raw EMG signals from dynamic contractions, as it identifies the rapid changes in the muscle activity during such contractions by using short duration sampling windows (Payton & Bartlett, 2008). Merletti et al. (2003) suggested that EMG analysis of dynamic contractions can make use of another processing method, the 'linear envelope', which uses a low pass filter to smooth the rectified EMG.

When a signal crosses the zero amplitude line, it is said to have made a 'zero-crossing'. When applied to sEMG data, the general idea is that an active muscle will produce more AP, and hence generate more zero crossings. However, at the onset of fatigue, the zero crossing rate drops dramatically due to the reduced conduction of electrical current in the muscle. Therefore zero-crossings are counted using geometric calculations to give an indication of the muscle status.

The total band power (TBP) of the sEMG signal can be estimated using the method by Welch (1967). This method has been used previously in several sEMG fatigue analyses (Cifrek et al., 2009; Helal et al., 1992) and has proved to be useful in quantifying the power of the EMG signals.

The frequency content of a signal can be determined by performing a Fourier transform to reveal its individual frequency components. The fast Fourier transform (FFT), a method for calculating the discrete Fourier transform, is suitable for use in stationary signals. EMG signals, which are non-stationary, should be represented in both the time and frequency domains. Therefore, the STFT, which analyses a small temporal section of the signal, can be used to determine the frequency and phase evolution of the EMG signal over time.

The time and frequency resolution depend upon the sampling rate and the temporal length of the signal section. Due to the inverse relationship between time and frequency in the Fourier transform, it follows that the higher the time resolution the lower the frequency resolution will be and *vice versa* (Merletti & Parker, 2004). The spectogram of the signal is the squared magnitude of the STFT.

Dimitrov et al. (2006) proposed a new spectral parameter with higher sensitivity than traditional indices for both dynamic and isometric contractions, which is a valid and reliable tool for the assessment of muscle fatigue. The parameter used the FFT to calculate ratios between different spectral moments measured over the power spectral density.

Following an FFT, this parameter represents the ratio between the low- and high-order spectral moments of the EMG power spectrum. Gonzalez-Izal, Malanda, Navarro-Amezqueta, Gorostiaga, Mallor, Ibanez & Izquierdo (2010) used this index to measure the changes in muscle power during a high-intensity dynamic protocol, and compared it to other frequency and amplitude parameters. It was found that the logarithm of this index detects the changes most accurately by assessing peripheral impairments.

EMG signals can be analysed in the time-domain using the PSD to describe how the power of a signal is distributed among its frequency components. Significant changes in the power spectrum indicate muscle fatigue (Ortengren et al., 1975), such that after fatigue onset the PSD is increased in the low frequency components and decreased in the higher frequency components.

Two of the most common frequency-dependent features in sEMG analysis are the MF and MDF. The MF is "the average frequency of the power spectrum and is defined as its first-order moment" (Asghari Oskœi et al., 2008), while the MDF is an index used in studies of spectral shifts and can be defined as "the frequency which divides the power spectrum in two parts with equal areas" (Kumar & Mital, 1996, p. 170). The power spectrum represents the MDF of the power, based on a continuous spectrum distribution. Hagberg (1981) stated that if the MDF decreases along with as the sEMG signal amplitude increases, which is a strong indication of fatigue.

The spectral frequency can be redefined to represent the non-stationary nature of the signal, or the instantaneous frequency, of the frequency content of the signal (Karlsson et al., 1999). The instantaneous median frequency (IMDF) was introduced by Roy et al. (1998). Studies by Asghari Oskœi et al. (2008) concluded that a significant decline in the IMDF of the signal is a significant manifestation of fatigue occurrence. In addition, Georgakis et al. (2003) demonstrated that the average instantaneous frequency is superior to the mean and median frequencies for the analysis of muscle fatigue during sustained contractions.

Some analysis methodologies use both the time and frequency domains to analyse the EMG signal. For example, the Cohen class transformation, a time-frequency representation applied in biomedical signal processing, is well-suited for analysis of signals from dynamic contractions. It is a distribution function introduced by Cohen (1995) using bilinear transformations, giving clearer results than the STFT. However, due to its use of bilinear transformations, the Cohen class is affected by cross-term contamination in its analysis of several functions, which can be avoided using window functions. The Wigner-Ville distribution function (WVD), proposed by Wigner in 1936 (Raez et al., 2006), was first used for corrections to classical statistical mechanics, however, it is also applicable as a transform in time-frequency analysis. This transform has higher clarity than the STFT and has more properties than most other time-frequency transforms, using all available information in the EMG signal. In 1948 Ville revised this function into a quadratic representation of the local time-frequency energy of a signal (Raez et al., 2006). It was discovered by Ricamato et al. (1992) that the WVD would detect the frequency ranges of the MUs, displaying recruitment patterns as muscles contract. However, Davies & Reisman (1994) found that the WVD joint density spectrum is noisy although its localisation properties are excellent and "generally concentrated around the instantaneous frequency of the signal". Another member of the Cohen's class functions is the Choi-Williams distribution (Davies & Reisman, 1994), which makes use of kernels to reduce the interference, something the Cohen's class distribution suffers from, although it is only possible for the kernel function to filter out the cross-term contamination.

The Gabor transform (named after Dennis Gabor) is a discrete Fourier transform utilising Gaussian windows, which is used in time-frequency analysis (Gabor, 1946). The transform determines the sinusoidal frequency and phase content of specific sections of a signal that changes over time, which is an advantage when representing local features. By using Gaussian windows, this function gives more weight to the signals near the time being analysed. Although this method is more precise than other methods, giving few errors, there are some major problems. The Gabor transform gives imaginary numbers with no physical meaning and it requires a lot of resources for full computation. Nevertheless, this transform guarantees energy conservation of the signal.

There are many time-frequency functions which can be used to analyse sEMG signals during localised muscle fatigue. Davies & Reisman (1994) showed that STFT can most precisely represent spectrum compression during muscle fatigue. Due to the cross-term contamination in the WVD, it is not possible to display the changes in the frequency components with muscle fatigue accurately. In a comparison between the STFT, the WVD, the continuous wavelet transform and the Choi-Williams distribution, Karlsson et al. (2000) found that the continuous wavelet transform resulted in a more precise estimation of EMG signals when applying various time-scale methods to analyse sEMG signals.

1.5.2 Wavelet analysis

By using a wavelet function (WF), the wavelet transform (WT) decomposes a signal into numerous multi-resolution components (Kleissen et al., 1998; Laterza & Olmo, 1997). It is used to detect and characterise the short time component within a non-stationary signal, providing information regarding the signal's time-frequency. The WF, being both dilated and translated in time and a linear function which does not suffer from cross-terms, undertakes a two-dimensional cross correlation with the time domain sEMG signal, making it an excellent alternative to other time-frequency parameters (Laterza & Olmo, 1997).

There are a number of so-called 'mother wavelets' that can be used for signal decomposition, including Symm-let, Coiflet, Haar, Morlet, Daubechies and Mexican Hat (Kumar et al., 2003). To select the most appropriate mother wavelet for a specific application and signal type, the properties of the WF and the characteristic of the signal should to be analysed and matched. Certain wavelets have somewhat established guidelines for their use, e.g., Db4 is said to be suited for signals using feature extractions and linear approximation with more than four samples, while Db6 is suited for signals that are approximated by a quadratic function over the support of six and finally coiflet6 is better suited for data compression results (Walker, 2000).

Guglielminotti & Merletti (1992) hypothesised that if the wavelet analysis is selected to fit with the shape of the MUAP, the WT would give the best energy location in a time-scale. Kumar et al. (2003) stated that the STFT does not give an optimal time or frequency resolution for the non-stationary signal, although the relatively short time windows may trace spectral variations with time. The WT, comprised of numerous WFs, can be used to decompose the sEMG signal. The output of the power transform domain is calculated and thus functions as a deciding parameter in selecting the most appropriate WF to give the highest contrast between sEMG cases. It has been shown that it is possible to detect muscle fatigue status by determining the Sym4 or Sym5 WFs and decomposing the signal at levels 8 and 9 (out of 10 levels). Kumar et al. (2003) discussed the effectiveness of decomposing the sEMG signal to measure its power in order to identify muscle fatigue as an automated process.

1.5.3 Autoregression analysis

Regression statistics is used to determine the relationship between an independent variable or variables and a dependent variable. An autoregressive (AR) model is a random process used in statistics and signal processing to model and predict natural phenomena. Graupe & Cline (1975) developed the AR moving average (ARMA) model to represent EMG signals, where the signals were split into short time intervals and the signal was considered to be stationary. However, Sherif (1980) replaced this model by a model using the AR integrated moving average (ARIMA) model, to be used on the non-stationary EMG signals. Hefftner et al. (1988) exploited the computational speed of the AR model for EMG feature discrimination.

Kim et al. (2005) measured fatigue in the trunk muscle using the first AR model, and concluded that the model was capable of assessing fatigue in static exercises, being sufficiently sensitive to detect fatigue at low force levels. Several authors have revised the AR parameters, adding a non-linear element (ARMA) (Bernatos et al., 1986) and a non-stationary identifier (Moser & Graupe, 1989). However, the ARIMA model is complex with a high computational cost and Tohru (1992) argued that more accurate models (ARMA and ARIMA) are not needed for studies on dynamic contractions.

1.5.4 Entropy

Entropy is a function that can be used in various fields, such as thermodynamics, communication and computer science. In physics, entropy is a statistical measure of disorder in a system, representing the probability that a certain outcome exists, while in information theory the basis of entropy relates to the randomness in a signal or in a random event (Jaynes, 1957). This is also applicable to a general probability distribution, rather than a discrete-valued event. Sung et al. (2008) argue that entropic measures reveal part of the sEMG signals that are not included in the power spectrum, and can be a useful tool in detecting muscle fatigue in gender differences.

1.5.5 Recurrence quantification analysis

Recurrence quantification analysis, a method of nonlinear data analysis which is used for the investigation of dynamical systems, is highly effective in detecting changes in the sEMG signal and is almost equivalent to the frequency domain analysis of the signal in non-isometric contractions (Filligoi et al., 2010). Morana et al. (2009) recently used recurrence quantification analysis in a study of muscle fatigue and stated that this method can be used to detect peripheral muscle fatigue.

1.5.6 Higher-order statistics

Higher-order statistics (HOS), a technique based on probability theory, characterises and analyses the nature of a random process, making it appropriate for use in the random time series produced by EMG signals. Due to the nature of the EMG signals, in particular when fatigue components are present in the signal, HOS will give more insight in terms of analysing the complexity of the EMG signal. In muscle fatigue HOS is used due to the increasing complexity of the EMG signal, the second order HOS (and higher orders) are used to detect non-gussian/non-linear properties of the signal. This is particularly useful method in muscle fatigue studies, which is an alternative of using the Gaussian/linear processes, such as the power spectrum of a signal giving the distribution of power among signal frequency. Moments and cumulants define the HOS of a signal. When analysing deterministic signals, moments are of great importance, while cumulants are useful for stochastic type signals (Gündoğdu et al., 2006). It has been used in sEMG studies to estimate the amplitude and the number of new MUAPs, as proposed by Kanosue et al. (1979). Several authors have studied HOS in sEMG signal processing, in particular testing it for Gaussianity and linearity, coherence and coupling of the signal. Their findings showed that during contractions at low- and high-force activity, HOS features are non Gaussian, while during the mid-level force the distribution is maximally Gaussian (Hussain et al., 2008; Raez et al., 2006; Shahid, 2007). HOS is also used to suppress Gaussian white noise in the sEMG signal (Hussain et al., 2008).

1.5.7 Composite features

The term 'composite features' relates to the use of a combination of common features to develop a new feature that aids in the analysis of sEMG signals. MacIsaac et al. (2006) presented a mapping function that maps segments of multiple myoelectrical signals for fatigue estimation of dynamic contractions, where the inputs are time domain features. This function is tuned by ANNs and is capable of use in real-time applications. Results show that this function better maps the sEMG signals than either the MF or the IMDF for different conditions.

Although combining features is a fairly new approach in the field of localised muscle fatigue research, there has already been work on multiple features utilised for myoelectric control of prosthetics. The concept of multiple features was introduced to overcome the stochastic nature of the the EMG signal, which makes it difficult for only one parameter to reflect the uniqueness of the EMG signal to a motion command. Hence various features are used for extraction at different times of the signal. Hudgins et al. (1993) used this method first for time domain features, such as mean absolute value, mean absolute value slope, wavelength form, zero crossings and slope sign changes, which were then classified using an ANN. This new method of control increased the number of prosthetic functions which can be controlled by a single channel of myoelectric signal without the amputee having to increase his/her effort. Other researchers have also applied this multiple function technique. Phinyomark et al. (2009) calculated two novel features by modifying the mean and median frequencies. Instead of calculating the power spectrum, they calculated the mean and median of the amplitude spectrum (MMNF). Then they used a combination of the MMNF, a histogram of EMG and Willison amplitude as a feature vector in a classification task, giving a better classification recognition result of the EMG in noisy environment than other features. Boostani & Moradi (2003) aimed at selecting the best features which would give a high rate of motion classification for controlling an artificial hand. Nineteen EMG signal features were taken into account, including combining the WT with other signal processing techniques. The results of this study showed that the best features for motion classification were wavelet coefficients of EMG signals in nine scales, and the cepstrum coefficients. Although the above-mentioned studies do not investigate muscle fatigue *per se*, they all use a combination of features of the EMG signal to improve the classification outcome.

2. Feature selection

Feature selection is an important process that ensures that the selected features contain class related information, since most features do not hold such information. In machine learning and statistics, as well as pattern recognition and data mining, feature selection is a technique whereby a subset of relevant features is selected from the data, which is then applied in a learning algorithm (Sewell, 2010). Feature selection typically creates a model that facilitates the generalisation of the unseen dimensions and may substantially enhance the comprehension of the classifier model which is produced (Kim & Street, 2010). In supervised learning, which has been thoroughly investigated, the aim is to select a feature subset which produces high classification accuracy (Kim & Street, 2010). However, for unsupervised learning the goal is to identify an optimal subset that produces high quality clusters for a set number of clusters. There are two main types of feature selection: the wrapper approach and the filter approach.

2.1 The wrapper approach

The wrapper approach uses a classification method to evaluate the most optimal feature or feature sub-set. This model, often used in machine learning, is excellent for improving the performance of the classifier due to using the same bias for both the feature selection and the learning of the classifier (Kohavi & John, 1997). The wrapper method searches for the optimal feature subset or a near-optimal subset that will best suit a certain algorithm and a domain, and it differs from other approaches as the measure of relevance is defined as the accuracy obtained by nonlinear regression (Kohavi & John, 1997). The wrapper approach goes through two phases (Liu & Motoda, 1998). In the first phase, which is the feature sub-set selection, the best sub-set is selected based on the classifier's accuracy. It is only the optimal features with highest accuracy which is kept for use in the second phase. Learning and testing is the second phase, where a classifier learns and trains from the optimal sub-set and then tests it on the test data to obtain its predictive accuracy. Cross-validation is then used to estimate the accuracy as the accuracy of the training data may not ensure accuracy in the testing data. Although cross-validation may help in the difficult task of estimating the true accuracy, it will lengthen the process of feature selection. Other disadvantages of the wrapper approach is linked to being unable to handle great sizes of data and to the limitation in choice of classifiers (Liu & Motoda, 1998). As the classifier is rebuilt for each feature sub-set in the first phase it eliminates the use of classifiers which requires great computational resources.

2.2 The filter approach

The filtering approach has been linked to data mining, when a classifier cannot be directly linked with the data set and where the aim is data reduction (Liu & Motoda, 1998). In this model the relevance measure is defined independently from the learning algorithm. In the filtering approach the subset selection procedure is like a preprocessing step (Kojadinovic & Wottka, 2000). Even this model consists of two phases. Firstly, the feature selection uses separation index or other measures such as distance, dependency, consistency and information to get the best feature sub-set. Secondly, the classifiers learns from the training data set and tests it on the testing data set. This model can handle huge data sets due to the feature selection process in phase one, which is a less complex and time consuming method. The filter approach also tend to be much faster and cheaper than the wrapper approach, however, the disadvantage is that the best subset of variables may not be independent of the representational biases of the algorithm used in the learning phase (Kojadinovic & Wottka, 2000).

In research on localised muscle fatigue, feature selection is used to facilitate the pattern recognition and classification of the features analysing the sEMG signals (Tamil et al., 2008; Yan et al., 2008). Various methods have been applied in this process, however, the DBI for measuring clustering selection is commonly used for EMG pattern recognition (Huang & Chen, 1999; Petrofsky, 1981; Wang et al., 2004)

Clustering is generally considered as an unsupervised algorithm for grouping a heterogeneous population into a set of homogeneous classes. However, this strategy does not always ensure grouping similar classes together.

2.2.1 Davies-Bouldin index

Cluster validity is an important measurement of how well clusters are related to other clusters generated by clustering algorithms. In most applications the clustering result needs validation. The number of clusters is determined as a user parameter in the majority of clustering algorithms. There are many methods of finding the best number of clusters, however Davies & Bouldin (1979) developed the Davies-Bouldin index (DBI), which measures the ratio of the sum of within-cluster scatter to between-cluster separation, so that it uses both the clusters and their sample means. The DBI evaluates the cluster quality by utilising the average error of each class, serving as a measure of cluster quality by calculating the distance of the cluster members to the cluster centroids and the distances between the cluster centroids. In the DBI small values indicate that clusters are compact with their centres far apart. Hence, the optimal number of clusters is considered as the number that minimises the DBI. The formulation of the modified DBI proposed by Sepulveda et al. (2004) can be used to measure cluster quality. For data based on real numbers, the DBI always yields a real value ≥ 0. The DBI is a measure of the standard deviation of the signal. A small DBI indicates well separated and grouped clusters, which means that the lower the DBI the more separable are the classes. There are several methods to measure cluster quality, but the DBI has been applied in research on muscle fatigue (Boostani & Moradi, 2003). The DBI is related to the performance of the linear Fisher discriminant classifier to pairwise clusters.

3. Classification methods

Classification methods, used in statistics and computational problem solving, are supervised machine learning procedures where individuals are grouped according to their characteristics, which can also be called traits, variables, characters, etc. This method bases its training set on previously labelled individuals. There are many ways of classifying a signal. Signal classification methods can be in continuous time or discrete time, analog or digital, periodic or aperiodic, finite or infinite, and deterministic or random. Discrete/continuous classification is determined by whether the signal is countable (discrete) or continuous.

There are numerous ways to classify the sEMG signals, although the non-stationary nature of the signals make classification more complicated (Khezri & Jahed, 2007). A number of classification methods used for sEMG fatigue related signals are described below.

One common method for sEMG classification is to measure the Euclidean distance between the waveform of an MUAP; where a shimmer is generated in the representation of time-triggered and non-overlapping MUAPs (Raez et al., 2006). The shimmer is influenced by external factors, such as background noise and noise from offsets. In addition, the shimmer of the MUAP is affected by the variance within a class as well as the distance between the classes.

Christodoulou & Pattichis (1995) suggested using an ANN as a classification method, which can be implemented in three phases. The first phase is unsupervised learning, which is built on competitive learning and on a one-dimensional self-organising feature map. In the second phase the learning vector is quantified, which is a self-supervised learning method which aids classification performance. Finally, the third phase is that of classification. The fuzzy approach has been compared with the ANN method on four subjects, and very similar classification results were obtained. It is superior to the latter in at least three points: slightly higher recognition rate, insensitivity to over-training and consistent outputs demonstrating higher reliability (Chan et al., 2000). Table 2 categorized some papers according to the classification methods used by authors.

Classification method	Refrence ID
GP	(Holland, 1975; Koza, 1994; Poli et al., 2008)
GA	(Koza, 1994; Michalewicz, 1996; Raikova & Aladjov, 2002; Wang, Yan, Hu, Xie & Wang, 2006)
ANN	(Bishop, 1995; Xie et al., 2010; 2009)
Fuzzy systems	(Chan et al., 2000; Kiryu & Yamashita, 2007; Takagi & Sugeno, 1985)
LDA	(Balakrishnama & Ganapathiraju, 2010; Fisher, 1936)
Support Vector Machine	(Gunn, 1998; Hsu et al., 2003)
One Clause at a Time	(Torvik et al., 1999)
Cross validation	(Kohavi, 1995; McLachlan et al., 2004)
Confusion matrix	(Kohavi & Provost, 1998)

Table 2. Classification Methods

3.1 Evolutionary computation

Genetic programming (GP), which implements a learning engine based on Darwin's theory of the natural selection of the fittest, was founded by Koza (1994). GP is based on the concept of evolutionary algorithms introduced in 1954 by Nils Aall Barricelli, who applied it to evolutionary simulations. GP optimises a computer program in order to solve tasks and creates computer programs as part of the solution (Holland, 1975). The optimal program (fittest) is selected from three standard genetic operators (crossover, mutation and reproduction), which modify the GP's structure and create new (and often improved) offspring (generations) (Michalewicz, 1996). GP is closely related to genetic algorithms (GAs) (Holland, 1975), however, GP actually creates computer programs as part of the solution. GP uses a tree structure to represent the computer programs it produces and reproduces when a genetic program is run (Koza, 1994). The tree structures represent the population and the new generations which are created and is similar in construction (and appearance) to what is commonly known as a family tree. Setting a maximum tree depth avoids excessive growth of (tree-based) individuals during the evolutionary process (Koza, 1994). GAs and GPs also work according to the strategy of the survival of the fittest, this time searching the solution space of a function. GAs have proved to be a useful means to solve linear and nonlinear problems, where the areas of the state space are explored through mutation, crossover and selection operations applied to individuals in the population (Michalewicz, 1996). GAs and GP use the determination of six fundamental components: solution representation, selection function, genetic operators, initialisation, termination and a fitness function. This will be explained in the following sub-sections.

3.1.1 Solution representation

In order to describe each individual in the population of interest, GAs us a chromosome (or individual) representation in which each individual is made up of a sequence of genes. This scheme decides which genetic operators it should use, in addition to determining the structure of the problem (Houck et al., 1996). Each individual consists of a sequence of genes from a specific alphabet. Binary digits, floating point numbers, integers, symbols etc. can make up the alphabet. In this thesis, GAs are utilised that use an alphabet consisting of floating point numbers. Research shows that better solutions are produced with a more natural problem representation, and it is also more efficient (Michalewicz, 1996). Hence, bounded floating point numbers are a useful representation of individuals for function optimisation.

3.1.2 Selection function

In a GA, individuals are selected to produce successive generations. The selection is based upon the fitness of an individual, where the fittest individuals have an increased probability of being selected and any individual can be selected more than once (Nordin & Banzhaf, 1996).

3.1.3 Genetic operator

Genetic operators are the basis for the search mechanism of GAs. Based on present solutions in the population, the operators are utilised to establish new solutions. The two main operators are crossover and mutation. Crossover uses two of the existing individuals to reproduce two new individuals, while mutation randomly changes the genes in one individual to get a single new solution (Michalewicz, 1996). A reproduction operator selects a parent based on its fitness and creates identical copies of that parent in the next generation (Koza, 1994). There are several options for applying genetic operators to a multi-tree representation. It is possible to apply a particular operator that is selected to all trees within an individual. Another possibility is to iterate over the trees in an individual and select a potentially different operator for each. Finally it is possible to constrain crossover to occur only between trees at the same position in the two parents or it was possible to let evolution freely crossover different trees within the representation.

3.1.4 GA Initialisation and GA termination

An initial population must be provided for the GA and it is common for it to be randomly generated. Since GAs have the ability to produce exciting solutions, the initial population may sometimes be seeded with specifically chosen individuals amongst the otherwise randomly generated individuals. To obtain a termination the GA goes from generation to generation to select parents and reproduce offspring, which then go on to become the next generation of parents (Houck et al., 1996). One possible termination strategy is to use the population convergence criteria, where most of the whole population is forced to converge to a single solution. However, the most popular termination strategy is to decide on a specified maximum number of generations.

3.1.5 Fitness function

The fitness function is an important concept of GAs as this is the indicator for how well a generated solution solves a specific problem; it evaluates the quality of the individuals and guides the evolution to uncover progressively improved solutions during a system run, while the fitness measure specifies what needs to be done (Koza, 1994). In order to select the best suited individuals, a fitness measure is determined by the user and the program will measure the fitness based on a fitness function. The fitness function is objective and quantifies the optimality in solutions. There are two main classes of fitness functions: one where the fitness function can mutate and one where it cannot. In order to calculate the fitness the program may need to run several times with a variety of parameters so that the output can be evaluated (Garner, 2010); this is termed 'training'. One common way to represent the fitness is to measure the difference between the theoretical or ideal value and the actual value, which means that a low fitness value indicates less error.

3.2 Artificial neural networks

An artificial neural network (ANN), also called neural network (NN), is an information processing model inspired by how biological neural networks process information (Bishop, 1995). The key element of ANN is its structure, consisting of interconnected groups of artificial neurons that processes information by a connectionist approach to computation, solving a specific problem. It is called an artificial neural 'network' as the network describes the basis of the system with inter-connected neurons in various layers. ANNs are adaptable systems where the structure is changeable depending on internal and external information flowing through the network in the learning phase, and are capable of modelling complex relationships. ANNs are used in classification, in particular for pattern recognition, but also in data processing (e.g. filtering, clustering, blind source separation and compression) as well as for robotics, and regression analysis.

One of the advantages of ANNs is their ability to find meaning in complicated data (Bishop, 1995). In pattern recognition, where trends are complex and cannot be derived by humans or linear computer models, they act as an expert analysing the problem. In addition, ANNs have other capabilities such as creating their own organisation of information given in the training phase and learning tasks simply by training experience. ANNs are also a useful method in real-time operations, where computations are executed in parallel, hence special hardware devices can be used in order to take advantage of this capability.

3.3 Fuzzy systems

Fuzzy logic, a form of logic that is tolerant to contradictory data, is used in biomedical signal processing and classification to overcome problems where signals are stochastic and therefore may be contradictory in nature (Chan et al., 2000). Fuzzy systems can be trained to identify patterns which are not identifiable by other methods. Fuzzy systems determine fuzzy operators, which may be unknown, on fuzzy sets, requiring the use of 'IF-THEN' rules. Fuzzy systems are used to model or classify problems with variables and rules that can be analysed by a human user. A fuzzy classifier is an algorithm that labels objects by class, and it is argued that the classifier can predict the class label. Kucheva et al. (2000) argued that any classifier that uses fuzzy logic in its training set can be considered to be a fuzzy classifier. A fuzzy system has a vector that contains the values of the features for a specific task, and the system runs a training algorithm and a training data set. Once the system is trained it can be applied to unseen objects. There are several models of fuzzy classifiers, and the simplest method is a rule-based approach that works as an 'IF-THEN' rule system, where the class label is the consequent part of the rule. If the consequent part of the rule contains linguistic values the output will be a soft label with values from the discriminant function. Takagi & Sugeno (1985) identified a fuzzy classifier where the function is the consequent. This method also works according to the IF-THEN rule, however, the rule is a regressor over the feature data space.

3.4 Linear discriminant analysis

Linear discriminant analysis, (LDA), also related to Fisher's linear discriminant, is a technique applied in statistics, pattern recognition and machine learning which finds a linear combination of features for the characterisation or separation of two or more classes. The result can be used as a linear classifier or for dimensionality reduction in later classification. This model is closely related to other techniques, e.g. regression analysis, analysis of variance and principal component analysis, however, in LDA the variance is categorical. LDA can easily execute cases with unequal within-class frequencies, whose performance is examined on randomly produced test data (Balakrishnama & Ganapathiraju, 2010). In this method the ratio of between-class variance to the within-class variance is maximised in any data set, which ensures optimal separability.

There are two different approaches for the transformation of data sets and classification of test vectors in the transformed space: class-dependent transformation and class-independent transformation (Balakrishnama & Ganapathiraju, 2010; Fisher, 1936). The class-dependent transformation involves maximising the ratio of between-class variance to within-class variance. The main aim is high class separability, which is obtained by maximising this ratio. The data sets are transformed independently by the use of two optimising criteria. The class-independent transformation maximises the ratio of overall variance to within-class variance. In this method, only one optimising criterion is used to transform the data sets, which means that data points are transformed regardless of their class identity. In this approach, each class is considered as a separate class against all other classes. LDA is often used for the characterisation of two classes. Here the sample set is considered to be a training set which will find a good predictor for the second class. The following linear transformation describes the classification where the LDA maps the data (feature vector) x:

$$y = w^t x + w_0, \tag{1}$$

where w and w_0 are determined by maximising the ratio of between-class variance to within-class variance to guarantee maximal separability. The LDA uses two classes that are classified at one time:

$$X \in \begin{cases} Class\ 1, & \text{if } y > 0, \\ Class\ 2, & \text{if } y < 0. \end{cases} \tag{2}$$

3.5 Support vector machine

A support vector machine (SVM) is essentially a supervised learning method which can be used in classification and regression. By undergoing training, the SVM uses an algorithm to develop a model that will predict which category the examples in the training set belongs to. SVMs are a useful technique of data classification (Gunn, 1998; Hsu et al., 2003).

3.6 One clause at a time

One clause at a time (OCAT) is a classification function developed by Torvik et al. (1999), where the aim was to create a flexible, but simple prediction function. In their study on predicting if a muscle is fatigued or rested by investigating the peaks and characteristics fractile frequencies in the EMG signals, they found, in their comparison with other classification methods, that OCAT achieved the highest accuracy. Although ANNs also showed great accuracy they need subjective fine tuning and are complex in their interpretation. Nevertheless, they acknowledged that the more classical methods might be more powerful as long as valid assumptions are made, which is why they stated that more research is needed. This is an interesting but fairly dated approach that attempts to predict localised muscle fatigue.

3.7 Research on classification of EMG signals

There are several approaches to signal classification, but for EMG signal processing, NNs, described in section 3.2, have often been suggested. More specifically, the dynamic recurrent NN, which has two different adaptive parameters using fully interconnected neuron-like units and which maps the relationship between arm movement and EMG muscle activity, was proposed by Cheron et al. (1996). Del Boca & Park (1994) suggested ANNs as a suitable technique for real-time applications of EMG. Their method can precisely identify the features of the EMG signals, and the EMG features are extracted by Fourier analysis, using a fuzzy algorithm for clustering. The operations are undertaken in real-time by an FFT performed by the multipliers in a digital signal processor. The use of fuzzy systems, as described in section 3.3, is also a classification method that has been used in muscle fatigue research as a fatigue index, showing better results than conventional fatigue indices (Kiryu & Yamashita, 2007). Xie et al. used a fuzzy approximate entropy analysis of sEMG signals (Xie et al., 2009) and a cross-fuzzy entropy (Xie et al., 2010) as means by which to assess muscle fatigue.

As mentioned in section 3.1, GP, a specialisation within the field of GAs (Holland, 1975) and based on Darwin's theory of evolution, finds the best suited computer program to perform a set task. Whereas GAs search the space of a function to find an optimum solution, GP creates computer programs as part of the solution. Raikova & Aladjov (2002) used hierarchical genetic algorithms (HGAs) to investigate the motor control for muscle forces during dynamic conditions. The HGA used genetic operators to find the moments of neural stimulation of all the MUs, which are the variables in genetic terms, so that the sum of MU twitches fulfills the set goals. Results showed that HGAs are a well suited method to examine motor control.

Wang, Yan, Hu, Xie & Wang (2006) have carried out several studies on classification of EMG signals using the wavelet packet method. One such study developed a classification method for sEMG signals based on discrete harmonic wavelet packet transform (DHWPT). Firstly, the relative energy of sEMG signals in each frequency band was extracted using DHWPT, and, secondly, a GA selected appropriate features that reduced the feature dimensionality. An NN would classify four types of prosthetic movement, utilising the selected features as the input vectors. This method produced high classification accuracy, in addition to saving computational time due to the fast algorithm in the DHWPT. In a similar study, Wang, Wang, Chen & Zhuang (2006) improved this sEMG signal classification method by using an optimal wavelet packet (OWP) method based on the DBI. Principle component analysis was applied for a reduction of the feature dimensionality of the outputs of the OWP decomposition. By using a neural network classifier to discriminate between the classes, the mean classification accuracy was 93.75%, outperforming the previous method developed by Wang, Yan, Hu, Xie & Wang (2006). Despite the fact that these two methods are based on EMG classification used for prosthetic movement, the classification methodologies are inventive and are of interest if they are applicable to sEMG signal classification of localised muscle fatigue.

3.8 Validation of classification

A statistical method for validation is cross validation, which evaluates how the classification results are applicable to an independent data set (Kohavi, 1995). Cross validation is based on an evaluation on the learning algorithm used for the applied classification technique. In cross validation the data is divided into two parts, out of which one is used for the training set and the other for the testing set (to validate the applied technique). There are several cross validation methods, such as repeated random sub-sampling validation, K-fold cross-validation, k x 2 cross-validation and leave-one-out cross-validation (Kohavi, 1995). Repeated random sub-sampling validation involves a random separation of the dataset into training and validation data. In every separation, the model fits the training set and predicts the outcomes for the data in the testing set (which is unseen). This strengths of this method are that it does not take long to compute compared to the other models and the proportion of the data set separation is not dependent upon the iterations (folds), however, some of the data may never be selected in the validation sub-sample while other data may be selected several times (Refaeilzadeh et al., 2008). K-fold cross validation partitions the original data set in for K sub-samples, out of which one subset is used for the validation process and the rest is used for the training set. This process is repeated K-times (iterations), ensuring that each of the K sub-samples are only used once in the validation and all of the observations are used for both training and validation (McLachlan et al., 2004). This is an advantage of this method, while the disadvantage is that the training algorithm needs to re-run several times, which means it requires a lot of time before it can make an evaluation. K × 2 cross validation is a variant of K-field validation, and this method is useful for large data sets, where the user randomly assign the data into two equal sets. Leave-one-out cross validation involves using a single observation from the original sample as the validation data, and the remaining observations as the training data. This is repeated such that each observation in the sample is used once as the validation data. This is the same as a K-fold cross-validation with K being equal to the number of observations in the original sample. Leave-one-out cross validation is also a method similar to K-fold classification, however, the number of iterations are equal to the number of data points in the sets, and each observation is used once as the validation data. This is an expensive method due to the number of times the training process is rerun.

4. Approaches in labeling the sEMG

In labelling the sEMG signal, only the kinematic data (the elbow angle and its standard deviation) were considered as they are reliable indicators in healthy individuals when assessing muscle fatigue onset (Barry, 1992; Guo et al., 2008; Herberts et al., 1980; James et al., 1995; Jarić et al., 1997; Taimela et al., 1999; Tho et al., 1997; Vedsted et al., 2006). The use of the kinematic variables defines the boundaries (Non-Fatigue, Transition-to-Fatigue and Fatigue) of the sEMG signal, providing the basis for training the sEMG classifier.

As the onset of muscle fatigue is diffuse, the use of fuzzy-logic classification is appropriate for setting the boundaries when labelling the sEMG. This study used both a fuzzy classifier to automate the labelling and human experts to verify the outcome of the fuzzy classifier. The two main criteria in labelling the sEMG signal are described below using fuzzy logic terms. The fuzzy classifier had two inputs (elbow angle and its standard deviation) and a single output. The labelling by the fuzzy classifier was verified by a human expert using Table 3 as a guide. The changes in the elbow angle and their indication of fatigue is based on a study by Van Roy et al. (2005). This study claims that changes in the elbow angle of 1.8 +/- 2.9 degrees in men indicates fatigue.

- Figure 1 indicates the fuzzy set input for the elbow angle provided by the goniometer (0 to 180°): Angles of 89° and above indicate Non-Fatigue, while angles below 86.5° indicate Fatigue. The figure also has a superimposed illustration of a single goniometer trial signal giving an example of how the fuzzy classifier identifies the boundaries to enable the labelling of the sEMG signal.

- Figure 2 indicates the fuzzy set input for the arm oscillations (Hristovski et al., 2010) (i.e., the standard deviation of the elbow angle), which was also provided by the goniometer: An increase in the standard deviation of the goniometer signals indicates either low angular oscillation or high angular oscillation. Calculation of the standard deviation was performed using a four-second non-overlapping window of the goniometer signal, then re-sampled to match the original signal size. Further examination of Figure 2, with the superimposed standard deviation signal, reveals that for this particular signal, at around 110 seconds, which resides at 0.6 standard deviations, the subject underwent the transition from the class of Non-Fatigue to that of Transition-to-Fatigue and at around 200 seconds indicates a Fatigue state at 1.0 standard deviations.

As with all fuzzy classifiers, only a single label was chosen as the final output (Slezak et al., 2005). Table 3 defines the rule base; the rule with the greatest firing strength was selected. The above fuzzy classifier inputs (elbow angle and amplitude of arm oscillation), when used in conjunction, were found to assist in finding the boundaries of the classes. Both inputs were used to define a 6 rule type-1 fuzzy classifier, using both triangular and trapezoidal antecedents and product inference.

Preliminary tests showed that the average sEMG signal in this data set was comprised of the muscle fatigue classes in the following estimated proportions: Non-Fatigue 54.5 %; Transition-to-Fatigue 43.18 % and Fatigue 2.32 %. These proportions varied between participants, with the only common feature being that the relative sizes and order of each

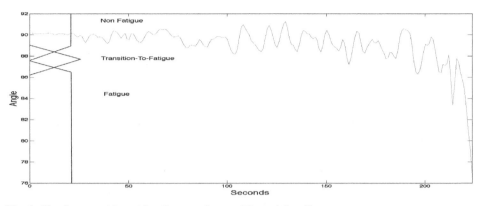

Fig. 1. The fuzzy set input for the angular position of the elbow.

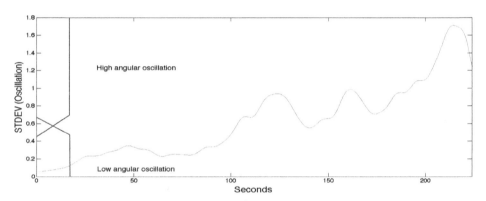

Fig. 2. The fuzzy set input for the angular oscillation (i.e., elbow angle standard deviation).

	IF		THEN
Rule	Input 1 (Elbow angle)	Input 2 (Oscillation)	Output
1	Non-Fatigue	Low	Non-Fatigue
2	Non-Fatigue	High	Transition-to-Fatigue
3	Transition-to-Fatigue	Low	Transition-to-Fatigue
4	Transition-to-Fatigue	High	Transition-to-Fatigue
5	Fatigue	Low	Fatigue
6	Fatigue	High	Fatigue

Table 3. Rule base for signal labelling.

signal component were always the same: Non-Fatigue component > Fatigue component > Transition-to-Fatigue component. For illustration purposes, Figure 3 shows an outcome of the labelling process for a single trial.

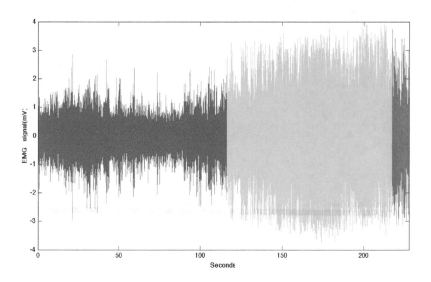

Fig. 3. An illustration of the sEMG signal after labelling (Blue=Non-Fatigue, Green=Transition-to-Fatigue and Red=Fatigue).

5. Conclusion

The defintion of localised muscle fatigue in the current litrutre has diffrent schools of thought, this chapter brought forward these definition to the reader. The chapter also looked at current state of the art in detecting, processing and calssification of sEMG for localized muscle fatigue. The novel concept of a three-phase approach to muscle fatigue(non-fatigue, transition-to-fatigue, and fatigue) was presented in this chapter.

6. References

Armstrong, W. J. (2010). Clinical applications of mechanomyography: technical brief, http://www.thefreelibrary.com/Clinical+applications+of+mechanomyography%3A+technical+brief-a0217771439.

Asghari Oskœi, M., Hu, H. & Gan, J. Q. (2008). Manifestation of fatigue in myoelectric signals of dynamic contractions produced during playing PC games, *Proceedings of the 30th annual international IEEE EMBS conference*, IEEE Engineering in Medicine and Biology Society, pp. 315–318.

Balakrishnama, S. & Ganapathiraju, A. (2010). Linear discriminant analysis -a brief tutorial, http://www.music.mcgill.ca/~ich/classes/mumt611_07/classifiers/lda_theory.pdf.

Barry, B. K. & Enoka, R. M. (2007). The neurobiology of muscle fatigue: 15 years later, *Integrative and Comparative Biology* 47(4): 465–473.

Barry, D. T. (1992). Vibrations and sounds from evoked muscle twitches, *Electromyography and clinical neurophysiology* 32: 35–40.

Basmajian, J. V. & De Luca, C. J. (1985). *Muscles alive: Their function revealed by electromyography*, Williams and Wilkins, Baltimore, MD, USA.

Bernatos, L., Crago, P. & Chizeck, H. (1986). A discrete-time model of electricity stimulated muscle, *IEEE Transactions on Systems, Man, and Cybernetics* pp. 829–838.

Bigland-Ritchie, B. & Woods, J. J. (1984). Changes in muscle contractile properties and neural control during human muscular fatigue, *Muscle Nerve* 7: 691–699.

Bills, A. G. (1943). *The psychology of efficiency*, Harper, New York, NY, USA.

Bishop, C. M. (1995). *Neural networks for pattern recognition*, Oxford University Press, New York, NY, USA.

Boostani, R. & Moradi, M. H. (2003). Evaluation of the forearm EMG signal features for the control of a prosthetic hand, *Physiological Measurement* 24: 309–319.

Borg, G. (1970). Perceived exertion as an indicator of somatic stress, *Scandinavian Journal of Rehabilitation Medicine* 2(2): 92–98.

Calder, K. M., Stashuk, D. W. & McLean, L. (2008). Physiological characteristics of motor units in the brachioradialis muscle across fatiguing low-level isometric contractions, *Journal of Electromyography and Kinesiology* 18: 2–15.

Chaffin, D. B. (1973). Localized muscle fatigue–definiton and measurement, *Journal of Occupational and Environmental Medicine* 15: 346–354.

Chan, F. H. Y., Yang, Y. S., Lam, F. K., Zhang, Y. T. & Parker, P. A. (2000). Fuzzy EMG classification for prosthesis control, *IEEE Transactions on Rehabilitation Engineering* 8(3): 305–311.

Cheron, G., Draye, J.-P. & Bourgeios, M. (1996). A dynamic neural network identification of electromyography and trajectory relationship during complex movements, *IEEE Transactions on Biomedical Engineering* 43(5): 552–558.

Christodoulou, C. I. & Pattichis, C. S. (1995). A new technique for the classification and decomposition of EMG signals, *IEEE international conference on neural networks (ICNN'95)*, Vol. 5, IEEE, Perth, Western Australia, pp. 2303–2308.

Cifrek, M., Medved, V., Tonkovi, S. & Ostoji, S. (2009). Surface EMG based muscle fatigue evaluation in biomechanics, *Clinical Biomechanics* 24: 327–340.

Cohen, L. (1995). *Time frequency analysis*, Prentice-Hall, Englewood Cliffs, NJ, USA.

Coorevits, P., Danneels, L., Cambier, D., Ramon, H., Druyts, H., Karlsson, S. J., Moor, G. D. & Vanderstraeten, G. (2008). Correlations between short-time Fourier- and continuous wavelet transforms in the analysis of localized back and hip muscle fatigue during isometric contractions, *Journal of Electromyography and Kinesiology* 18: 637–644.

Courteville, A., Gharbi, T. & Cornu, J. Y. (1998). MMG measurement: a high-sensitivity microphone-based sensor for clinical use, *IEEE Transactions on Biomedical Engineering* 45: 145–150.

Davies, D. L. & Bouldin, D. W. (1979). A cluster separation measure, *IEEE Transactions on Pattern Analysis and Machine Intelligence* 1(4): 224–227.

Davies, M. & Reisman, S. S. (1994). Time frequency analysis of the electromyogram during fatigue, *Proceedings of the 20th annual northeast bioengineering conference*, pp. 93–95.

Day, S. (2010). Important Factors in Surface EMG Measurement, http://www.bortec.ca/Images/pdf/EMG20measurement20and20recording.pdf.

De Luca, C. J. (1979). Physiology and mathematics of myoelectric signals, *IEEE Transactions on Biomedical Engineering* 26: 313–325.

De Luca, C. J. (1997). The use of surface electromyography in biomechanics, *Journal of Applied Biomechanics* 13: 135–163.

Del Boca, A. & Park, D. C. (1994). Myoelectric signal recognition using fuzzy clustering and artificlal neural networks in real time, *IEEE international conference on neural networks (ICNN'94)*, IEEE, Orlando, FL, USA, pp. 3098–3103.

Dimitrov, G. V., Arabadzhiev, T. I., Mileva, K. N., Bowtell, J. L., Crichton, N. & Dimitrova, N. A. (2006). Muscle fatigue during dynamic contractions assessed by new spectral indices, *Medicine and Science in Sports and Exercise* 38: 1971–1979.

Duchene, J. & Goubel, F. (1993). Surface electromyogram during voluntary contraction: processing tools and relation to physiological events, *Critical Reviews in Biomedical Engineering* 21: 313–397.

Eberstein, A. & Beattie, B. (1985). Simultaneous measurement of muscle conduction velocity and EMG power spectrum changes during fatigue, *Muscle Nerve* 8: 768–773.

Edwards, R. (1981). Human muscle function and fatigue, *Ciba Foundation Symposium* 82.

Farina, D. (2006). Interpretation of the surface electromyogram in dynamic contractions, *Exercise and Sport Sciences Review* 34: 121–127.

Filligoi, G., Felici, F., Vicini, M. & Rosponi, A. (2010). Recurrence quantification analysis of surface electromyograms, http://library.med.utah.edu/cyprus/proceedings/medicon98/medicon98.filligoi.giancarlo.pdf.

Fisher, R. A. (1936). The use of multiple measurements in taxonomic problems, *Ann. Eugenics* 7: 179–188.

Gabor, D. (1946). Theory of communication, *Journal of the Institution of Electrical Engineers - Part III: Radio and Communication Engineering* 93: 422–457.

Garner, Z. (2010). An introduction to genetic programming, http://www.generation5.org/content/2000/ga00.asp.

Georgakis, A., Stergioulas, L. K. & Giakas, G. (2003). Fatigue analysis of the surface EMG signal in isometric constant force contractions using the averaged instantaneous frequency, *IEEE Transactions on Biomedical Engineering* 50: 262–265.

Gerdle, B., Karlsson, S., Day, S. & Djupsbacka, M. (1999). *Acquisition, processing and analysis of the surface electromyogram. Modern techniques in neuroscience*, Springer Verlag, Berlin, Germany.

Gonzalez-Izal, M., Malanda, A., Navarro-Amezqueta, I., Gorostiaga, E. M., Mallor, F., Ibanez, J. & Izquierdo, M. (2010). EMG spectral indices and muscle power fatigue during dynamic contractions, *Journal of Electromyography and Kinesiology* 20: 233–240.

Gonzalez-Izal, M., Rodriguez-Carreno, I., Malanda, A., Mallor-Gimenez, F., Navarro-Amezqueta, I., Gorostiaga, E. M. & Izquierdo, M. (2010). sEMG wavelet-based indices predicts muscle power loss during dynamic contractions, *Journal of Electromyography and Kinesiology* 20: 1097–1106.

Gordon, G. & Holbourn, A. H. (1948). The sounds from single motor units in a contracting muscle, *The Journal of Physiology* 107: 456–464.

Graupe, D. & Cline, W. K. (1975). Functional separation of EMG signals via ARMA identification, *IEEE Transactions on Systems, Man, and Cybernetics* 5: 252–259.

Gregori, B., Galie, E. & Accornero, N. (2003). Surface electromyography and mechanomyography recording: a new differential composite probe, *Medical and Biological Engineering and Computing* 41: 665–669.

Gross, D., Ladd, H. W., Riley, E. J., Macklem, P. T. & Grassino, A. (1980). The effect of training on strength and endurance of the diaphragm in quadriplegia, *American Journal of Medicine* 68: 27–35.

Guglielminotti, P. & Merletti, R. (1992). Effect of electrode location on surface myoelectric signal variables: a simulation study, *9th international congress of The International Society of Electrophysiological Kinesiology*, Florence, Italy.

Gündoğdu, U., Sayin, A., Akan, A., Arslan, Y., Orhan, E. & Baslo, M. (2006). Investigation of muscle fatigue using temporal and spectral moments, *Proceedings of the 5th WSEAS*

international conference on Signal processing, SIP'06, World Scientific and Engineering Academy and Society (WSEAS), Stevens Point, Wisconsin, USA, pp. 10–14.
URL: *http://portal.acm.org/citation.cfm?id=1983937.1983941*

Gunn, S. R. (1998). Support vector machines for classification and regression, *Technical report*, University of Southanpton, Southampton, UK.
URL: *http://eprints.ecs.soton.ac.uk/6459/*

Guo, J. Y., Zheng, Y. P., Huang, Q. H. & Chen, X. (2008). Dynamic monitoring of forearm muscles using one-dimensional sonomyography system, *Journal of Rehabilitation Research and Development* 45: 187–195.

Hagberg, M. (1981). Work load and fatigue in repetitive arm elevations, *Ergonomics* 24: 543–555.

Hefftner, G., Zucchini, W. & Jaros, G. G. (1988). The electromyogram (EMG) as a control signal for functional neuromuscular stimulation–Part I: autoregressive modeling as a means of EMG signature discrimination, *IEEE Transactions on Biomedical Engineering* 35: 230–237.

Helal, J.-N., Van Hoecke, J., Garapon-Bar, C. & Goubel, F. (1992). Surface myoelectric signals during ergocycle exrcises at various mechanical powers and pedalling rates, *Journal of Electromyography and Kinesiology* 2(4): 242–251.
URL: *http://www.sciencedirect.com/science/article/B6T89-4CDHXXY-5/2/e121acb16d3fc8c 8480ee3e64fee8e18*

Herberts, P., Kadefors, R. & Broman, H. (1980). Arm positioning in manual tasks. An electromyographic study of localized muscle fatigue, *Ergonomics* 23: 655–665.

Hermens, H. J., Boon, K. L. & Zilvold, G. (1986). The clinical use of surface EMG, *Acta Belgica. Medica Physica* 9: 119–130.

Holland, J. H. (1975). *Adaptation in natural and artificial systems*, The University of Michigan Press, Ann Arbor, MI, USA.

Hong, Y. & Bartlett, R. (2008). *Routledge handbook of biomechanics and human movement science*, Routledge, New York, NY, USA.

Houck, C. R., A., J. J. & Kay, M. G. (1996). Comparison of genetic algorithms, random restart and two-opt switching for solving large location-allocation problems, *Computers and Operations Research* 23(6): 587–596.
URL: *http://dx.doi.org/10.1016/0305-0548(95)00063-1*

Hristovski, R., VenskaitytÆŠÂş, E., Vainoras, A., Balague, N. & Vazquez, P. (2010). Constraints-controlled metastable dynamics of exercise-induced psychobiological adaptation., *Medicina (Kaunas)* 46(7): 447–453.

Hsu, C. W., Chang, C. C. & Lin, C. J. (2003). A practical guide to support vector classification, *Technical report*, National Taiwan University, Taipei, Taiwan.
URL: *http://www.csie.ntu.edu.tw/ cjlin/papers/guide/guide.pdf*

Huang, H.-P. & Chen, C.-Y. (1999). Development of a myoelectric discrimination system for a multi-degree prosthetic hand, *IEEE International Conference on Robotics and Automation*, pp. 2392–2397.
URL: `http:{//dblp.uni-trier.de/db/conf/icra/icra1999-3.htmlHuangC99}`

Hudgins, B., Parker, P. & Scott, R. N. (1993). A new strategy for multifunction myoelectric control, *IEEE Transactions on Biomedical Engineering* 40: 82–94.

Hussain, M. S., Reaz, M. B. I. & Ibrahimy, M. I. (2008). SEMG signal processing and analysis using wavelet transform and higher order statistics to characterize muscle force, *ICS'08: Proceedings of the 12th WSEAS international conference on systems*, World

Scientific and Engineering Academy and Society WSEAS, Stevens Point, WI, USA, pp. 366–371.

James, C., Sacco, P. & Jones, D. A. (1995). Loss of power during fatigue of human leg muscles, *The Journal of Physiology* 484 (Pt 1): 237–246.

Jarić, S., Radovanović, S., Milanović, S., Ljubisavljević, M. & Anastasijević, R. (1997). A comparison of the effects of agonist and antagonist muscle fatigue on performance of rapid movements, *European Journal of Applied Physiology and Occupational Physiology* 76: 41–47.

Jaynes, E. T. (1957). Information theory and statistical mechanics, *Physical Review* 106(4): 620–630.

Jorgensen, K., Fallentin, N., Krogh-Lund, C. & Jensen, B. (1988). Electromyography and fatigue during prolonged, low-level static contractions, *European Journal of Applied Physiology and Occupational Physiology* 57: 316–321.

Kadefors, R., Kaiser, E. & Petersen, I. (1968). Dynamic spectrum analysis of myo-potentials and with special reference to muscle fatigue, *Electromyography* 8: 39–74.

Kanosue, K., Yoshida, M., Akazawa, K. & Fujii, K. (1979). The number of active motor units and their firing rates in voluntary contraction of human brachialis muscle, *The Japanese Journal of Physiology* 29: 427–443.

Karlsson, S., Yu, J. & Akay, M. (1999). Enhancement of spectral analysis of myoelectric signals during static contractions using wavelet methods, *IEEE Transactions on Biomedical Engineering* 46: 670–684.

Karlsson, S., Yu, J. & Akay, M. (2000). Time-frequency analysis of myoelectric signals during dynamic contractions: a comparative study, *IEEE Transactions on Biomedical Engineering* 47: 228–238.

Khezri, M. & Jahed, M. (2007). Real-time intelligent pattern recognition algorithm for surface EMG signals, *Biomedical Engineering Online* .

Kim, J.-Y., Jung, M.-C. & Haight, J. (2005). The sensitivity of autoregressive model coefficient in quantification of trunk muscle fatigue during a sustained isometric contraction, *International Journal of Industrial Ergonomics* 35: 321–330.

Kim, Y. & Street, W. N.and Filippo Menczer, F. (2010). Feature selection in data mining, http: //dollar.biz.uiowa.edu/~street/research/dmoc.pdf.

Kiryu, T. & Yamashita, K. (2007). A ubiquitous wearable unit for controlling muscular fatigue during cycling exercise sessions, *Conference Proceedings - IEEE Engineering in Medicine and Biology Society*, pp. 4814–4817.

Kleissen, R. F., Buurke, J. H., Harlaar, J. & Zilvold, G. (1998). Electromyography in the biomechanical analysis of human movement and its clinical application, *Gait Posture* 8: 143–158.

Kohavi, R. (1995). A study of cross-validation and bootstrap for accuracy estimation and model selection, *Proceedings of the 14th international joint conference on artificial intelligence - Volume 2*, Morgan Kaufmann Publishers Inc., San Francisco, CA, USA, pp. 1137–1143.
URL: *http://portal.acm.org/citation.cfm?id=1643031.1643047*

Kohavi, R. & John, G. H. (1997). The wrapper approach.

Kohavi, R. & Provost, F. (1998). Editorial for the special issue on applications of machine learning and the knowledge discovery process, *Machine Learning* 30: 271–274.

Kojadinovic, I. & Wottka, T. (2000). Comparison between a filter and a wrapper approach to variable.

Komi, P. V. & Tesch, P. (1979). EMG frequency spectrum, muscle structure, and fatigue during dynamic contractions in man, *European Journal of Applied Physiology and Occupational Physiology* 42: 41–50.

Koza, J. R. (1994). *Genetic programming II: automatic discovery of reusable programs*, MIT Press, Cambridge, MA, USA.

Kramer, C. G., Hagg, T. & Kemp, B. (1987). Real-time measurement of muscle fatigue related changes in surface EMG, *Medical and Biological Engineering and Computing* 25: 627–630.

Kucheva, L. I., Whitaker, C. J., Shipp, C. A. & Duin, R. P. W. (2000). Is independence good for combining classifiers?, *Proc. of ICPR2000, 15th Int. Conference on Pattern Recognition, Barcelona, Spain*, Vol. 2, pp. 168–171.

Kumar, D. K., Pah, N. D. & Bradley, A. (2003). Wavelet analysis of surface electromyography to determine muscle fatigue, *IEEE Transactions on Neural Systems and Rehabilitation Engineering* 11: 400–406.

Kumar, S. & Mital, A. (1996). *Electromyography in ergonomics*, Taylor and Francis Ltd., London, UK.

Laterza, F. & Olmo, G. (1997). Analysis of EMG signals by means of the matched wavelet transform, *Electronic Letters* 33(5): 357–359.

Lindstrom, L., Kadefors, R. & Petersen, I. (1977). An electromyographic index for localized muscle fatigue, *Journal of Applied Physiology* 43: 750–754.

Linssen, W. H., Stegeman, D. F., Joosten, E. M., van't Hof, M. A., Binkhorst, R. A. & Notermans, S. L. (1993). Variability and interrelationships of surface EMG parameters during local muscle fatigue, *Muscle Nerve* 16: 849–856.

Liu, H. & Motoda, M. (1998). *Feature selection for knowledge discovery and data mining*, Kluwer Academic Publishers, Norwell, MA, USA.

MacIsaac, D. T., Parker, P. A., Englehart, K. B. & Rogers, D. R. (2006). Fatigue estimation with a multivariable myoelectric mapping function, *IEEE Transactions on Biomedical Engineering* 53: 694–700.

Marras, W. (1990). Industrial electromyography (EMG), *International Journal of Industrial Ergonomics* 6: 89–74.

Masuda, K., Masuda, T., Sadoyama, T., Inaki, M. & Katsuta, S. (1999). Changes in surface EMG parameters during static and dynamic fatiguing contractions, *Journal of Electromyography and Kinesiology* 9: 39–46.

Maton, B. & Gamet, D. (1989). The fatigability of two agonistic muscles in human isometric voluntary submaximal contraction: an EMG study. II. Motor unit firing rate and recruitment, *European Journal of Applied Physiology and Occupational Physiology* 58: 369–374.

McLachlan, G. J., Do, K. A. & Ambroise, C. (2004). *Analyzing microarray gene expression data*, Wiley, New York, NY, USA.

Merletti, R. (1999). Standards for Reporting EMG data., *Journal of Electromyography and Kinesiology* 9(1).

Merletti, R., Farina, D. & Gazzoni, M. (2003). The linear electrode array: a useful tool with many applications, *Journal of Electromyography and Kinesiology* 13: 37–47.

Merletti, R. & Parker, P. A. (2004). *Electromyography: physiology, engineering and non-invasive applications*, John Wiley and sons, Inc, New York.

Michalewicz, Z. (1996). *Genetic Algorithms + Data Structures = Evolution Programs*, Springer-Verlag, New York, NY, USA.

Minning, S., Eliot, C. A., Uhl, T. L. & Malone, T. R. (2007). EMG analysis of shoulder muscle fatigue during resisted isometric shoulder elevation, *Journal of Electromyography and Kinesiology* 17: 153–159.

Morana, C., Ramdani, S., Perrey, S. & Varray, A. (2009). Recurrence quantification analysis of surface electromyographic signal: sensitivity to potentiation and neuromuscular fatigue, *Journal of Neuroscience Methods* 177: 73–79.

Moser, A. T. & Graupe, D. (1989). Identification of nonstationary models with application to myoelectric signals for controlling electrical stimulation of paraplegics, *IEEE Trans Acoust Speech Sig Proc* ASSP-37(5): 713.

Moshou, D., Hostens, I., Papaioannou, G. & Ramon, H. (2005). Dynamic muscle fatigue detection using self-organizing maps, *Applied Soft Computing* 5: 391–398.

Naik, G. R., Kumar, D. K., Wheeler, K. & Arjunan, S. P. (2009). Estimation of muscle fatigue during cyclic contractions using source separation techniques, *Proceedings of the 2009 digital image computing: techniques and applications (DICTA 2009)*, IEEE Computer Society, pp. 217–222.

Nordin, P. & Banzhaf, W. (1996). Programmatic compression of images and sound, *in* J. R. Koza, D. E. Goldberg, D. B. Fogel & R. L. Riolo (eds), *Proceedings of the first annual conference on genetic programming*, MIT Press, Boston, MA, USA, pp. 345–350. URL: *ftp://lumpi.informatik.uni-dortmund.de/pub/biocomp/papers/gp96.ps.gz*

Ortengren, R., Andersson, G., Broman, H., Magnusson, R. & Petersen, I. (1975). Vocational electromyography: studies of localized muscle fatigue at the assembly line, *Ergonomics* 18: 157–174.

Payton, C. & Bartlett, R. (2008). *Biomechanical evaluation of movement in sport and exercise: The British Association of Sport and Science*, Routledge, New York, NY, USA.

Petrofsky, J. S. (1981). Quantification through the surface EMG of muscle fatigue and recovery during successive isometric contractions, *Aviation, Space, and Environmental Medicine* 52: 545–550.

Petrofsky, J. S., Glaser, R. M., Phillips, C. A., Lind, A. R. & Williams, C. (1982). Evaluation of amplitude and frequency components of the surface EMG as an index of muscle fatigue, *Ergonomics* 25: 213–223.

Phinyomark, A., Limsakul, C. & Phukpattaranont, P. (2009). A novel feature extraction for robust EMG pattern recognition, *Journal of Computing* 1(1).

Poli, R., Langdon, W. B. & McPhee, N. F. (2008). *A field guide to genetic programming*, Published via http://lulu.com. (With contributions by J. R. Koza). URL: *http://www.gp-field-guide.org.uk*

Raez, M. B., Hussain, M. S. & Mohd-Yasin, F. (2006). Techniques of EMG signal analysis: detection, processing, classification and applications, *Biological Proceedings Online* 8: 11–35.

Raikova, R. T. & Aladjov, H. T. S. (2002). Hierarchical genetic algorithm versus static optimization-investigation of elbow flexion and extension movements, *Journal of Biomechanics* 35: 1123–1135.

Refaeilzadeh, P., Tang, L. & Liu, H. (2008). Cross-validation, http://www.public.asu.edu/~ltang9/papers/ency-cross-validation.pdf.

Ricamato, A., Absher, R. G., M.T., M. & Tranowski, J. P. (1992). A time-frequency approach to evaluate electromyographic recordings, *Proceedings of the 5th annual IEEE symposium on computer-based medical system*, pp. 520–527.

Roy, S. H., Bonato, P. & Knaflitz, M. (1998). EMG assessment of back muscle function during cyclical lifting, *Journal of Electromyography and Kinesiology* 8: 233–245.

Samet, H. (2006). *Foundations of multidimensional and metric data structures*, Morgan Kaufmann, USA.

Sato, H. (1982). Functional characteristics of human skeletal muscle revealed by spectral analysis of the surface electromyogram, *Electromyography and Clinical Neurophysiology* 22: 459–516.

Sepulveda, F., Meckes, M. & Conway, B. (2004). Cluster separation index suggests usefulness of non-motor eeg channels in detecting wrist movement direction intention, *IEEE conference on cybernetics and intelligent systems*, pp. 943–947.

Sewell, M. (2010). Feature selection, http://machine-learning.martinsewell.com/feature-selection/feature-selection.pdf.

Shahid, S. (2007). *Higher order statistics techniques applied to EMG signal analysis and characterization of skeletal muscles*, PhD thesis, University of Limerick, Limerick, Ireland.

Sherif, M. F. (1980). *Stochastic model of myoelectric signals for movement pattern recognition in upper limb prostheses*, PhD thesis, School of Engineering and Applied Sciences, University of California at Los Angeles, Los Angeles, CA, USA.

Singh, V. P., Kumar, D. K., Polus, B. & Fraser, S. (2007). Strategies to identify changes in SEMG due to muscle fatigue during cycling, *Journal of Medical Engineering and Technology* 31: 144–151.

Slezak, D., Yao, J. T., Peters, J. F., Ziarko, W. & Xiaohua Hu, X. (2005). *Rough sets, fuzzy sets, data mining, and granular computing*, Springer, Berlin, Germany.

Soo, Y., Nishino, M., Sugi, M., Yokoi, H., Arai, T., Kato, R., Nakamura, T. & Ota, J. (2009). Evaluation of frequency band technique in estimating muscle fatigue during dynamic contraction task, *Proceedings of the 2009 IEEE International Conference on Robotics and Automation (ICRA'09)*, IEEE, pp. 933–938. URL: *http:{//dx.doi.org/10.1109/ROBOT.2009.5152845}*

Stulen, F. B. & De Luca, C. J. (1982). Muscle fatigue monitor: a noninvasive device for observing localized muscular fatigue, *IEEE Transactions on Biomedical Engineering* 29: 760–768.

Sung, P. S., Zurcher, U. & Kaufman, M. (2008). Gender differences in spectral and entropic measures of erector spinae muscle fatigue, *Journal of Rehabilitation Research and Development* 45: 1431–1439.

Taimela, S., Kankaanpaa, M. & Luoto, S. (1999). The effect of lumbar fatigue on the ability to sense a change in lumbar position. A controlled study, *Spine* 24: 1322–1327.

Takagi, T. & Sugeno, M. (1985). Fuzzy identification of systems and its application to modeling and control, *IEEE Transactions on Systems, Man, and Cybernetics* 15(1): 116–132.

Tamil, E. M., Bashar, N. S., Idris, M. Y. I. & Tamil, A. M. (2008). Review on feature extraction and classification techniques for biosignal processing part III: electromyogram, *in* N. A. Abu Osman, F. Ibrahim, W. A. B. Wan Abas, H. S. Abdul Rahman & H.-N. Ting (eds), *4th Kuala Lumpur international conference on biomedical engineering*, Vol. 21 of *IFMBE Proceedings*, Springer Berlin Heidelberg, Germany, pp. 117–121.

Tepavac, D. & Schwirtlich, L. (1997). Detection and prediction of FES-induced fatigue, *Journal of Electromyography and Kinesiology* 7: 39–50.

Tho, K. S., Nemeth, G., Lamontagne, M. & Eriksson, E. (1997). Electromyographic analysis of muscle fatigue in anterior cruciate ligament deficient knees, *Clinical Orthopaedics and Related Research* pp. 142–151.

Tohru, K. (1992). Investigation of parametric analysis of dynamic EMG signals by a muscle-structured stimulation study, *IEEE Transactions on Biomedical Engineering* 39(3): 280–288.

Torvik, G. I., Triantaphyllou, E., Liao, T. & Waly, S. (1999). Predicting muscle fatigue via electromyography: A comparative study, `http://arrowsmith.psych.uic.edu/torvik/papers/iccie25_1999_torvik.pdf`.

Van Roy, P., Baeyens, J., Fauvart, D., Lanssiers, R. & Clarijs, J. (2005). Arthro-kinematics of the elbow: study of the carrying angle., *Ergonomics* 48(11): 1645–1656.

Vedsted, P., Blangsted, A. K., Søgaard, K., Orizio, C. & Sjøgaard, G. (2006). Muscle tissue oxygenation, pressure, electrical, and mechanical responses during dynamic and static voluntary contractions, *European Journal of Applied Physiology* 96: 165–177.

Viitasalo, J. H. & Komi, P. V. (1977). Signal characteristics of EMG during fatigue, *European Journal of Applied Physiology and Occupational Physiology* 37: 111–121.

Walker, J. S. (2000). *A primer on wavelets and their scientific applications*, Chapman and Hall/CRC, Boca Raton, FL, USA.
  URL: *http://millenium.itesm.mx/record=i566853&searchscope=0*

Wang, G., Wang, Z., Chen, W. & Zhuang, J. (2006). Classification of surface emg signals using optimal wavelet packet method based on davies-bouldin criterion, *Medical and Biological Engineering and Computing* 44: 865–872. 10.1007/s11517-006-0100-y.
  URL: *http://dx.doi.org/10.1007/s11517-006-0100-y*

Wang, G., Yan, Z., Hu, X., Xie, H. & Wang, Z. (2006). Classification of surface EMG signals using harmonic wavelet packet transform, *Physiological Measurement* 27: 1255–1267.

Wang, J., Yang, H. C. & Liu, J. H. (2004). Studies on the non-fatigue specificity of the fatigue-related sEMG signal parameters, *Space medicine and medical engineering Beijing* 17: 39–43.

Watakabe, M., Itoh, Y., Mita, K. & Akataki, K. (1998). Technical aspects of mechnomyography recording with piezoelectric contact sensor, *Medical and Biological Engineering and Computing* 36: 557–561.

Welch, P. D. (1967). The use of fast Fourier transform for the estimation of power spectra: a method based on time averaging over short, modified periodograms, *IEEE Transactions on Audio and Electroacoustics* 15: 70–73.

Xie, H.-B., Zheng, Y.-P., Guo, J.-Y. & Chen, X. (2010). Cross-fuzzy entropy: a new method to test pattern synchrony of bivariate time series, *Information Sciences* 180(9): 1715–1724.

Xie, H. B., Zheng, Y. P., Guo, J. Y., Chen, X. & Shi, J. (2009). Estimation of wrist angle from sonomyography using support vector machine and artificial neural network models, *Medical Engineering and Physics* 31: 384–391.

Yan, Z., Wang, Z. & Xie, H. (2008). The application of mutual information-based feature selection and fuzzy LS-SVM-based classifier in motion classification, *Computer Methods and Programs in Biomedicine* 90(3): 275–284.

Zhang, Z. G., Liu, H. T., Chan, S. C., Luk, K. D. & Hu, Y. (2010). Time-dependent power spectral density estimation of surface electromyography during isometric muscle contraction: methods and comparisons, *Journal of Electromyography and Kinesiology* 20: 89–101.

10

Clinical Application of Silent Period for the Evaluation of Neuro-Muscular Function in the Field of the Sports Medicine and Rehabilitation

Shinichi Daikuya[1], Atsuko Ono[1], Toshiaki Suzuki[2],
Tetsuji Fujiwara[3] and Kyonosuke Yabe[4]
[1]*Kishiwada Eishinkai Hospital*
[2]*Kansai University of Health Sciences*
[3]*Kyoto University*
[4]*Nagoya University*
Japan

1. Introduction

A transient suppression of muscle activation was produced by electric stimulation to the innervating nerve during continued effort. This period of electrical inactivity, designated the mixed nerve silent period, results from several physiologic mechanisms (Kimura, 2001). On the other hand, the silent period during tonic muscle contraction demonstrated on electromyography is due to the rapid voluntary movement during tonic and mild muscle contraction (Ikai, 1955) and is elicited by cutaneous electrical stimulation of supplying nerve during muscle contraction (Higgins & Lieberman, 1968). In many previous studies about silent period, it was generally classified into three categories: (1) the quiet period of bursting wave activity on electromyography, recorded before the rapid motion in response to visual, auditory, light and/or sound stimulation (Yabe, 1976); (2) a transient suppression of muscle activation following electric stimulation of the mixed nerve innervating that muscle during continued effort (Kimura, 2001); (3) a pause of the muscle activity following the motor potential elicited by cortical magnetic stimulation during voluntary target muscle contraction (Calancie et al, 1987). In this study, we used the second category, according to which the silent period consists of several waves, including M wave, F wave and Long Latency Reflex (LLR).

The silent period in this article, which classified in the second category, is the duration of the inhibitory period of muscle contraction detected on surface electromyography, which is due to electrical stimulation at the innervating nerve during tonic muscle contraction (Figure 1). We have considered that the silent period of lower extremity is the total circuit time from the peripheral nerve stimulus point to the central nervous system (i.e., brainstem or motor cortex), because the M wave, F wave and LLR are included in the silent period on evoked electromyography. M wave is affected by the conductive condition of peripheral nerve and the muscle state (i.e. rest or contraction, length, volume and so on) (Fuglevand et al, 1993, Cupido et al, 1992, Behm & St-Pierre, 1997). F wave is influenced by the excitability of the spinal motor neuron function (Suzuki et al, 1993). LLR in the lower extremities is affected by the excitability of the spinal cord, brainstem or motor cortex (Roby-Brami & Bussel, 1987, Upton et al, 1971, Kuroiwa, 1986). Therefore, it has been thought that a variation of the silent period may be able to become an index of the degree of facilitation of the brainstem or motor cortex. So, the origin of silent period that we used in this study is thought to be influenced by muscle spindle function, afferent inhibited impulse from Golgi tendon organ or Ia fiber, recurrent inhibition in the spinal cord, inhibitive mechanism of cerebral cortex (Higgins & Lieberman, 1968, Upton et al, 1971, Anastasijevic & Vuco, 1980). And we have tried to apply the silent period to clarify the magnitude of facilitation of the brainstem or motor cortex in the field of physical therapy. In previous study, we had studied the neuromuscular function of healthy subjects in various conditions (i.e. control of degree of muscle contraction and alteration of postural condition) with a silent period using an electro-physiological method (Daikuya et al, 2003.). Though LLR may be included in silent period, LLR was usually distinguished under the supra-maximal stimulation, which was used to record the silent period. In addition, if the fluctuation of silent period was large, it was thought that it shown the possibility of having arrived in the level where electric stimulus differs every stimulus.

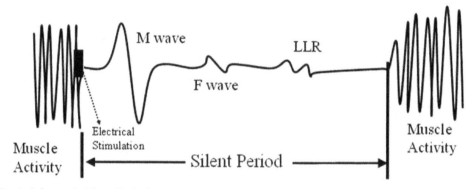

Fig. 1. Schematic Silent Period.

While, the state of improvement process after reconstruction of anterior cruciate ligament of the knee (ACL), following parameters were usually used as the index of recovery of physical function; muscle strength, range of motion (ROM), quality of sports performance, and so on. However, it is thought that results of their index and ability or disability of sports competition have little correlation, because we have experienced some cases with instability and/or a strange sensation of the knee during sports activity, although their muscle strength and ROM were good enough. Whereas, we have also experienced some cases without any problems, although their muscle strength and ROM were not enough. Therefore, we considered that as the index of recovery degree after reconstruction of ACL, only their parameters were not sufficient. And, we emphasized the necessity of evaluation of neuromuscular function after reconstruction of ACL. So, we had considered the neuromuscular function of healthy subjects in various conditions (i.e. control of degree of muscle contraction and alteration of postural condition.) with a mixed nerve silent period using an electro-physiological method (Daikuya et al, 2003.) and have attempted to apply the alteration of silent period aspects for the evaluation of the neuromuscular function of a lower extremity after reconstruction of ACL.

Clinical Application of Silent Period for the Evaluation of Neuro-Muscular Function in the Field of
the Sports Medicine and Rehabilitation

189

2. Silent period in healthy subjects; its aspects in relation to strength of tonic muscle contraction and postural alteration

Silent period aspects in healthy subjects were displayed as preliminary findings, which demonstrated the tendency of the change of the duration of silent period with an alteration of the strength of tonic muscle contraction, and the relationship between the duration of silent period and postural change in upper and lower extremity for application in the field of sports medicine.

2.1 Effect of electric stimulating condition on silent period recording

The effect of electric stimulation on silent period measurement was studied, in non-athlete, 9 healthy subjects with a mean age of 25.1 years (9 healthy subjects, 18 extremities, 8 males and 1 female). The experimental landscape was shown in Figure 2. The silent period was recorded from the opponens pollicis muscle under the following 3×3 electric stimulation conditions: 0.2Hz, 0.5Hz and 1.0Hz of frequency; 80%, 100% and 120% of intensity in maximal amplitude of M-wave. In this article, we defined the silent period as the duration from artifact produced by electrical stimulation of the muscle re-bursting on EMG, and the silent period was calculated the duration from the artifact due to electrical stimulation to reappearance or uninterrupted voluntary tonic muscle activity under the 200 or 500µV/div on a screen. The duration of silent period was expressed as the average of the latencies of all waves recorded.

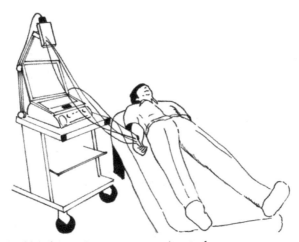

Fig. 2. Experimental landscape in upper extremity study.

The results were as follows; when the electric intensity was changed, the duration of silent period did not vary significantly. However, the silent period was become clearly with increase of intensity of the stimulation (Figure 3) and this mechanism was involved the "collision" effect. And more, with a faster frequency of stimulation, the duration of silent period became significantly shorter (Table 1). The present findings suggested that in silent period measurement, supra-maximal electric stimulation is most suitable. However, for frequency of electric stimulation, 1.0Hz stimulation is not suitable because there is the possibility that CNS is facilitated by the electric stimulation.

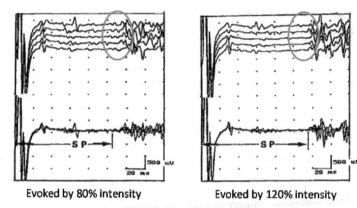

| Evoked by 80% intensity | Evoked by 120% intensity |

Fig. 3. Silent period due to 80% and 120% electric stimulus of intensity evoked the maximal amplitude of M-wave.

The upper shows typical 5 raw waves and the lower demonstrated the overlaid them.When the weak stimulus was provided, the starting point of muscle bursting was not clear (part of the circle on left figure) compared with providing the strong stimulus (part of the circle on right figure).

Frequency / intensity	80%	100%	120%
0.2Hz	105.3±5.3	107.2±6.5	106.4±6.4
0.5Hz	103.1±5.3	103.6±4.4	102.9±5.5
1.0Hz	102.2±4.6	101.9±4.3	101.8±5.5

(n=9, Average±SD ms)

Table 1. Effect of electric stimulating condition on silent period recording.
Silent period was shortened with increasing stimulation frequency (ANOVA and Tukey: $p < 0.05$).

2.2 Silent period aspects in the strength change of background tonic muscle contraction
2.2.1 Upper extremity

We studied the silent period and its relation to isometric contraction in 15 healthy subjects, who were not athletes. Their mean age was 21.4 years. The silent period was recorded from opponens pollicis muscle by electrical stimulation followed by 25%, 50%, 75% and 100% of strength of tonic contraction with the maximal voluntary effort (MVE) under following conditions: subjects were in supine position at rest. The experimental landscape was also shown in Figure 2. Electrical stimulation (intensity: supra-maximal; duration: 0.2ms; frequency: 0.5Hz) was administered to median nerve at wrist. Recording electrode was placed on the opponens pollicis muscle and the reference electrode was put on the distal part of the first proximal phalanx, and samplings were repeated 20 times.

The acquired typical waveforms were demonstrated on Figure 4. Overall average, dominant side average and non-dominant side average in all subjects, the duration of silent period

Clinical Application of Silent Period for the Evaluation of Neuro-Muscular Function in the Field of
the Sports Medicine and Rehabilitation

191

showed significant differences in all combinations. In particular, the duration of silent period at 75%MVE was shortest (paired t-test; p<0.05, Table 2). This suggests that CNS may be more facilitated during 75%MVE of isometric contraction compared to other levels, and that the 75% level may be most suitable for preparing some types of movements.

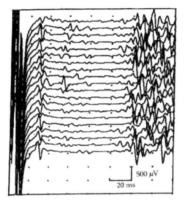
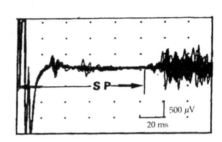

Fig. 4. Typical waveforms of silent period in upper extremity study.
The left figure shows typical 20 raw waves and the right figure demonstrates the overlaid them. Silent period on this figure was recorded at 25%MVE (Maximal Voluntary Effort).

Contraction level	25%MVE	50%MVE	75%MVE	100%MVE
Bilateral	108.8±6.4	106.9±7.2	105.8±6.6	107.6±8.0
Dominant	110.1±5.9	106.7±6.2	105.0±6.5	107.4±7.6
Non-dominant	107.5±6.6	107.1±8.1	106.7±6.6	107.8±8.4

Average±SD ms
MVE: Maximal Voluntary Effort

Table 2. The duration of silent period in the strength change of background tonic muscle contraction in upper extremity.

2.2.2 Lower extremity

The study was performed on the soleus muscles of 10 healthy non-athletes (20 lower extremities of healthy 8 males and 2 females, their mean age 25.2±2.7 years). The silent period was recorded from soleus muscle with same conditions of muscle contraction and sampling numbers as upper extremity. Subjects were in supine position with the hip and knee joints of the recorded side flexed at 45 degrees, and with the ankle joint kept 0 degree (Figure 5). Electrical stimulation was administered to tibial nerve at popliteal fossa with same condition as upper extremity. Recording electrode was placed on the soleus muscle and the reference electrode was put on the ipsilateral Achilles tendon.

The acquired typical waveforms were demonstrated on Figure 6. Similar to the results of upper extremity, the results indicated that the duration of silent period was the shortest during 75% of maximal effort (paired t-test; p<0.05, Table 3). It was considered that the supra-spinal inhibition was remarkably released during sub-maximal effort level; in other words, CNS was most facilitated during sub-maximal effort.

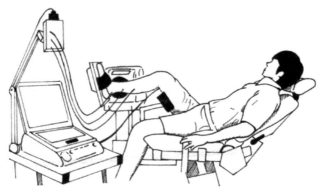

Fig. 5. Experimental landscape in lower extremity study.

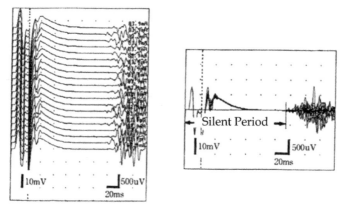

Fig. 6. Typical waveforms of silent period in lower extremity study.
The left figure shows typical 20 raw waves and the right figure demonstrates the overlaid them. Silent period on this figure was recorded at 25%MVE (Maximal Voluntary Effort).

Contraction level	25%MVE	50%MVE	75%MVE	100%MVE
Bilateral	153.0±15.4	142.3±14.2	127.6±14.5	144.3±13.7
Dominant	150.3±14.5	141.2±15.6	127.6±17.5	144.1±13.6
Non-dominant	155.7±16.5	143.4±13.5	127.6±11.7	144.5±14.6

Average±SD ms
MVE: Maximal Voluntary Effort

Table 3. The duration of silent period in the strength change of background tonic muscle contraction in lower extremity.

Clinical Application of Silent Period for the Evaluation of Neuro-Muscular Function in the Field of
the Sports Medicine and Rehabilitation

193

2.3 Silent period aspects in relation to postural change
2.3.1 Creeping posture

We measured the silent period in 10 healthy right-handed subjects (9 males and 1female),
who were not athletes. Their mean age was 24.9±2.6 (range; 21-31) years and mean height
was 169.7±7.8 (range; 152-182) cm. The silent period was recorded in the abductor pollicis
brevis muscles (APB) of the dominant side. The subjects were asked to adapt 3 positions as
follows in a shielded room. The 3 positions were all fours with bilateral elbows not bent
(position 1), all fours with bilateral elbows bent at 45 degrees (position 2) and all fours with
using the only dominant upper extremity (position 3).

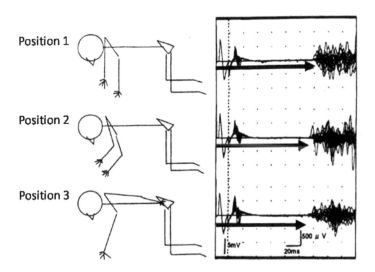

Fig. 7. Typical waveforms of silent period in relation to creeping posture.
The left figure shows the schematic three kinds of creeping postures and the right figures
demonstrates the overlaid waveforms of the silent period on each posture.

And we confirmed that amplitudes of background EMG of APB were almost same in all
positions. The silent period was recorded at APB with electrical stimulation of the median
nerve in each position. The position sequence was randomized, and we let subjects take
sufficient inter-test intervals to exclude the influence of contraction and electric stimulation
of the previous test or muscle fatigue. Monopolar electrodes were used to measure surface
EMG on median nerve stimulation at the wrist, and the sweep lime was 200ms. Electrodes
were attached to the APB (recording), and the distal part of the proximal phalanx 1
(reference). The stimulus conditions were as follows; intensity: 1.2 times that which evoked
maximum M wave, frequency: 0.5Hz, duration: 0.2ms, and number of recordings: 20 limes.
A representative pattern of the silent period is shown in Figure 7.
Table 4 summarizes the duration of silent period data in each position. The duration of
silent period changed with alterations in posture. The duration of silent period in position 3
was the shortest. This finding indicates that the amount of weight bearing has an effect on
the silent period and CNS function, because the amount of weight borne by the upper-
extremity was the most in position 3.

	Position 1	Position 2	Position 3
Duration of silent period	124.3±15.2	119.6±13.7	112.0±13.9

(Average±SD ms)

Table 4. The duration of silent period from APB in the alteration of creeping postures. The duration of silent period in position 3 was the shortest. And the one in position 2 is shorter than in position 1 and longer than in position 3 (Paired t-test, p<0.05).

2.3.2 Standing posture

Subjects were 8 healthy males, with a mean age of 23.5±2.2 (21-27) years and a mean height of 170.8±2.4 (167-175) cm. Every subject's dominant leg was the right leg. The silent period by single stimulation to tibial nerve at the popliteal fossa was recorded from the dominant side soleus and gastrocnemius muscles during ten kinds of standing postures regulated by visual information, supporting or not by a finger and a width of base of support (Figure 8). And the silent period of each muscle was recorded during above ten kinds of standings under the following stimulus and recording conditions. The stimulating condition for

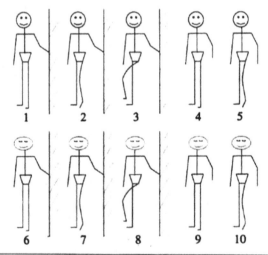

Eyes	Supporting by finger	Base of support	Posture No.
Open	With	Bilateral	1
		Toe	2
		Semi lateral	3
	Without	Bilateral	4
		Toe	5
Close	With	Bilateral	6
		Toe	7
		Semi lateral	8
	Without	Bilateral	9
		Toe	10

Fig. 8. Ten kinds of standing postures.

Clinical Application of Silent Period for the Evaluation of Neuro-Muscular Function in the Field of
the Sports Medicine and Rehabilitation

195

recording the silent period was as follows; intensity of supra-maximum, duration of 0.2ms, frequency of 0.5Hz and numbers of 30 times. As to the recording conditions of silent period, recording electrodes were placed on soleus and gastrocnemius (lateral head) muscles and reference electrode was put on the ipsilateral Achilles tendon. Sweep time on recording was 200ms. The raw data were amplified with a band pass between 20Hz and 2000Hz and averaged 30 times by a Nicolet Viking IIe. The silent period was calculated the duration from the artifact due to electrical stimulation to reappearance of uninterrupted voluntary tonic muscle activity under the 100μV or 200 μV/div on a screen. The difference of soleus and gastrocnemius silent periods was compared with the postural alteration as the ten kinds of standings. And a one-way analysis of variance (one-way ANOVA) was used as the statistical method to compare the data.

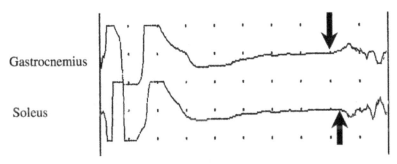

Gastrocnemius

Soleus

Fig. 9. Typical waveform of silent period on natural standing (posture 1).
Each arrow shows the re-bursting of the muscle activity. Each silent period was calculated the duration from starting of a waveform to a point demonstrated by arrow (22 y.o., male. Gain of amplitude: 100 μ V /div, Sweep: 200ms, Averaged: 30 times.).

Typical wave forms on natural standing of soleus and gastrocnemius silent periods were demonstrated on Figure 9. The duration of silent period on each standing was demonstrated on the Table 5. Both soleus and gastrocnemius silent periods did not change among 10 kinds of standing (One-way ANOVA, F = 1.797, F = 1.786). It is thought that a variation of the duration of silent period may reflect the magnitude of facilitation or disinhibition of the CNS including spinal, brainstem or motor cortex. As the result of this study in healthy persons, it was suggested that the degree of facilitation or disinhibition of CNS related to silent period from soleus and gastrocnemius was not different on ten kinds of standings regulated by visual information and a width of base of support.

3. Silent period application in the field of sports medicine - Silent period from soleus muscle as an index in a neuro-muscular function after reconstruction of anterior cruciate ligament

To clarify that silent period from soleus muscle may become an index expressed neuro-muscular function after reconstruction of anterior cruciate ligament (ACL), we studied the alteration of silent period from the soleus muscle in the patient with ACL reconstruction. Subjects of this study were three patients with anterior cruciate ligament (ACL) reconstruction, with two male athletes (case A and B) and one female sport instructor (case C). They have consented to be performed an electrophysiological study and to report their

	Gastrocnemius	Soleus
Position 1	160.5±27.3	165.9±26.7
2	135.5±28.9	144.0±28.3
3	129.3±18.9	143.8±18.8
4	146.5±21.3	157.8±17.8
5	130.1±20.4	135.6±20.9
6	157.0±22.2	164.9±19.5
7	136.7±21.8	148.5±24.5
8	121.3±15.9	129.7±14.3
9	147.1±25.1	157.7±21.7
10	137.1±23.3	147.1±23.9

(Average±SD ms)

Table 5. The duration of silent period on each standing.

own data in this study. Case A was a college soccer player for competition level. In rehabilitation process, he remarkably brought his nonl0Perative side lower extremity into the practice of running and cutting. Case B was a high school basketball player for competition level. Much instruction was need to alter his incorrect motion image related to sports activity on time, when his activity was growing in his rehabilitation process. Both case A and B was performed the left side ACL reconstruction immediately after the injury, and they reached to competition level in 6 months after operation. Case C was a sports instructor, and ACL reconstruction was provided to bilateral knee followed a conservative therapy for a few years after ACL tear. Rehabilitation after the operation was focused to acquired ability of her daily life, and she had no trouble when she returned to her occupation.

Rehabilitation protocol after ACL reconstruction was following (Figure 10). Hard type knee brace have been used for two weeks. Four weeks after, full weight bearing was permitted. Following the permission of full weight bearing, such various activities were trained as ambulation, jogging, running, cutting, splinting, jumping, and landing and so on with an adequate graded acquisition of sports activities. For the time of acquisition of sports activities, adequate grading was very important and was emphasized from the point of a dynamic energy and/or an Injury mechanism. Concretely, we have set the rehabilitation protocol as follows; stepping exercise for all direction and slow and fast stamping without sway for up and/or down and left or right were introduced at post eight weeks. From three to four months later, jogging and running without neither starting dash nor sudden stop, and side step cutting were started. At five months, exercises for jumping and landing were introduced. Post six months, which was final stage, following activities were acquired; a pursuit, a flight, a hopping and a contact under a therapist's control.

Clinical Application of Silent Period for the Evaluation of Neuro-Muscular Function in the Field of
the Sports Medicine and Rehabilitation

197

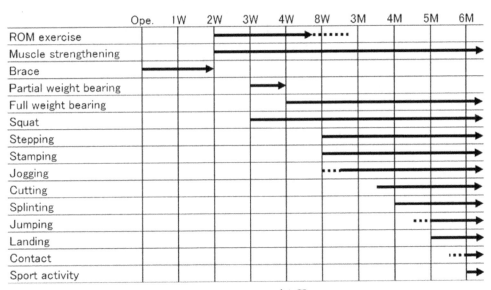

Fig. 10. Rehabilitation protocol after reconstruction of ACL.

Silent period from soleus muscle were recorded at every month after ACL reconstruction
from post one month after operation (see Table 6). Silent period from soleus muscle were
evoked by single stimulation to tibial nerve at the popliteal fossa on prone position with a
tonic slight voluntary contraction of ankle plantar flexion. The stimulating conditions for
recording the silent period were as follows; Intensity of supra-maximum, duration of 0.2 ms,
frequency of 0.5 Hz and numbers of 16 times. As to the recording conditions of silent period,
recording electrodes were placed on soleus muscle (leg medial and 4 or 5cm upper from
ankle joint) and reference electrode was put on the ipsilateral attachment of Achilles tendon
(calcaneus). Sweep time on recording was 200 ms. The raw data were amplified with a band
pass between 20 Hz and 2000 Hz by a Nicolet Viking quest. And we determined a
coefficient of variation of the duration of silent period in each recording.

	Post-surgery					
	1 m	2 m	3 m	4 m	5 m	6 m
Case A		Record	Record	Record	Record	
Case B	Record	Record	Record	Record	Record	Record
Case C	Record		Record	Record		Record

Table 6. Recording sessions of silent period in Case A, B and C.
Silent period was recorded for each subject at monthly intervals after ACL reconstruction as
frequently as possible from one to six months post-surgery.
All subjects were able to return to sporting competition or her occupation at six months after
their operations. (m: months)

Acquired raw waveforms, and the duration and the coefficient of variation of silent period in every subject were demonstrated in Figure 11-16. With case A, silent period of non-operative side shortened and a coefficient of variation of silent period increased in time of 2 months and 4months after the ACL reconstruction. In case B, bilateral silent period had no tendency in the mean value, however as for a coefficient of variation of silent period, it was little on non-operative side and it was large on operative side. Also, on operative side from one month to four months after ACL reconstruction, the fluctuation of silent period became large, and after four months it became the same as one of non-operative side. Furthermore, from one month after the operation, the long latency reflex (LLR) appeared in silent period

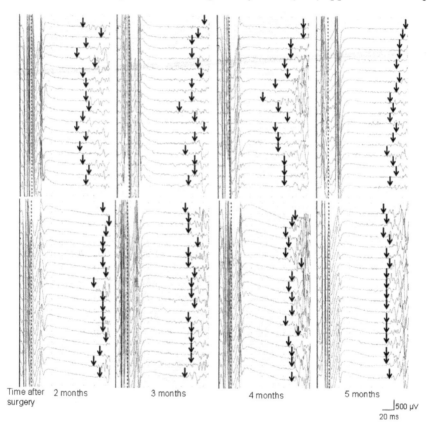

Time after   2 months   3 months   4 months   5 months
surgery   ⏜500 µV
                                                                              20 ms

Fig. 11. Typical waveform of silent periods in Case A (Upper: non-operative side, Lower: operative side).
In non-operative side, a shortening of the duration and an increase in the coefficient of variation of the silent period were observed at 2 and 4 months post-surgery, when his overuse of the non-operative lower extremity was detected during sporting activity.
In operative side, no remarkable finding was observed and it was clarified that his neural functions related to soleus on the operative side did not change during the course of rehabilitation (Arrows show re-bursting points of voluntary muscle activation. The silent period was identified by the duration after the arrow).

Clinical Application of Silent Period for the Evaluation of Neuro-Muscular Function in the Field of
the Sports Medicine and Rehabilitation

199

recording, and it became most remarkable in four months and disappeared in six months after ACL reconstruction. With case C, remarkable and characteristic finding was not obtained in both duration and coefficient of variation of silent period.

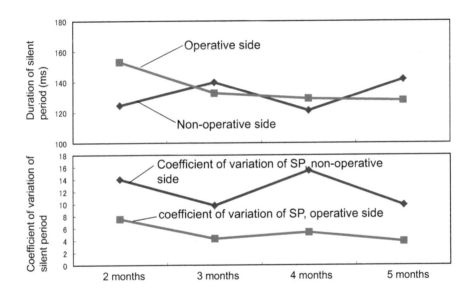

Fig. 12. The duration and coefficient of variation of silent period in Case A.
Coefficient of variation of the silent period increased at two and four months after ACL reconstruction.

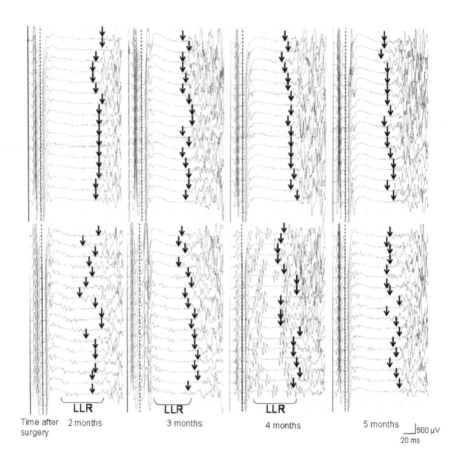

Time after   2 months   3 months   4 months   5 months   ‾‾|500 µV
surgery   20 ms

Fig. 13. Typical waveform of silent periods in Case B (Upper: non-operative side, Lower: operative side).
In non-operative side, no remarkable finding of the silent period was not observed.
In operative side, the appearance of LLR was the most clearest at 4 months post-surgery. After 4 months was the period when the patient had to re-acquire various activities at a higher rate and involved rapid step cutting in various directions. Large silent period variations indicated that this activated various neural functions (i.e., polysynaptic reflex on spinal and/or supra-spinal nervous system).
Arrows show re-bursting points of voluntary muscle activation. The silent period was identified by the duration after the arrow.

Clinical Application of Silent Period for the Evaluation of Neuro-Muscular Function in the Field of
the Sports Medicine and Rehabilitation

201

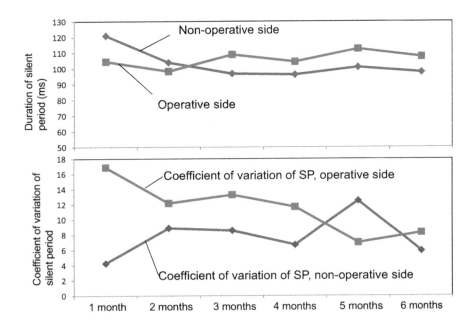

Fig. 14. The duration and coefficient of variation of silent period in Case B.
The large variation in the silent period from one to five months after operation needed to
activate various neural functions (i.e., polysynaptic reflex on spinal and/or supra-spinal
nervous system) for ankle plantar flexion in the prone position.

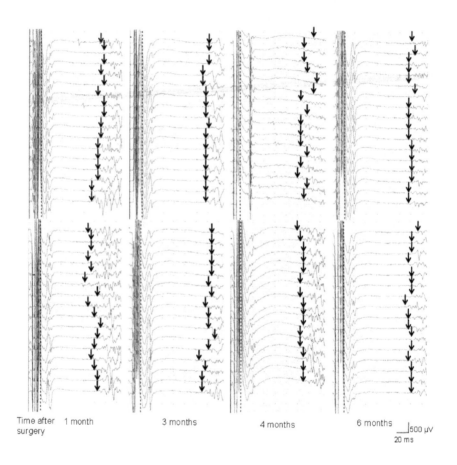

Time after   1 month   3 months   4 months   6 months   ⌐500 μV
surgery   20 ms

Fig. 15. Typical waveform of silent periods in Case C (bilateral reconstruction, Upper: right side, Lower: left side).
No remarkable findings of the silent period were observed on the non-operative side (Arrows show re-bursting points of voluntary muscle activation. The silent period was identified by the duration after the arrow.)

Clinical Application of Silent Period for the Evaluation of Neuro-Muscular Function in the Field of
the Sports Medicine and Rehabilitation

203

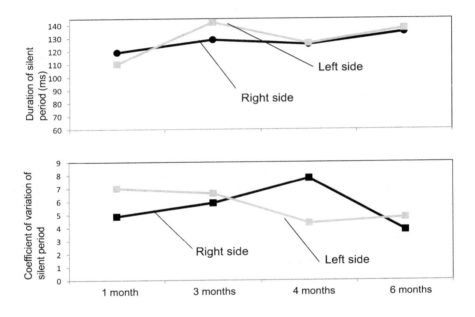

Fig. 16. The duration and coefficient of variation of the silent period in Case C.
There was no typical finding.

From a result of this experiment, non-operative side silent period in case A presented a shortening of the duration and an increase of coefficient of variation of silent period when we could see his overusing activity of non-operative lower extremity in the sports activity. From the results of the shortening of the duration of silent period in case A, following speculation about neuro-muscular function of case A was acquired. When his overusing activity of non-operative side was observed, the excitability of spinal neural function has increased and supra-spinal neural function also has affected by his overuse. In operative side of case B, the appearance of LLR and the increase of coefficient of variation of silent period in simultaneous period were observed when much guidance was required in order to correct motion image in operative side. The appearance of LLR in operative side was most remarkably four months after the operation. As for the rehabilitation for the patient with ACL reconstruction, from operation to four months later, various activities has to be acquired; i.e., from no to full weight-bearing ambulation, squatting, jogging, and cutting. Therefore, they have to acquire the various activities rapidly within four months after the operation. With case B, his large silent period variation within four months after the operation indicated that it needed to activate various neural functions (i.e., polysynaptic reflex on spinal and/or supra-spinal nervous system) for ankle plantar flexion on prone position, which is easy and simple task. In case C, remarkable problem related to acquire the activity of daily life and to return her occupation did not appear, and she did not have any clinical findings in silent period. As for this, it was thought that neurological function related to silent period from soleus muscle did not affect with ACL reconstruction due to a long term conservative therapy and a sequential reconstruction in both side. Like above, it has been verified that silent period from soleus muscle has the possibility of reflecting the neural function according to recovery situation after the ACL reconstruction from three cases findings. Concretely, it has been cleared that silent period can become an index expressed neuro-muscular function during a process of acquisition the various activity, the motor learning and the adaptation after ACL reconstruction with a recovery state from injury and operation.

4. Conclusion

4.1 Clinical findings from healthy subject
From the examination in the healthy person, following findings were existed;
1. The duration of silent period was changed by strength of tonic muscle contraction.
2. The duration of silent period was also altered by intensity of muscle contraction of remote parts.
3. The duration of silent period was affected with amount of load of weight to extremity including recording muscle.
4. The duration of silent period was also affected with amount of load of weight to remote part.

4.2 Clinical application of silent period in the field of sports medicine
About the clinical application of silent period for the evaluation of neuro-muscular function in the field of the sports medicine and rehabilitation, we mention like below based on the experiment aimed at healthy subjects and its application to the patient with ACL reconstruction.

Clinical Application of Silent Period for the Evaluation of Neuro-Muscular Function in the Field of
the Sports Medicine and Rehabilitation

205

The silent period from soleus muscle has become an index expressed neuro-muscular function of lower extremity and supra-spinal function in the patient after reconstruction of ACL. From the examination in cases after the reconstruction of ACL, following findings were existed;

1. The duration and aspects of silent period have become the proof of observation view of case's sports activity and were able to become the index of the neuro-muscular function in the recovery phase after ACL reconstruction.

2. Silent period can apply to the evaluation of CNS function in the field of sports science, because the fluctuation of silent period was useful to search the adequate condition of readiness of sports activity and was able to clear the clinical and observational impression about athletes' sports activity.

5. References

Anastasijevic R & Vuco J (1980): Renshaw cell discharge at the beginning of muscular contraction and its relation to the silent period. *Experimental Neurology*, Vol.69, No.3, (Sep 1980), pp.589-598, ISSN 0014-4886.

Behm DG & St-Pierre DM (1997): Effects of fatigue duration and muscle type on voluntary and evoked contractive properties. *Journal of Applied Physiology*, Vol. 82, No.5, (May 1997), pp.1654-1661, ISSN 8750-7587.

Calancie B.; Nordin M, Wallin U & Hagbarth KE (1987): Motor-unit responses in human wrist flexor and extensor muscles to transcranial cortical stimuli. *Journal of Neurophysiology*, Vol.58, No.5, (Nov 1987), pp.1168-1185, ISSN 0022-3077.

Cupido CM.; Hicks AL & Martin J (1992): Neuromuscular fatigue during repetitive stimulation in elderly and young adults. *European Journal of Applied Physiology and Occupational Physiology* Vol.65, No.6, (1992), pp.567-572, ISSN 0301-5548.

Daikuya S.; Tanino Y, Nishimori T, Takasaki K & Suzuki T (2003): The silent period from soleus and gastrocnemius muscles in relation to conditions of standing. *Electromyography and Clinical Neurophysiology*, Vol.43, No.4, (June 2003), pp.217-222, ISSN 0301-150X

Fuglevand AJ.; Zackowski KM, Huey KA & Enoka RM (1993): Impairment of neuromuscular propagation during human fatiguing contraction at submaximal force. *Journal of Physiology*, Vol.460, (Jan 1993), pp.549-572, ISSN 0022-3751.

Higgins DC & Lieberman JS (1968): The muscle silent period and spindle function in man. *Electroencephalography and Clinical Neurophysiology*, Vol.25, No.3, (Sep 1968), pp.238-243, ISSN 1388-2457.

Ikai M (1955): Inhibition as an accompaniment of rapid voluntary act (Summary in English). *Nippon Seirigaku Zasshi (Journal of the Physiological Society of Japan)*, Vol. 17, (1955), pp.292-298, ISSN 0031-9341.

Kimura J (2001): *Electrodiagnosis in diseases of nerve and muscle: principles and practice. Ed 3.*, Oxford university press, ISBN 0-19-512977-6, NY, USA.

Kuroiwa Y (1986): Long-loop reflex. *Rinsho Nouha (Clinical electroencephalography)*, Vol.28, (1986), pp.353-362, ISSN 0485-1447. (Abstract in English)

Roby-Brami A & Bussel B (1987): Long-latency spinal reflex in man after flexor reflex afferent stimulation. *Brain*, Vol.110, No.Pt3, (Jun 1987), pp.707-725, ISSN 0006-8950.

Suzuki T.; Fujiwara T & Takeda I (1993): Excitability of the spinal motor neuron pool and F-waves during isometric ipsilateral and contralateral contraction. *Physiotherapy Theory and Practice*, Vol.9, (1993), pp.19-24, ISSN 0959-3985.

Upton AR.; McComas AJ & Sica RE (1971): Potentiation of 'late' responses evoked in muscles during effort. *Journal of Neurology, Neurosurgery & Psychiatry*, Vol.34, No.6, (Dec 1971), pp.699-711, ISSN 0022-3050.

Yabe K (1976): Premotion silent period in rapid voluntary movement. *Journal of Applied Physiology*, Vol.41, No.4, (Oct 1976), pp.470-473, ISSN 8750-7587.

Part 3

Diagnostics

11

Non-Invasive Diagnosis of Neuromuscular Disorders by High-Spatial-Resolution-EMG

Catherine Disselhorst-Klug
Department of Rehabilitation & Prevention Engineering
Institute of Applied Medical Engineering, RWTH Aachen University
Germany

1. Introduction

Neuromuscular diseases are defined as pathological changes of the peripheral nerves (neuronal disorders), the neuromuscular junctions or the muscle fibres (muscular disorders). Since they are accompanied by weakness commonly, they have essential impact on the patient's movement performance. Especially in childhood, the consequences are serious and early diagnosis is essential for an adapted and task orientated therapy. The main aim in diagnostics of neuromuscular diagnosis is to distinguish between patients without any morbid changes in the MUs, patients with muscular disorders, and patients with neuronal disorders. Here, diagnostics avail on the fact that changes in the skeletal muscles, which take place during the progress of the disorder, are mostly on the level of single motor units (MUs). The MU is the smallest unit of the muscle, which can be activated independently by the central nervous system [Basmajian 1985]. Muscular disorders, for example, are characterised by a loss of single muscle fibres. This results in the fact that less muscle fibres contribute to an affected MU than to a healthy one. This is in contrast to neuronal disorders in which the motor neuron is destroyed. Consequently, complete MUs are affected. In this case the number of muscle fibres contributing to a MU is unchanged but the number of MUs available for force generation is reduced [Jerusalem 1979, Dubowitz 1991].

In human movement and locomotion the voluntary and active contraction of a muscle is initiated by the electrophysiological excitation of a pool of MUs. Since Electromyography (EMG) detects the electrophysiological signal generated by the muscle during excitation, it is a well established procedure utilised in studies of muscle function [Basmajian 1985]. During the last years surface electromyography (sEMG) has become more and more important. It offers a number of advantages when compared to invasive EMG procedures, like needle- or wire-EMG. For example, it causes no discomfort or risk of infection due to the insertion of the needle or the wire and it does not require the supervision by a physician. Compared to invasive measurements, the repeatability of surface EMG measurements is superior, and long term monitoring is possible, [Jonsson 1968]. In addition, the conventional needle-EMG is not suitable for investigations of the excitation spread. Compared to the needle EMG the wire EMG is less painful and allows the detection of the excitation spread. But after insertion the wire electrode tends to migrate within the muscle tissue even during isometric contraction [Jonsson 1968, Komi 1970]. Consequently, the reproducibility of the EMG signal detected with wire electrodes is limited.

The conventional sEMG has a limited spatial resolution and detects, therefore, a superposition of a large number of MUs. The separation of the activity of single MUs from simultaneously active adjacent ones is hard to achieve with surface electrodes. This task still needs highly specialised acquisition techniques, [Merletti 1989]. Consequently, sEMG is mainly used to obtain 'global' information about the muscle activation, like timing or intensity of the muscle activation. Therefore, for diagnostic purpose of neuromuscular disorders, the conventional sEMG techniques are not suitable, since information about the single MUs is needed to distinguish between patients without any morbid changes in the MUs, patients with muscular disorders, and patients with neuronal disorders. This is why in clinical practice still invasive Needle-EMG techniques are used, which gain the needed information about the single MU activity. The diagnostic selectivity of the commonly used Needle-EMG-procedures has been determined by comparing the Needle-EMG diagnosis and the result of a muscle biopsy [Hausmanova 1971, Black 1974, Buchtal 1982]. The most significant work is that of Buchtal and Kamieniekwa, which establishes a diagnostic selectivity of the Needle-EMG procedure of 77% in muscular disorders and 91% in neuronal disorders. However, in addition to the non-convincing diagnostic selectivity, the Needle-EMG methods are invasive and, consequently, painful for the patient.

2. High-spatial-resolution-EMG

In contrast to the conventional surface EMG techniques, the High-Spatial-Resolution EMG (HSR-EMG) allows the non-invasive detection of the single MU activity even during maximal voluntary contraction of the muscle. The methodology is based on the use of a multi-electrode array in combination with a spatial filter processing [Disselhorst-Klug 1998, Disselhorst-Klug 2000].

During a voluntary excitation of the muscle by the central nervous system, a time variable potential distribution is generated on the skin surface. Multi-electrode arrays can be beneficially used for the detection of the spatial potential distribution generated. From this information about the localisation of the source and its movement in time can be gained. Multi-electrode arrays are commonly used in electroencephalography and are recently becoming more popular in sEMG. In sEMG they have been described first by Rau [Rau1985], Masuda et al. [Masuda1985], De Luca et al. [de Luca 1987] and Reucher et al. [Reucher1987] and have been advantageously used in the fields of neurology, ergonomics, and biomechanics during the last years [Disselhorst-Klug 2000, Rau 2004]. Commonly used multi-electrode arrays consist of several (up to 240) pin-electrodes arranged either in a row or two-dimensionally with an inter-electrode distance of only a few millimetre. A multi-electrode array consisting of 16 gold-covered pin-electrodes (Figure 1) for example is used for the diagnostics of neuromuscular disorders. In this case the electrodes have a diameter of 0.5 mm and are springing-fitted to provide optimal contact with the skin surface. They are arranged two-dimensionally and have an inter-electrode distance between 2.5 mm and 5 mm depending on the muscle being investigated [Disselhorst-Klug 2000].

The potentials detected by the different electrodes of the array can be regarded as instantaneous spatial samples of the potential distribution generated on the skin surface by the excitation of the muscle fibres. To this potential distribution contribute different MUs in a different way. A small number of MUs, which are located very close to the skin surface, contribute to the resulting potential distribution with a spatially steep and high potential. On the contrary, MUs which are located more far away from the skin surface contribute

HSR-EMG

• 2dim Laplace Filter

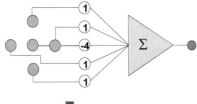

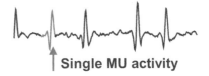

Single MU activity

• Multi-Elektroden Array

- • 2D- Array
- • 16 Electrodes
- • Inter-electrode distance 2.5 –5 mm
- • Electrode diameeter0.5 mm

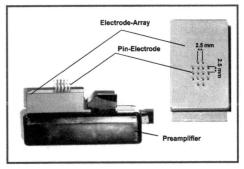

Fig. 1. HSR-EMG.
Multi-electrode array for the detection of the single motor unit activity during maximum voluntary contractions of the m. abductor pollicis brevis. By using an NDD-filter the single MU activity can be isolated in the signal. Adapted from [Disselhorst-Klug 2000].

lower and spatially more widened potential (Figure 2) [Disselhorst-Klug 1998]. This is due to the fact that caused by the electrical characteristic of the tissue between the source and the skin surface spatially high frequencies in the signal are more suppressed the deeper the source is located in the body [Lynn 1978]. Figure 2 shows an example of the potential distribution generated on the skin surface by two MUs located in different depth. If both MUs are excited at the same time. The potential distribution generated on the skin surface is equal to the superposition of the contributions of both MUs. Conventional sEMG applications are based on a bipolar lead with an inter-electrode distance of about 20 mm [Hermens 2000]. Due to this relatively large inter-electrode distance such an electrode arrangement detects the absolute value of the superimposed potential distribution, to which both MUs contribute in the same manner (Figure 2).

The volume conductor between the excited MU and the skin surface acts like a spatial low-pass filter. On the other hand, a spatial high-pass filter with an adequate cut-off frequency would transmit spatial frequencies higher than its cut-off frequency and would suppress spatially lower ones. Thus, by using a spatial high-pass filter the spatially high frequency contribution of MUs located close to the skin surface will be amplified and the contribution of MUs located more distantly will be reduced.

In a first approach, the simplest spatial high-pass filter - a bipolar lead with an inter-electrode distance in the mm-range and arranged in parallel to the muscle fibres - was used to improve the spatial selectivity of the non-invasive EMG-recording techniques (Figure 2) [Lynn 1978]. The bipolar lead differentiates the spatial potential distribution in the direction of the electrode arrangement. Due to this differentiation the bipolar lead enhances spatially steep components and reduces more flat ones (Figure 2). However, particularly at high force levels the bipolar lead with a small inter-electrode distance is not sufficient to discriminate the single MU activity in the signal course. Therefore, the principle of spatial filtering has been extended to more complex electrode arrangements.

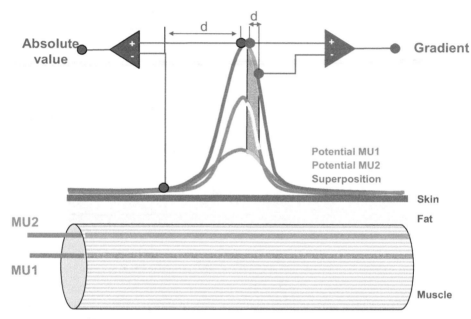

Fig. 2. Potential Distribution.
Potential distribution generated on the skin surface by two MUs located in differed distances from the skin surface. By using electrode distances d in the mm-range the contribution of the MU located close to the skin surface can be emphasised and the contribution of the more distantly located MU can be suppressed. Adapted from [Disselhorst-Klug 2000].

From image-processing it is known, that Laplace filters - which give the second spatial derivative - are well suited for the detection of edges perpendicular to the direction of differentiation. A one-dimensional Laplace filter can be realised with three electrodes arranged in a row. The central electrode has to be weighted with a factor of –2 and the two outer electrodes with a factor of 1. Such double differentiating filters have been first used in sEMG by Broman et al., [Broman 1985], and are now frequently used by different other groups. A higher spatial selectivity of the recording set-up can be achieved with two-dimensional Laplace filter arrangements [Reucher 1987, Disselhorst-Klug 1998]. It has been shown that a weighted summation of five cross-wisely arranged EMG leads forms the second spatial derivative of the potential distribution in two orthogonal directions (**Normal-Double-Differentiating-Filter**). To perform a NDD-Filter the central electrode is weighted with a factor of –4 and the surrounding electrodes with a factor of +1. The NDD-Filter amplifies only the activity of MUs located directly below the centre electrode of the filter and reduces the signals of more distantly located sources. In this way, the activity of single MUs becomes clearly distinguishable in the signal course (Figure 1). Thus, the HSR-EMG allows the non-invasive detection of the single MU activity and seems, consequently, to be suitable for a non-invasive diagnosis of neuromuscular disorders [Disselhorst-Klug 1994, Farina 2003].

In initial clinical investigations the HSR-EMG has been validated in children suffering from Duchenne Muscle Dystrophy (Duchenne) or Spinal Muscle Atrophy (SMA) [Ramaekers 1993, Huppertz 1995, Rau 1997, Disselhorst-Klug 2000]. The investigations show that the HSR-EMG allows the detection of changes in the electrical activity of the muscle which are typical for each disorder and which might allow a reliable distinction between healthy volunteers and patients with neuromuscular disorders as well as between patients with muscular disorders and patients with neuronal disorders (Figure 3). In contrast to the HSR-EMG of healthy volunteers, the HSR-EMG pattern of patients with neuronal disorders shows high and isolated peaks within the signal course. However, the HSR-EMG pattern of patients with muscular disorders is characterised by low and wide MU action potentials, which are hard to distinguish within the signal course.

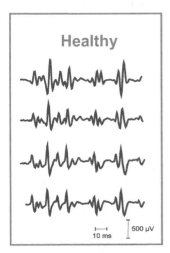 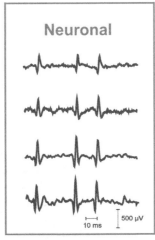 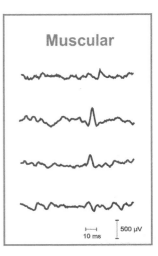

Fig. 3. Pathodological Changes.
Typical pathological changes in the HSR-EMG signal. Represented are four spatially filtered channels.

3. Quantitative evaluation of pathological changes in the HSR-EMG

Due to the first clinical experience with the HSR-EMG the question arises, whether the methodology allows a reliable distinction between healthy volunteers and patients with neuromuscular disorders as well as between patients with muscular disorders and patients with neuronal disorders. For that purpose a set of parameters has to be introduced, which allow a quantitative evaluation of the changes in the HSR-EMG pattern typical for each disorder. This can be understood as a classical feature extraction process. By an adapted classification procedure, which is based on extracted features, each patient can be assigned to one of the three disorder groups. In this way, the diagnostic selectivity of the non-invasive HSR-EMG can be determined.

Altogether seven parameters have been used for the validation of the typical differences in the HSR-EMG pattern of healthy volunteers, patients with muscular disorders and patients with neuronal disorders. The parameters can be divided into three groups regarding the excitation spread, the entire signal course in time as well as the shape of isolated peaks within the signal [Huppertz 1997]. Most of the parameters are well established in the field of signal processing and data analysis.

3.1 Parameters characterising the HSR-EMG signal in time

This group of parameters describes the entire signal course in time. In this way, the interaction of all MU located within the recording area of the spatial filter is regarded. The parameters belonging to this group are the signal **entropy (H)**, the **first zero crossing of the auto-correlation function (ACF_{zero})**, the **Chi-value (χ)** as well as the number of **values exceeding the RMS (T_{RMS})**.

The signal **entropy (H)** is a parameter well known in the field of signal processing. It describes the relation between the amplitude values of each sample within one measurement. Thus the entropy quantifies the predictability of the next measured amplitude value and characterises, in this way, the stochastic variability of the signal.

$$H = 1 - \sum_{i=\min}^{\max} \frac{p(x_i) \cdot \ln p(x_i)}{\ln(2)}$$

x_i = measured value
$p(x_i)$ = occurrence probability of x_i
min = smallest measured value
max = largest measured value

Comparable to the signal entropy the **first zero crossing of the auto-correlation function (ACF_{zero})** quantifies the stochastic variability of the signal too. The auto-correlation function (ACF) describes how similar different signal parts are. In the case of non-deterministic signals, like the HSR-EMG signal, the first zero crossing takes at higher values place, if the signal becomes more equal to itself.

$$ACF_{zero} = \frac{1}{2T} \sum_{t=-T}^{T} s(t) \cdot s(t + \tau)$$

$s(t)$ = HSR-EMG signal
τ = time variable
T = smallest measuring duration
t = time

The **Chi-value (χ)** is based on the frequency distribution of the sample values. The frequency corresponds in this case to the probability that a sample with an amplitude within a given range is appears in the signal. The shape of the frequency distribution can be quantified by means of the χ^2-test which checks the probability that the frequency distribution is Gaussian. Here, as a quantifying parameter the Chi-value has been introduced. It corresponds not to the probability but to the absolute deviation to a Gaussian distribution.

$$\chi = \sum_{i=1}^{K} \frac{(X_i - N_i)^2}{N_i}$$

K = Number of different amplitude values
X_i = Frequency of a certain amplitude in the HSR-EMG signal
N_i = Frequency of a certain amplitude, when a Gaussian distribution is assumed
The parameter **values exceeding the RMS (T_{RMS})** has been defined as the number of samples with amplitude higher than the root mean square of the signal. To be independent from the recording time the parameter has been normalised to the total number of samples belonging to the signal.

$$T_{RMS} = \frac{1}{T}\sum_{i=1}^{n} t_i \quad \text{with} \quad \begin{array}{l} t = 1 \quad x_i > RMS \\ t = 0 \quad x_i < RMS \end{array}$$

n = number of samples
T = measuring duration
t = time

3.2 Parameters regarding the isolated peaks

The excitation of a single MU can be identified in the signal by isolated peaks. Therefore, to the second group belong parameters describing the shape of isolated peaks. A signal part has been identified as a peak, if the following criteria are satisfied:

- The maximum amplitude must be higher than three times the RMS of the signal.
- Between the peak maximum and the adjacent minima the signal has to be continuous increasing respectively decreasing.
- The signal part identified as a peak is limited by the first crossing of the baseline before the minimum left to the peak maximum and by the first zero crossing of the baseline after the minimum right to the peak maximum

In initial investigations it has been shown that two parameters are sufficient to characterise the changes in the HSR-EMG pattern [Huppertz 1997]. These parameters are the **slope of the peak (S)** and the **peak amplitude frequency distribution (PAFD)**.
The parameter **slope of the peak** has been defined as the amplitude difference between the left minimum of the peak and its maximum divided by the time delay between both points. The parameter has been calculated for each peak detected within the HSR-EMG signal. The median value of all slops has been used standing in for all peaks which occur in the signal.

$$S = median\left[\left|\frac{x_{min} - x_{max}}{t_{min} - t_{max}}\right|\right]_P$$

P = number of peaks

The **peak amplitude frequency distribution (PAFD)** counts the number of peaks which have maximum peak amplitude within in a given interval. Similar to the frequency distribution of sample values the peak amplitude frequency distribution corresponds to the probability that a peak with maximum amplitude in a given interval can be found in the HSR-EMG signal. The PAFD of patients with muscular disorders shows high values for low amplitude peaks and low values for high amplitude peaks. This is in contrast to patients with neuronal disorders in which a typical biphasic shape of the PAFD can be found [Ramaekers 1993]. As a parameter describing the shape of the peak frequency distribution, the centroid of area has been calculated. The centroid of area is defined as the amplitude interval which divides the peak frequency distribution in two areas of the same size.

$$\sum_{i=1}^{a-1} N_i \Delta a \ < \frac{\sum_{i=1}^{A} N_i \Delta a}{2} < \sum_{i=a}^{N} N_i \Delta a$$

N_i = Frequency of maximum peak amplitudes within the interval i
A = Number of intervals
Δa = interval width
a = PAFD = bound which satisfies the inequality

3.3 Parameters regarding the excitation spread
The most significant parameter describing the excitation spread along the muscle fibres is **the conduction velocity in single MU (MUCV)**. The MUCV can be determined from the delay between the maximum amplitude of one peak in two adjacent and parallel to the muscle fibres orientated channels and their spatial distance (Figure 4). Since the conduction velocity depends on the temperature of the muscle, all MUCV values have been normalised to a temperature of 33°C [Rau 1997]. It has been shown earlier by Ramaekers et al. that the conduction velocity in single MUs is decreased in muscular disorders but unchanged in neuronal disorders [Ramaekers 1993].

3.4 Classification process
The parameter set can be used as a basis for the classification of the patients in healthy volunteers, patients with muscular disorders, and patients with neuronal disorders. Therefore, a classification procedure has been introduced based on a Fuzzy-approach [Kamel 1991].
Since the parameters have different diagnostic selectivity, the classification procedure has to be adapted to this specific classification task. This has been done by introducing weighting factors between 0 and 50 for each parameter. The weighting factors regard the contribution of each parameter to the classification result. They have been optimised by classifying a training data set generated with an especially developed muscle model [Disselhorst-Klug 1998]. This was to separate the training data set from the data set used for validation. The training data set consists of different simulated HSR-EMG signals regarding muscle structures with no pathological changes, muscle structures where a loss of muscle fibres takes place (muscular disorders), and muscle structures where a loss of entire MUs takes place (neuronal disorders) [Disselhorst-Klug 1998].
Performing the Fuzzy classification process, in a first step, all parameter values have been normalized to mean zero and variance 1. Starting the classification process, three clusters have been defined using a hierarchical cluster process like the nearest neighbourhood

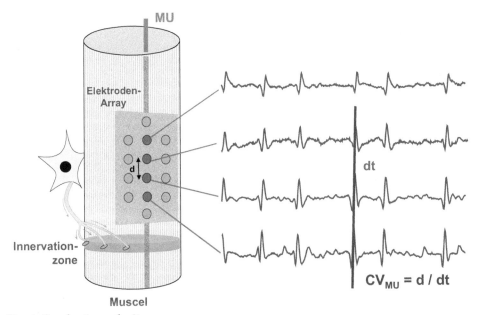

Fig. 4. Conduction velocity.
The conduction velocity of single motor units MUCV can be detected by several NDD-filtered channels arranged parallel to the muscle fibres.

algorithm. These three clusters represent the groups "neuronal disorder", "muscular disorder" and "healthy". The centroid of each cluster has been used to characterise its position in the feature space. After that, the Euclidian distances between the features of each HSR-EMG signal and the centroid of each cluster have been calculated. According to the Fuzzy classification process introduced by Kamel et al. [Kamel 1991], membership-values v_{ij} have been calculated:

$$v_{ij} = \frac{1}{\sum\limits_{k=1}^{z} \left(\dfrac{d_{ij}}{d_{ik}} \right)^{\frac{1}{m-1}}}$$

v_{ij} = membership-values
m = 2: controlling the degree of fuzzyfication
d_{ij} = Euclidian distance between the HSR-EMG$_i$ and the centroid of the cluster$_j$
d_{ik} = Euclidian distance between the HSR-EMG$_i$ and the centroid of the cluster$_k$
z = 3: Number of clusters
Afterwards a new centroid for each cluster Z_j has been has been determined following:

$$\vec{Z}_j = \frac{\sum\limits_{i=1}^{n} v_{ij} \vec{x}_i}{\sum\limits_{i=1}^{n} v_{ij}}$$

n = 7: Number of parameters

x_i = set of parameter values calculated from the HSR-EMG$_i$

Due to the weighting of the set of parameter values calculated from the HSR-EMG signals with the membership-values, this iteration converges. The iteration process has been stopped when the following abort criterion is fulfilled:

$$\sum_{j=1}^{z}\sum_{k=0}^{n}\left|Z_{jk}^{(s)} - Z_{jk}^{(s-1)}\right| < \varepsilon$$

s = Number of iteration

ε = 0.9: defined value

Next the membership-ship values have to be normalised with:

$$\overline{v}_{ij} = \frac{v_{ij}}{\sum_{k=1}^{z} v_{ik}}$$

And finally, each HSR-EMG signal has been assigned to the cluster with the highest membership-value.

The training data set, consisting of simulated HSR-EMG signals and representing the different types of disorders, has been classified with all possible combinations of weighting factors. The optimal combination of weighting factors was found when a maximum number of simulated HSR-EMG signals were classified correctly. The weighting factor combination as a result of the optimisation process is shown in Table 1.

Parameter	Weighting-factor
Signal entropy	2
First zero crossing of ACF	1
Values exceeding the RMS	19
Chi-value	19
Slope of the peak	2
Peak frequency distribution	9
MUCV	40

Table 1. Weighting of the parameter.

Optimised weighting factors for each parameter. The weighting-factors take the diagnostic selectivity of each parameter into consideration. [Disselhorst-Klug 1998]

The same classification algorithm can be used to classify HSR-EMG signals recorded in patients suffering from neuromuscular disorders. Here, in a first step the parameter values have to be multiplied by the related weighting-factor. Afterwards the classification procedure has to be executed as described above.

4. Clinical validation

The HSR-EMG has been recorded at isometric, maximum voluntary contraction of the m. abductor pollicis brevis. The used electrode array consists of 16 gold covered pin electrodes

(0.5 mm diameter) in a two-dimensional arrangement. Due to the low distance between the m. abductor pollicis brevis and the recording side, the inter-electrode distance has been chosen to 2.5 mm. Directly at the electrode array, each of the 16 EMG-leads has been amplified and, later, transmitted to a recording unit. It consists of a band-pass filter (1 – 500 Hz) and a second amplifier. All 16 EMG-leads have been stored on a PC with a sampling frequency of 4000 HZ each. The spatial filtering of the EMG-data has been performed on the PC by specially developed software. From each spatially filtered channel, all evaluation parameters have been calculated. The value of each parameter has been averaged over all NDD-filtered channels. After determination of the parameter values, the HSR-EMG signal of each patient has been assigned to one of the three groups by the described Fuzzy classification process.

For the quantitative evaluation of the typical HSR-EMG patterns altogether 97 subjects, healthy volunteers (41) and patients with neuromuscular disorders (56), aged between the infancy and 25 years, have been investigated. The group of patients investigated consists of 35 patients with Duchenne Muscle Dystrophy (muscular disorder) and 21 patients with Spinal Muscle Atrophy (neuronal disorder). The diagnosis of the patients has been proofed by muscle biopsy. The parameters have been calculated in three different HSR-EMG recordings of each child. Afterwards, the median value of each parameter has been used, accounting for the typical HSR-EMG pattern. Some of the parameters, such as the conduction velocity in single MUs depend significantly on the age of the investigated child [Huppertz 1997]. Those parameters have been normalised to an age of eight.

Diagnostic selectivity of the HSR-EMG: 97%			
	Duchenne	Healthy	SMA
classified as muscular disorder	35	0	0
classified as healthy	0	41	3
classified as neuronal disorder	0	0	18
sensitivity	100%	100%	90%
specificity	100%	95,1%	100%
positive prediction	100%	93,2%	100%

Table 2. Diagnostic selectivity of the non-invasive HSR-EMG in children with Duchenne muscle dystrophy and spinal muscle atrophy. Shown, are the numbers of patients which have been classified in each group. Adapted from [Disselhorst-Klug 2000]

The result of the classification which was based on the weighted evaluation parameters is summarised in Table 2. With the classification, 100% of all investigated healthy children, 100% of all investigated patients with muscular disorders, and 87% of all investigated patients with neuronal disorders have been correctly identified. That mean, that on the average, in 97% of all investigated children the diagnosis by means of the non-invasive HSR-EMG was correct.

5. Conclusions

The High-Spatial-Resolution EMG provides information about the single MU activity in a non-invasive way even during maximum voluntary contraction of the muscle. Therefore, the methodology could be suitable for a non-invasive diagnosis of neuromuscular disorders. Earlier investigations of healthy children and children with Duchenne Muscle Dystrophy or Spinal Muscle Atrophy have shown, that there is a typical change in the HSR-EMG signal course in each patient group. These typical changes in the HSR-EMG pattern can be evaluated by seven parameters regarding the signal course in time, the shape of isolated peaks, and the excitation spread in single MUs. Based on these evaluation parameters and an especially developed classification procedure, it is possible to classify correctly 97% of all investigated children. That means, in this patient group, the diagnostic selectivity of the HSR-EMG is in the same range or even better than the commonly used needle-EMG techniques. This result could be reached, though the HSR-EMG methodology is limited to superficial muscles and MUs. Therefore, the HSR-EMG promises to be a suitable tool for a non-invasive diagnosis of neuromuscular disorders in clinical application.

6. References

Basmajian J.V. and De Luca C.J. (1985) Muscle Alive; Their Functions Revealed by Electromyography, *William & Wilkins 5th edition*

Black J.T:, Bhatt G.P., Dejesus P.V., Scotland D.L., Rowland L.P., (1974) Diagnostic accuracy of clinical data, quantitative electromyography and histochemistry in neuromuscular disease. *J. Neurol Science*, 21, 59-70.

Broman H., Bilotto G., and De Luca C. (1985) A note on non-invasive estimation of muscle fibre conduction velocity. *IEEE Tras. Biomed. Eng.*, 32, 311-319

Buchtal F., Kamieniecka Z. (1982) The diagnostic yield of quantitative electromyography and quantitative muscle biopsy in neuromuscular disorders. *Muscle Nerve*, 5, 265 – 280.

De Luca C., and Merletti R. (1987) Surface myoelectric signal cross-talk among muscles of the leg. *Electroencephalography. and Clin. Neurophysiol.* 69, 568-575

Disselhorst-Klug C., Bahm J., Ramaekers V., Trachterna A., Rau G. (2000): Non-invasive approach of motor unit recording during muscle contractions in humans. *European Journal of Applied Physiology*, 83: 144 – 150.

Disselhorst-Klug C., Silny J., Rau G. (1997): Improvement of spatial resolution in surface EMG: A theoretical and experimental comparison of different spatial filters. *IEEE Trans. Biomed. Eng.*, 44,7,567-574.

Disselhorst-Klug C., Silny J., Rau G. (1998): Estimation of the Relationship between the non-invasively Detected Activity of Single Motor Units and their Characteristic Pathological Changes by Modelling. *J. of Electromyography and Kinesiology*, Vol. 8/5, 323 – 335.

Dubowitz V. (1991) Atlas der Muskelerkrankungen im Kindesalter. *Hippokrates Verlag.*

Farina D, Schulte E, Merletti R, Rau G, Disselhorst-Klug C. (2003): Single motor unit analysis from spatially filtered surface electromyogram signals. PartI: spatial selectivity. *Med Biol Eng Comput.*, 41(3):330-7. IF 0,744

Hausmanova-Petusewicz I., Jedrezejowska H. (1971) Correlation between electromyographic findings and muscle biopsy in cases of neuromuscular disease. *J. Neurol. Science*, 13, 85-106.

Hermens H., Freriks B., Disselhorst-Klug C., Rau G. (2000): Development of recommendations for sensors and sensor placement procedures. *Journal of Electromyography and Kinesiology*, Vol. 10, 5, 361 – 374.

Huppertz H.-J. Disselhorst-Klug C., Silny J., Rau G., Heimann G. (1997) Diagnostic yield of non-invasive High-Spatial-Resolution-EMG in Neuromuscular Disease. *Muscle and Nerve*, in press.

Jerusalem F. (1979) Muskelerkrankungen, Klinik – Therapie – Pathologie. *Thieme Verlag Stuttgart.*

Jonsson B., Bagge U.E. (1968) Displacement, deformation and fracture of wire electrodes for electromyography. *Electromyography. 8. 328 - 347.*

Kamel M.S. (1991) A threshold Fuzzy c.means algorithm for semi-fuzzy clustering. *Pattern Recognition, 27,9,*

Komi P.V., Buskirk E.R. (1970) Reproducibility of electromyographic measurements with inserted wire electrodes and surface electrodes. *Electromyography, 10, 357 - 367*

Lynn P.A., Bettkes N.D., Hugh A.D. and Johnson S,W. (1978) Influence of electrode geometry on bipolar recordings of the surface electromyogram. *Med. Biol. Eng. Comput., 16, 651-660.*

Masuda T., Miyano H., Sadoyama T. (1985) A surface electrode array for detecting action potential trains of single motor units. *Electroenceph. Clin. Neurophysiol. 60, 435-443.*

Merletti R. and De Luca C.J. (1989) New Techniques in surface electromyography. *In Desmedt J.E, (ed): Computer-Aided electromyography and expert systems., Elsevier, Amsterdam, 115-124.*

Papoulis A. (1965) Probability, random variables, and stochastic processes. *McGraw Hill, New York.*

Ramaekers V., Disselhorst-Klug C., Schneider J., Silny J., Forst J., Forst R., Kotlarek F., Rau G. (1993) Clinical Application of a non-invasive multi-electrode array EMG for the recording of single motor unit activity. *Neuropaediatrics, 24, 134-138.*

Rau G., Disselhorst-Klug C. (1997): Principles of high spatial resolution EMG (HSR-EMG): Single motor unit detection and the application in the diagnosis of neuromuscular disorders. *J. of Electromyography and Kinesiology*, Vol.7, No.4, 233-239.

Rau G., Disselhorst-Klug C., Silny J. (1997a) Non-invasive approach to motor unit characterization: muscle structure, membrane dynamics and neuronal control. *J. of Biomechanics*, Vol. 30, No. 5, 441 – 446.

Rau G., Reucher H. (1985) Muscular activity and surface EMG. In Perren S.M. and Schneider E. (ed.): Biomechanics: Current Interdisciplinary research, 27 - 35.

Rau G., Schulte E., Disselhorst-Klug C. (2004): From cell to movement: To what answers does EMG really contribute? *J. of Electromyography and Kinesiology*, 14, 611–617.

Reucher H., Rau G. and Silny J. (1987a) Spatial filtering of non-invasive multi-electrode EMG: Part I – Introduction to Measuring Technique and Applications. *IEEE trans. Bio-Med. Eng.*, BME-34,2, 98-105.

Reucher H., Silny J. and Rau G. (1987b) Spatial filtering of non-invasive multi-electrode EMG: Part II - Filter performance in theory and modelling. *IEEE Trans. Bio-Med. Eng.*, BME-34,2, 106-113.

12

EMG vs. Thermography in
Severe Carpal Tunnel Syndrome

Breda Jesenšek Papež and Miroslav Palfy
University Clinical Centre Maribor,
Slovenia

1. Introduction

Carpal tunnel syndrome (CTS) is one of the most common compressive neuropathies in the upper extremities (Bland, 2007) and a frequent cause of pain, paresthesias and impaired hand function. A syndrome is, by definition, a collection of signs and symptoms. Its clinical symptoms depend on duration and degree of the compression of the median nerve (MN). At first the sensory nerve fibres are affected, but as the compression persists, large calibre myelinated nerve fibres (sensory and motor) undergo damage as well. Clinical symptoms and signs alone are not sufficient to confirm the diagnosis and surgical release, electrodiagnostic methods are needed for this purpose (Rosenbaum & Ochoa, 2002).

Within the last decades, CTS reached epidemic proportions in many occupations and industries. It represents a large expense because of absence from work and wage compensation due to temporary incapacity for work. For this reason numerous researches, not only in the field of medicine, are looking for a non-invasive diagnostic method for determining those loads in workplaces that facilitate the development of CTS (Ammer, 1999, 2003; R.T. Herrick & S.K. Herrick, 1987; Schartelmüller & Ammer, 1996; Tchou et al., 1992).

Intelligent systems have turned out to be useful and successful aids in medicine for determining, classifying, sample searching, data analysis, and new knowledge discovery (Haas & Burnham, 2008). But thermography, on the contrary, did not receive due attention (American Academy of Neurology, 1990) in the area of determining entrapment neuropathies, despite its advantages (completely safe, passive investigation, without contact, painless and can be easily repeated with low costs of use) (Hackett, 1976).

1.1 Thermography

Thermography is a procedure for remote determination of temperature of objects, based on the detection of infrared radiation that the observed objects emit. As the name itself implies, thermographic or infrared cameras detect electromagnetic radiation below the frequency of red light. The range of wave lengths of infrared radiation includes lengths ranging from 700 nm to 1 mm, while thermographic cameras operate within an even narrower spectre, ranging from approx. 900 nm and 14 µm. As all objects emit infrared radiation, thermographic camera can determine an object's temperature on the basis of object's energy flux density. In this manner it can create a thermal image of observed objects (Fig. 1), where warmer objects usually appear in a warmer and lighter colour (light red to white) and colder objects appear in a colder and darker colour (blue to black) (Gaussorgues, 1994).

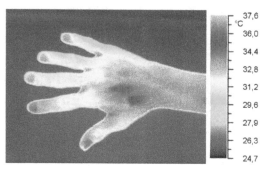

Fig. 1. Thermographic image of a patient's hand.

The possibility of detection of warmer objects on a colder background resulted in the development of thermography primarily for military and surveillance purposes, but with the decrease in prices of (initially very expensive) cameras, thermography established its position in numerous other areas too, such as industry, medicine, meteorology, and archaeology (Ring, 1995b).

Thermography, as we know it today, started to develop as late as the second half of the 20th century. Before this, remote temperature measurement was not possible, so surface measurements performed with various thermometers were used. The invention of the first thermometer is ascribed to the Venetian scientist Santorio Santorio, who improved Galileo's thermoscope in the beginning of the 17th century and equipped it with a scale, whereby enabling reading of ambient temperature. The precision of this thermometer was poor, because it was filled with air, and the effect of air pressure on the thermometer was not taken into account. The following improvement occurred in the mid 17th century – the use of alcohol in a closed bottle somewhat improved precision. The first mercury thermometer was made in 1714 by Gabriel Fahrenheit, who also takes credit for the first standardized temperature scale. He used the recently discovered freezing point and boiling point as reference values, and divided the intermediate interval to 180 degrees. He also added additional 32 degrees for values below the freezing point and set the lowest temperature 0, because this was the lowest temperature, which he achieved in his laboratory with a mixture of ice, water, and salt. In 1742, a Swedish scientist Anders Celsius developed his own scale by dividing the interval between the boiling point and the freezing point to 100 degrees. Interestingly enough, 0° was used to mark the boiling point, and 100° for the freezing point. The following year, Jean Pierre Cristin reversed the Celsius's scale and called it the hundred-degree scale. This name was in use until 1948, when it was renamed into the Celsius scale by international agreement. In 1848, a Scot William Thomson, later known as Lord Kelvin, proposed an absolute temperature scale with absolute zero at the lowest theoretical temperature the body can have -273.15°C. The standard unit for temperature is named after him – Kelvin (K).

At the end of the 16th century, a Neapolitan Giambattista della Porta was the first to notice the consequences of thermal radiation. In working on experiments with the concave glass he established that warmth or coldness can also reflect from glass, after placing candle flame and snowball in front of the glass. Almost two decades later, in 1790, a Swiss physicist, Pierre Prevost, introduced a theory, according to which all bodies, both warm and cold, thermally radiate, and that the quantity of radiation depends on body temperature. Only a few years later, a British astronomer of German descent, William Herschel, while diverting

EMG vs. Thermography in Severe Carpal Tunnel Syndrome

225

sunrays by means of prism discovered radiation beyond a still visible, red part of the light spectrum (Ring, 1987). With the thermometer he detected higher temperature beyond the red part of the spectrum and predicted that there is invisible light.

Herschel published his results in 1800, and named the invisible radiation "heat rays". The name infrared radiation was established as late as the second half of the 19th century. This was followed by the period of new developments in the area of thermodynamics. Firstly, in 1859, Gustav Kirchhoff introduced his law of thermal radiation, followed by Stefan (1879, by means of experiments) and Boltzmann (1884, with theoretical derivation) with the black body radiation law. In 1893, Wilhelm Wien introduced his relation between the wave length of the strongest radiation of black body and its temperature, which lead to Planck's black-body radiation law published in 1901. These laws represent physical background, which serves as the basis for the functioning of thermographic cameras.

One of the first steps in the development of the measurement of thermal radiation was the discovery of thermoelectric effect or the Seebeck's effect, named after his inventor, Thomas Johann Seebeck, Estonian physicist of German origin. In 1821 he discovered that voltage exists between two ends of metal rods, when these ends are at different temperatures. This resulted in the discovery of thermocouple. For measuring the created voltage he had to connect a metal rod to a conductor, which resulted in voltage opposite to the initial one. By using a different metal he was able to take advantage of the difference in both voltages, since it depends on the material used. He measured the created voltage and with it, indirectly, the temperature difference. Increase in temperature difference also increased the measured voltage, and this enabled him to calibrate the thermocouple and use it as a thermometer. Italian physicists Leopoldo Nobili and Macedonio Melloni increased the precision of temperature measurement by connecting several thermocouples. But in 1878, Samuel Pierpont Langley, an American astronomer, took a step further, as he invented a bolometer.

Langley used two platinum strips, covered with soot, as the ends of the Wheatstone bridge or the electrical resistance meter, equipped with a sensitive galvanometer and battery. One of the strips was exposed to infrared radiation, which caused the strip to warm up. This altered its resistance, which he was able to measure with his circuit. Thus he created the first temperature sensor, which exploits predictable variations of platinum resistance as the result of temperature variations. In the 20th century, the discovery of new combinations of materials lead to increasingly more precise and smaller bolometers, which in the mid 1980s resulted in the invention of the microbolometer – fields of temperature sensors made of silicon or vanadium oxide or amorphous silicon (Fig. 2). It was invented by the American corporation Honeywell for the US Department of Defense. After 1992 the technology became available to the wider public and is now used as the detection field in thermographic cameras of numerous producers (Cuthbertson, 1995).

Thermographic camera is an infrared camera, which generates a thermal image on the basis of measured values of infrared radiation of observed objects. Unlike a thermovision camera, which is used for watching in dark or under poor visibility conditions, a thermographic camera also determines actual values of surface temperatures of observed objects. The activity of thermographic camera can basically be compared to the activity of an ordinary digital videocamera, whereby the role of CCD sensors is assumed by the field of thermal IR sensors (microbolometers or semi-conductors with a narrow passage). By taking into account emissivity, distance, ambient temperature, and other factors, the camera calculates temperatures, which are detected by individual sensors, and generates thermal image on the basis of these temperatures. For the display of individual temperatures it uses a non-linear palette of so-called "non-primary colours", ranging from white for the highest temperature through red and yellow shades for higher temperatures to blue for lower, and black for the lowest temperatures (Fig. 1). The resolution of a thermal image rarely exceeds 320x240 pixels and is determined by the number of IR sensors (Fig. 2).

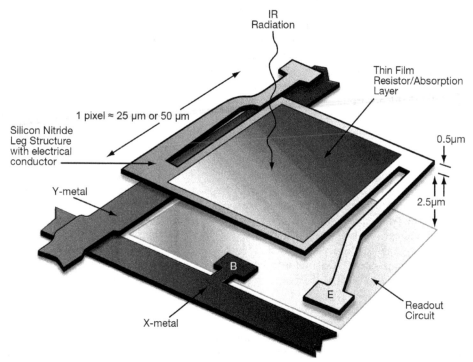

Fig. 2. The basis structure of a microbolometer (uncooled IR camera pixel).

Despite the initial development solely for military purposes, today thermographic cameras are used in different areas. Thermography is an excellent method of examination, also useful in the field of medicine for its safety (passive, no touch examination), lack of pain and invasiveness, easy reproducibility and low running costs (Hackett, 1976). Despite its advantages TG is not useful for routine diagnosis of CTS, since unmyelinated fibres remain intact until late in the severe nerve entrapment (American Academy of Neurology, 1990). Many patients with EMG diagnosed CTS have normal thermographic studies; however TG may show abnormalities in median nerve distribution in severe cases of CTS (Rosenbaum & Ochoa, 2002). To ensure reliability of TG pattern recognition we introduced a novel approach to thermal image analysis by using an artificial neural network (ANN).

1.2 Artificial neural networks

Data mining techniques provide a variety of different approaches for data analysis. ANNs are one of them (Larose, 2005). They are increasingly used in problem domains involving classification and are capable of finding shared features in a set of seemingly unrelated data.

An ANN is an abstract computational model of the human brain. Similar to the brain, an ANN is composed of artificial neurons and interconnections. When we view such a network as a graph, neurons can be represented as nodes and interconnections as edges (Fig. 3). There are many known variations of ANNs, differing in their topology, orientation of connections and approaches to learning (Kasabov, 1996). Probably the most established are "feed-forward backpropagation" neural networks (a.k.a. multilayer perceptrons). Due to its efficiency and relatively simple training process this type of ANN was chosen for our classification (diagnosis of CTS, based on collected data).

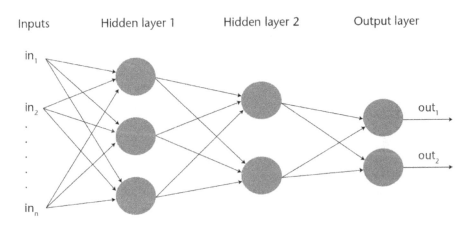

Fig. 3. Example of an ANN (multilayer perceptron).

A multilayer perceptron consists of layers of neurons, more specifically an input layer, an output layer and at least one hidden middle layer. Neurons on the same layer are not connected; all interconnections are directed from the input layer towards the output layer. The input layer is represented by normalized numerical values or inputs, passed on to the neurons on the 1st hidden layer. These neurons generate their own numerical outputs and pass them on to the next layer. This process continues until the last (output) layer and resembles the transmission of impulses inside the brain. Each connection in a network is weighted. The weights are internal parameters of an ANN and simulate the biological synaptic strengths in a natural neuron (McCulloch & Pitts, 1943).

An artificial neuron generates its output through an activation function (Fig. 4) which accepts as its input the sum of weighted outputs from neurons on the previous layer and an externally applied bias, denoted by b_k (1). The bias has the effect of increasing or lowering the net input of the activation function, depending on whether it is positive or negative. Weights and biases directly affect the importance of individual connections.

$$net_k = x_1 w_{k1} + x_2 w_{k2} + \cdots + x_m w_{km} + b_k \tag{1}$$

Different activation functions are commonly used. We chose the log-sigmoid function (2).

$$f(net_k) = \frac{1}{1+e^{-net}} \tag{2}$$

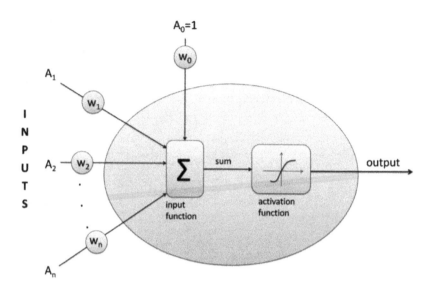

Fig. 4. Model of an artificial neuron.

The output of a multilayer perceptron consists of numerical values, generated by the last (output) layer. It is usually mapped into a binary value, identifying the class of the object, represented by its numerical descriptors at the input level. In order to successfully classify input objects an ANN must go through a thorough process of supervised learning. It consists of applying a large number of training examples to the inputs of an ANN and adjusting the parameters (weights) according to a highly popular algorithm known as the "error back-propagation algorithm".

First, numerical descriptors of an object from the training set are applied to the inputs of the ANN. The network classifies the object by calculating the output values. The output is compared to the desired (correct) result and an error value is calculated. If this error exceeds the defined threshold value, the sequence of corrective adjustments to the weights is started. Adjustments are done from the output towards the input layer as the error signal travels backwards. After the corrections are done, the network generates a smaller error when classifying the same object, thus improves itself through learning. A more detailed description of the error back-propagation algorithm is beyond the scope of this chapter and is well documented in literature (Rojas, 1996). More knowledgeable readers might find it interesting that weight adjustments were done under *generalized delta rule* which included a *momentum* constant, increasing the rate of learning while avoiding the danger of instability (Kantardzic, 2003).

In theory, if the training set is large and diverse enough, an ANN can accumulate enough knowledge to reliably classify unknown objects.

To test the reliability of an ANN the data to be classified is usually divided into two sets. The first set consists of cases used for the learning process through which an ANN adapts itself and the second set consists of cases, previously unknown to trained ANN. These cases are then classified and the results are compared to actual class values.

2. Background

There have been several studies published that have used thermography as a diagnostic tool for determining various entrapment neuropathies (Ammer, 1999, 2003; R.T. Herrick & S.K. Herrick, 1987; Schartelmüller & Ammer, 1996; Tchou et al., 1992). There is a generally accepted opinion that thermography is not appropriate for routine diagnostics of CTS and other entrapment neuropathies, as they predominantly affect thick myelinated fibres, while thermography (indirectly through the arrangement of temperature changes) enables only an assessment of the functional status of thin, mostly unmyelinated, nociceptor and sympathetic, vasomotor nerve fibres (Rosenbaum & Ochoa, 2002). However, since MN contains motor, sensory and sympathetic fibres, we can justifiably expect involvement of the autonomous nervous system and consequently thermoregulation of hand, when entrapment occurs. A quick, precise, dynamic, very sensitive, and non-invasive surface detection of temperature changes of the skin is within the domain of thermography (Jones & Plassmann, 2002).

3. Methods

Monitoring the dynamics of thermographic changes in CTS aided by artificial intelligence, represented the basic research challenge. We asked ourselves if the artificial intelligence system can identify the typical CTS pattern from the thermogram of a hand, and, if so, at what stage of entrapment. Much like in other entrapment neuropathies, the myelinated fibres are the ones that are primarily affected, but chronic or extremely severe acute entrapment also captures thin sympathetic (autonomous) nerve fibres (Benaroch, 2007). However, it is necessary to point out that the latter have the capacity of improving much faster (Marotte, 1974).

In 1976, for the purposes of thermographic diagnostics in the area of entrapment neuropathies, researchers developed the provocative cold stress test (Ring, 1995a). In this test the patient's hands wrapped in thin plastic gloves are submerged in cold water (in different researchers temperature varies from 1°C to no more than 20°C) for 1 minute. After a 10 to 15-minute adaptation to the room temperature the temperature changes of the hand are determined using an IR camera. Thermographic images are taken before and after the stress test, in specific time intervals. During this process the patient should not touch anything.

According to a theory, provocation excites sympathetic autonomous nerve fibres of the hand and induces vasoconstriction. Quantitative thermography (measurement of hand temperature after a specific time interval) is used for estimating the response of the autonomous nervous system. It is expressed as vasodilation or reactive hyperthermia, which consequently normalizes hand temperature. A healthy person develops reactive hyperthermia relatively early (within 10 minutes) and equally on all fingers. But in CTS, by using thermography, we discovered different temperature changes. Neurophysiologic basis of the procedure is the measurement of the response of the sympathetic nervous system. Autonomous nerve fibres, which innervate the skin, run together with sensory fibres of peripheral nerves and also have the same arrangement within an individual nerve (Kline & Hudson, 1990). The autonomous, vegetative, nervous system of the hand controls sweat secretion and vasomotorics. The latter is responsible for the control of skin circulation required for maintaining body temperature. In vasodilation body temperature is diverted from the body and, vice versa, in vasoconstriction the temperature is retained. The initial response of the body to the provocation cold stress test is vasoconstriction.

We believe that the provocation stress test is more useful for research purposes. In our previous clinical practice the method did not stand the test. We often tried with different water temperatures. We have used ice cold water, in line with the published standard and protocol for clinical thermography (International Academy of Clinical Thermology, 2002), as well as warmer water, up to 20°C, which is recommended by Ring (Ring, 1995a). The latter claims that in the case of cold water the regeneration period is (too) long, while the Guidelines advise against water that is warmer than ice cold, as otherwise sympaticus stimulation would not be sufficient. The basic deficiencies of the test we have come across in clinical use are: it is too time consuming, unpractical (requires putting on and taking off thin plastic gloves with as little contact as possible), "old-fashioned" (the majority of patients thought it was too banal holding hands in a vessel with usually cold water, and for this reason they were not very cooperative), and unpleasant (people with impaired autonomous nervous system experience holding hands in cold water as pain). Numerous volunteers have declared that they would rather undergo EMG investigation again than the provocation cold stress test. Clear and simple instructions not to touch the wall or bottom of the vessel have frequently been breached. Constant supervision was required for a very simple test. Obviously, other clinicians have also come across similar problems, because we found no literature sources on published clinical (just research) studies using the provocation stress test on a sufficiently large population, which would provide enough data for a reliable statistical analysis. For the reasons described above our attention has been directed to finding a method that would enable us to abandon the stress test.

In currently published studies, thermographic images were analysed by means of commercial computer programmes and manual definition of fields of interest (Ammer, 1999, 2003; R.T. Herrick & S.K. Herrick, 1987; Schartelmüller & Ammer, 1996; Medical Imaging Research Group, University of Glamorgan, 2004). The analysis of thermographic images is a demanding and time-consuming task, because the precision in determining the fields of interest of images is the decisive factor for a proper diagnosis. We often require measurements with a precision of 0.1°K.

For this purpose we have developed software tool, which provided us with an exact analysis of thermographic images and automated the CTS diagnosis procedure, while eliminating the need for the preliminary provocation cold stress test (Fig. 5).

We have used the well-known advantages of machine learning by using data mining (Kantardzic, 2002). We have developed a neural network, which is capable of diagnosing CTS on the basis of very discrete temperature differences that are invisible to the eye on a thermographic image.

Patients were selected from a pool of clinically suspect CTS patients referred by general practitioners and various specialists to our department. The exclusion criteria for participation was: previous operation for CTS, negative electrodiagnostic test for CTS, abnormal hand anatomy (amputations, injuries, other anomalies) preventing the acquisition of standard images of hands. Volunteers who did not exhibit symptoms of CTS and were subsequently diagnosed by electromyography as not having the syndrome were used to acquire images of healthy hands (dorsal and palmar views).

For our pilot study 112 images were examined: 23 patients (15 females, eight males; mean age 51.4 years, range 26-71 years) were used to acquire 60 images depicting 30 hands (dorsal and palmar views) at different stages of CTS; 13 volunteers (eight females, five males; mean age: 48.3 years, range 28-66 years) who did not exhibit symptoms of CTS and who were subsequently diagnosed by EMG as not suffering from the syndrome were used to acquire 52 images of healthy hands (dorsal and palmar views of 26 hands).

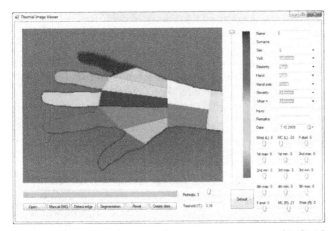

Fig. 5. Computer software for identification of mean temperatures of individual hand segments.

The results of a pilot study were very promising. In the majority of performed measurements classification exceeded the 77% effectiveness (Table 1).

The most important segments turned out to be fingers, especially the index finger and the little finger (which also coincides with the anatomic distal innervation area for the median or ulnar nerve (ulnaris). The results also coincided with a similar study carried out by Schartelmüller and Amer in relation to the thoracic syndrome pathology by means of manual analysis of thermograms (Schartelmüller & Ammer, 1996). Successful classification of our neural network was supported by the fact that whenever we excluded the majority of fields of interest of MN (thumb, index finger, and middle finger), the efficiency was not better, only accidental.

Included segments	Success rate (%)
All dorsal segments (reference case)	80.6
All segments	74.3
All palmar segments	65.6
All dorsal but thumb	81.8
All dorsal but index finger	77.3
All dorsal but middle finger	81.8
All dorsal but ring finger	79.2
All dorsal but little finger	75.2
All dorsal but index and little finger	70.8
All dorsal but thumb, index and middle finger	64.5
All dorsal without wrist segments	82.5
All dorsal without metacarpal segments	78.4

Table 1. Pilot study CTS classification success rates (each success rate percentage is the mean of five repeat runs on 22 randomly selected hands).

The findings of our pilot study spoke in favour of the applicability of the intelligent system for discerning CTS from thermovision images. In a smaller number of study and test cases (n = 112) the efficiency of classification exceeded our expectations. We were aware of the fact that a small set of elements can lead to misleadingly good (or bad) results. Therefore, for a realistic evaluation of efficiency of classification we have collected a significantly larger data base. In total we acquired 502 images of 251 hands (dorsal and palmar side of each hand). 71 patients (52 females and 19 males with mean age 56.8 years, range 23 – 90 years) contributed 274 images of 137 hands (in 5 patients only one hand met the inclusion criteria) and 57 volunteers (35 females, 22 males; mean age 47.6 years, range 25 – 74 years) contributed 228 images of 114 healthy hands.

3.1 Statistical analysis

All statistical analyses were performed using the R Project for Statistical Computing, a software language and environment for statistical computing, available as free software under the terms of GNU General Public License. Where appropriate, data are presented as mean ± SD or as percentages. Comparisons between patient and volunteer groups regarding segment temperatures were analysed by non-parametric Mann-Whitney-Wilcoxon test since it is used to compare two independent groups of sampled data and unlike the parametric t-test, makes no assumptions about the distribution of the data (e.g., normality). A p-value < 0.05 was considered to be statistically significant.

4. Study results

The prevailing opinion in literature states that for determining CTS by using thermography dorsal segments of the hand are more important than the palmar ones (R.T. Herrick & S.K. Herrick, 1987). Even more so, we have confirmed that palmar segments are not useful for detecting CTS by means of IR thermography (Fig. 6).

The finding was a surprise to us, because we have initially expected palmar changes, considering the distal innervation sample of MN. Our explanation is that obvious temperature differences on the dorsal or palmar side are the result of hand complexity. They originate both from anatomical and physiological and functional features of the hand. In anatomical terms, the skin on the hand is thinner and contains essentially more sweat glands (>450/cm²) than on the dorsal side (Tortora & Derrickson, 2008). In physiological terms, the emotional stress is initially reflected by palm sweating (next to feet and armpits). In the majority of basic hand functions (grasping, leaning, carrying) the palmar side of palms and fingers is burdened. Everything we have described above has an important influence on local temperature changes even in a healthy person, which is in our opinion a sufficient reason why the palmar side of hands is not the most appropriate for a credible analysis of thermograms in CTS cases.

One of our further objectives, after having expanded our data base, was the attempt of classifying CTS with thermography, while considering neurophysiological levels of MN entrapment. For this purpose we have developed a neural network, which is capable of classifying data into four classes (no entrapment, mild, moderate, severe). However, the results of this classification were even weaker. We have also tried using other methods of machine learning (Podgorelec et al., 2002), but they did not produce favourable results either, so we abandoned the idea. On the basis of statistical data processing (Table 2), which has shown significant difference among healthy patients and the severe level of CTS entrapment, we have decided to use only the latter for classification.

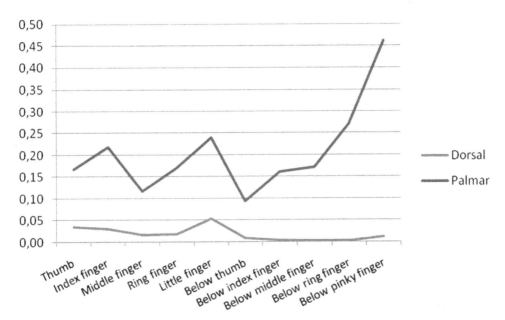

Fig. 6. Statistical significances of differences between segment temperatures in patients' and volunteers' hands (Mann-Whitney-Wilcoxon test, p=0.05), for dorsal and palmar side.

Segment	Mild-Normal	Moderate-Normal	Severe-Normal	All CTS-Normal
Whole hand	0,237400	0,285800	1,79E-006	0,007162
Thumb	0,244800	0,509300	5,07E-005	0,034990
Index finger	0,295100	0,449800	6,19E-005	0,029850
Middle finger	0,470900	0,397900	4,90E-005	0,017270
Ring finger	0,550600	0,557500	3,49E-005	0,017840
Little finger	0,473400	0,619200	4,03E-004	0,053060
Below thumb	0,111200	0,165400	2,32E-006	0,008782
Below index finger	0,166000	0,218600	3,36E-007	0,004250
Below middle finger	0,175600	0,228700	1,42E-007	0,003147
Below ring finger	0,176200	0,279400	1,24E-007	0,003551
Below pinky finger	0,132300	0,318200	1,69E-006	0,011470

Table 2. Statistical significances of differences between dorsal segment temperatures in different NCS severity levels (Mann-Whitney-Wilcoxon test, p=0.05).

After repeated learning and testing of the neural network on the basis of these reduced results (dorsal images of the severe CTS and healthy hands; n = 185), we have achieved our best results. The efficiency of classification has exceeded 83% (Table 3).

Classification run	Incorrectly classified	Correctly classified	Success rate (%)
1	6	31	83,78
2	5	32	86,49
3	8	29	78,38
4	5	32	86,49
5	7	30	81,08
Mean	6.2 ± 1.30	30.8 ± 1.30	83.24 ± 3.52

Table 3. CTS diagnosis success rate when only dorsal segments of severe cases and healthy hands were used (n=37, 20% of all hands, each success rate percentage is the mean of five repeat runs).

5. Discussion

On the basis of such results, we can claim that thermography is a useful method for assessing severe CTS levels, even without using a preliminary stress test. Our attention has to be directed to the interpretation of thermograms in relation to the clinical picture, because pathological thermographic samples can be a result of neuropathic changes, local inflammation, or vascular diseases.

In terms of pathophysiology, we differentiate between four basic thermographic patterns of neuropathic origin (Rosenbaum & Ochoa, 2002):

1. Warm pattern I: sympathoparalytic vasodilatation;
   It occurs due to the loss of vasoconstrictor activity of sympaticus, (such as blockade of sympaticus or local blockade of somatic nerve). The skin is warm. Mechanism of action: the result of reduced vasomotor tonus of arteriolesis vasodilation, which is expressed as increased blood flow to the skin.

2. Cold pattern I: Denervation supersensitive vasoconstriction;
   The result of chronic interruption of postganglionic sympathetic neuron, which supplies the skin, leads to hypothermia of denervated area (sympathetic denervation supersensitivity). The skin is cold. Postsynaptic abnormality in the smooth muscles. Mechanism of action: the result of increased vasomotor tonus of arterioles is vasoconstriction, which is expressed as reduced blood flow to the skin.

3. Cold pattern II: Somatosympathetic reflex vasoconstriction;
   It is the result of the excitation of sensory receptors from the skin or irritation of sensory nerve, which is reflected as sudden cooling of skin on the area, where afferent impulses originate from. It is a reflex action, and afferent sensory fibres in this case are sympathetic.

4. Warm pattern II: Antidromic vasodilatation;
   Hyperthermia occurs due to vasodilatation, which does not depend on sympathetic activity, but on neurosecretion of vasodilatatory substances. Every stimulus, which reaches sufficient intensity to stimulate noniceptive nerve endings, can induce neurosecretory functions and consequently antidromic vasodilatation. The skin, which is cold due to symptomatic vasodilatation, retains the capacity for reflex sympathetic vasoconstriction.

In CTS, including rare cases of painful MN entrapment, we can come across any of the pathological samples mentioned above. However, further attention is required for the interpretation of results, because changes in vasomotor tonus are not exclusively the result of stimulation of sympathetic nerve fibres (Aminoff, 1979; Ochoa & Verdugo, 1995; Ochoa, 2002). And namely:

1. Reflex sympathetic activity can merely be physiological response to pain;
2. Vasoconstriction is often the result of denervation supersensitivity rather than of sympathetic hyperactivity;
3. Antidromic vasodilatation can also be caused by stimulation of sensory nociceptors;
4. Vasomotor disorders can simply be a result of the non-use of hand (Ochoa & Yarnitsky, 1994).

Giordano and others (Giordano et al., 1992) examined 40 patients with idiopathic CTS by applying electroneurography and thermography, and compared them to 30 healthy volunteers. Abnormal hypothermia and hyperthermia were attributed to changes in vasoconstrictor tonus caused by the compression of thin non-myelinated sympathetic fibres. With regard to complex thermoregulation mechanisms, autonomous activity of vegetative nervous system and individual reaction of individuals, the interpretation of thermograms is not uniform and must be done in conjunction with anamnesis, clinical picture and/or electrodiagnostics. It is commonly known that clinical signs for CTS are highly specific, but also not sensitive (Gunnarsson et al., 1997; Kuhlman & Hennessey, 1997; Kuntzer, 1994; Seror, 1993; Uncini et al., 1993). D`Arcy and Mc Gee have published work in which they present an overview of literature covering the period from April 1966 to December 2000, which discuss symptoms and signs for CTS diagnostics, in comparison to electrodiagnostic testing. They have established that sensitivity and specificity of clinical investigation vary considerably (D'Arcy & McGee, 2000). As part of our research we decided to compare thermograms with electrodiagnostics, since the latter is considered the most specific, sensitive (over 90%), and objective test for CTS diagnostics (Cassvan et al., 1988; Hennessey & Johnson, 1996; Hilburn, 1996; Jackson & Clifford, 1989; Johnson, 1993; Lew et al., 2005; Seror, 1987).

Rosenbaum and Ochoa warn that thermography cannot simply be equated with the CTS diagnostics, because it does not say much about the patophysiological basis of thermographic changes and entrapment, other than presenting changes in body temperature in a very precise and spectacular manner (Rosenbaum & Ochoa, 2002). In currently published clinical studies on CTS it has been reported that many patients with the clinically and electrodiagnostically confirmed CTS had normal thermographic samples (So et al., 1989; Myers et al., 1988). Thermograms were manually read. Y.T. So and others registered pathological samples in no more than 55% (So et al., 1989. In 1992 Tchou and others compared thermograms of 61 patients with CTS and 40 volunteers. Thermograms were considered abnormal, if at least 25% of distal median area was affected by temperature increase by more than 1°C. They have noted 93% sensitivity and 98% specificity of the thermographic method in impaired MN in the carpal tunnel, but only in the case of unilateral CTS (Tchou et al., 1992).

Our study also includes use of artificial intelligence, because we wanted to avoid the provocation cold stress test and manual interpretation of thermograms. By using neural networks of the multi-level perceptron type, we have, after preliminary supervised training, automated the analysis of thermograms and the CTS diagnosis procedure. As it turned out, by using a new software tool we were able to register very discrete temperature changes, which are not perceived macroscopically on the thermogram, and which the neural network successfully classified into the pathological sample. By using artificial intelligence we were able to abandon the need for contralateral comparison with the "healthy" side, which represented reference values in currently manually analysed thermograms. With regard to the findings of our research we can claim that the use of thermography in detecting CTS is useful even in the case of bilateral impairment. Considering this, the method achieved wider indication area, as by its definition CTS is more frequently bilateral (Rosenbaum & Ochoa, 2002). Our neural network was used on a group of patients with predominantly bilateral impairment, and the threshold for successful classification was set at 80%.

The assessment of the autonomous nervous system, in MN entrapment, was evidenced only by few authors (Aminoff, 1979; Verdugo et al., 2004; Verghesse et al., 2000). As a matter of fact, the incidence of these symptoms is not completely clear both in healthy people and in people with some other hand pathology. Burke and other discuss that more than a half of all patients with electrodiagnostically confirmed CTS, and also approximately two thirds of those without CTS, mentioned hand sweating. The entrapment of autonomous median fibres in the carpal tunnel was assessed with the sympathetic skin response, which was pathological in one third of all those patients with CTS, who stated symptoms, consistent with vegetative symptomatics (Burke et al., 1999). Yarnitsky and Ochoa claim that symptoms, which potentially belong to the autonomous nervous system disorder (finger sweating, dry palms, Raynaud's phenomenon, and finger pallor), can only be noticed in 17% to 32% of patients with CTS, and don't have high diagnostic value (Yarnitsky & Ochoa, 1991). But on the contrary, Verghese and others point out that the involvement of autonomous nervous system in CTS is frequent (55%), especially in the group of people with severe neurophysiological level of entrapment (Verghesse et al., 2000).

The results of our research are in line with the latter; as a matter of fact, the classification was by far the most successful in the group with the most severe level of entrapment in terms of electrodiagnostics (Table 3). In this group, even pathophysiologically, we can already expect impairment of thin, non-myelinated, autonomous, nerve fibres.

6. Conclusion

After an in-depth deliberation we believe that a pathophysiologically-substantiated doubt, with regard to the mechanism of the incidence of temperature changes in CTS, doesn't diminish the applicability of thermography in diagnosing MN entrapment by using artificial intelligence. As is often the case in medicine, temperature is a symptom and reflects a certain condition. By using artificial intelligence, considering reliable electrodiagnostic criteria, we have succeeded in classifying the discussed condition on hands as the result of severe level of MN entrapment in the carpal tunnel. Doctrinally, even though this is the best and the most frequently researched entrapment neuropathy on hands, there is currently no consensus reached with regard to treatment (Gerritsen et al., 2002; Gunnarsson et al, 1997; Hui et al., 2005; Kanaan & Sawaya, 2001; O'Gradaigh & Merry, 2000; Padua et al., 2001). Usually, mildly expressed CTS symptomatics in clinical terms is initially treated conservatively. With regard to the decision when and which type of operative relaxation of MN is the most appropriate, there are no uniform scientifically-supported evidences (Chang et al., 2008; Finsen & Russwurm, 2001; Iida et al., 2008; Mondelli et al., 2001). In patients, who refuse surgical procedures, neurophysiological investigation with a very clear clinical picture makes no sense, because it doesn't change their treatment in any way. Not taking into account results of neurophysiological measurements, it is conservative (disburden, braces), which means cheap, non-invasive, and completely reversible. Likewise, it also does not make sense to refer patients with CTS symptoms, which last less than six months, to neurophysiological measurements, because the probability of spontaneous healing is

EMG vs. Thermography in Severe Carpal Tunnel Syndrome

237

particularly high in the early period (Padua et al., 2001). Considering the described doctrine, recommendation, and clinical practice, we can diagnose CTS in cases of severe entrapment with a high level of reliability by using thermography and appropriate software tool. Simultaneously, critical interpretation of thermograms, considering anamnesis and clinical picture, is also sufficient for the beginning of CTS treatment. Patients with severe level of entrapment (where typical thermogram is registered), if they consent to the operative procedure, are referred to EMG investigation and then to decompression; all others are treated conservatively for the next six months.

On the basis of the conducted study, IR thermography cannot be recommended as an equal diagnostic method to the already established EMG investigation. However, we are determining that it can be used as a successful, non-invasive method for detecting severe CTS cases. It could also be useful in preventive examinations of a wider population, such as in different industries, where ergonomic conditions of work represent a major risk for the development of CTS (repeating hand and wrist movements, work with vibration machines, work in extreme wrist positions along with simultaneous pressure on palms, work in cold atmosphere, professional drivers, etc.), as well as in pregnant women and children and those symptomatic patients, who as a principle reject EMG and operative therapy.

Considering good results we have obtained by using neural networks in the group of severe entrapments we recommend thermography as a screening method for determining CTS. Indirectly, the method can also be useful in reducing long waiting periods for EMG investigation, which is the major deficiency of this generally established, standard diagnostics. By using non-invasive thermography we would focus on the group of patients most at risk, who would be given priority for EMG investigation.

The method we have developed with a clear indication for or restriction only to severe cases of entrapment is recommended as a screening method for determining CTS and as pre-level of EMG investigation, which otherwise still remains the most reliable standard in the area of diagnostics of entrapment neuropathies.

7. References

American Academy of Neurology [AAN]. (1990). Report of the American Academy of Neurology and Therapeutics and Technology Assessment Subcommittee. Assessment: Thermography in neurologic practice. *Neurology*, Vol. 40, No.3, pp. 523-525, ISSN 0028-3878

Aminoff, MJ. (1979). Involvement of peripheral vasomotor fibers in carpal tunnel syndrome. *J Neurol Neurosurg Psychiatry*, Vol.42, No.7, pp. 649-55, ISSN 0022-3050

Ammer, K. (1999). Diagnosis of nerve entrapment syndromes by thermal imaging, *Proceedings of the First Joint BMES/EMBS Conference*, Vol.2, p. 1117, ISBN 0-7803-5674-8, Atlanta, Georgia, USA, October 13-16, 1999

Ammer, K. (2003). Nerve entrapment and skin temperature of the human hand, In: *A case book of infrared imaging in clinical medicine*, A. Jung, J. Zuber, F. Ring, (Eds.), 94-96, Medpress, ISBN 83-916116-2-0, Warsaw, Poland

Benaroch, EE. (2007). The Autonomic nervous system: Basic anatomy and physiology. *Continuum Lifelong Learning Neurol*, Vol.13, No.6, pp. 13-32, ISSN 10802371

Bland, JDP. (2007). Carpal tunnel syndrome, BMJ, Vol.335, No.7615, pp. 343-346, ISSN 0959-8138

Burke, DT.; Burke, MA.; Bell, R.; Stewart, GW.; Mehdi, RS. & Kim, HJ. (1999). Subjective swelling: a new sign for carpal tunnel syndrome. *Am J Phys Med Rehabil*, Vol.78, No.6, pp. 401-405, ISSN 0894-9115

Cassvan, AA.; Ralescu, S.; Shapiro, E.; Moshkovski, FG. & Weiss, J. (1988). Median and radial sensory latencies to digit 1 as compared with other screening tests in carpal tunnel syndrome. *Am J Phys Med Rehabil*, Vol.67, No.5, pp. 221-224, ISSN 0894-9115

Chang, MH.; Wei, SJ. & Chen, LWA. (2008). Practical electrophysiological guide for non-surgical and surgical treatment of carpal tunnel syndrome. *J Hand Surg Eur Vol*, Vol.33, No.1, pp. 32-37, ISSN 1753-1934

Cuthbertson, GM (1995). The development of IR imaging in the United Kingdom, In: *The Thermal Image in Medicine and Biology*, Ammer, K. & Ring, EFJ. (Eds.), pp. 21-32, Uhlen-Verlag, ISBN 3-900466-57-2, Vienna, Austria

D'Arcy, CA. & McGee, S. (2000). The rational clinical examination. Does this patient have carpal tunnel syndrome?. *JAMA*, Vol.283, No.23, pp. 3110-3117, ISSN 0098-7484

Finsen, V. & Russwurm, H. (2001). Neurophysiology not required before surgery for typical carpal tunnel syndrome, *J Hand Surg Br*, Vol.26, No.1, pp. 61-64, ISSN 0266-7681

Gaussorgues, G. (1994). Infrared Thermography, Chapman & Hall, ISBN 0412479001, Cambridge, UK

Gerritsen, AA.; de Krom, MC.; Struijs, MA.; Scholten, RJ.; de Vet, HC. & Bouter, LM. (2002). Conservative treatment options for carpal tunnel syndrome: a systematic review of randomised controlled trials. *J Neurol*, Vol.249, No.3, pp. 272-280, ISSN 0340-5354

Giordano, N.; Batissti, E.; Franci, A.; Magaro, L.; Marcucci, P.; Cecconami, L. & Marcolongo, R. (1992). Telethermographic assesment of carpal tunnel syndrome. *Scand J Rheumatolo*, Vol.21, No.1, pp. 42-45, ISSN 0300-9742

Gunnarsson, LG.; Amilon, A.; Hellstrand, P.; Leissner, P. & Philipson, L. (1997). The diagnosis of carpal tunnel syndrome. Sensitivity and specificity of some clinical and electrophysiological tests. *J Hand Surg Br*, Vol.22, No.1, pp. 34-37, ISSN 0266-7681

Haas, OCL. & Burnham, KJ. (Eds.)(2008). Intelligent and Adaptive Systems in Medicine, Taylor & Francis, ISBN 978-0-7503-0994-3, London, UK

Hackett, MEJ. (1976). The place of thermography in medicine. *Acta thermographica*, Vol.1, pp. 176–180, ISSN 0391-9846

Hennessey, WJ. & Johnson, EW. (1996). Carpal tunnel syndrome, In: *Practical electromyography*, 3rd ed., Johnson EW., Pease WS. (Eds.), 195-216, Williams and Wilkins, ISBN 0683044575, Baltimore, USA

Herrick, RT. & Herrick, SK. (1987). Thermography in detection of carpal tunnel syndrome and other compressive neuropathies. *J. Hand Surg Am*, Vol.12, No.5, Pt.2, pp.943-949, ISSN 0363-5023

Hilburn, JW. (1996). General principles and use of electrodiagnostic studies in carpal and cubital tunnel syndromes. *Hand Clin*, Vol.12, No.2, pp. 205-221, ISSN 0749-0712

Hui, ACF.; Won, SG.; Leung, CH.; Tong, P.; Mok, V.; Poon, D.; Li-Tsang, CW.; Wong, LK. & Boet, R. (2005). A randomized controlled trial of surgery vs steroid injection for carpal tunnel syndrome. *Neurology*, Vol.64, No.12, pp. 2074-2078, ISSN 0028-3878

Iida, J.; Hirabayashi, H.; Nakase, H. & Sakaki, T. (2008). Carpal tunnel syndrome: electrophysiological grading and surgical results by minimum incision open carpal tunnel release. Neurol Med Chir (Tokyo), Vol.48, No.12, pp. 554-559, ISSN 0470-8105

EMG vs. Thermography in Severe Carpal Tunnel Syndrome

239

International Academy of Clinical Thermology. (2002). *Thermography guidelines: Standards and protocols in clinical thermographic imaging.* June 2011, Available from: http//www.iact-org.org/professionals/thermog-guidelines.html#/imaging

Jackson, DA. & Clifford, JC. (1989). Electrodiagnosis of mild carpal tunnel syndrome. *Arch Phys Med Rehabil*, Vol.70, No.3, pp. 199-204, ISSN 0003-9993

Johnson, EW. (1993). Diagnosis of carpal tunnel syndrome. The gold standard. *Am J Phys Med Rehabil*, Vol.72, No.1, p. 1, ISSN 0894-9115

Jones, BF. & Plassmann, P. (2002). Digital Infrared thermal imaging of human skin. *IEEE Eng Med Biol Mag*, Vol.21, No.6, pp. 41-48, ISSN 0739-5175

Kanaan, N. & Sawaya, RA. (2001). Carpal tunnel syndrome: modern diagnostic and management techniques. *Br J Gen Pract*, Vol.51, No.465, pp. 311-314, ISSN 0960-1643

Kantardzic, M. (2002). *Data Mining: Concepts, Models, Methods, and Algorithms.* Wiley-Interscience, ISBN 0471228524, Hoboken, New Jersey, USA

Kasabov, NK. (1996). *Foundations of Neural Networks, Fuzzy Systems, and Knowledge Engineering.* MIT Press, ISBN 0262112124, Cambridge, Massachusetts, USA

Kline, DG. & Hudson, A. (1990). Acute injuries of peripheral nerves. In: *Neurological Surgery*, Youmans RJ., (Ed.), 2423-2510, WB Saunders Co, ISBN 0721620949, Philadelphia, USA

Kuhlman, KA. & Hennessey, WJ. (1997). Sensitivity and specificity of carpal tunnel syndrome signs. *Am J Phys Med Rehabil*, Vol.76, No.6, pp. 451-457, ISSN 0894-9115

Kuntzer, T. (1994). Carpal tunnel syndrome in 100 patients: sensitivity, specificity of multi-neurophysiological procedures and estimation of axonal loss of motor, sensory and sympathetic median nerve fibers. *J Neurol Sci*, Vol.127, No.2, pp. 221-229, ISSN 0022-510X

Larose, DT. (2005). *Discovering Knowledge in Data: An Introduction to Data Mining.* John Wiley, ISBN 978-0-471-66657-8, Hoboken, New Jersey, USA

Lew, HL.; Date, ES.; Pan, SS.; Wu, P.; Ware, PF. & Kingery, WS. (2005). Sensitivity, specificity, and variability of nerve conduction velocity measurements in carpal tunnel syndrome. *Arch Phys Med Rehabil*, Vol.86, No.1, pp. 12-16, ISSN 0003-9993

Marotte, LR. (1974). An electrone microscope study of chronic median nerve compression in guinea-pig. *Acta Neuropathol*, Vol.27, pp. 69-82, ISSN 0001-6322

McCulloch, WS. & Pitts, W. (1943). A Logical Calculus of the Ideas Immanent in Nervous Activity. *Bulletin of Mathematical Biophysics* , Vol.5, pp.115-133, ISSN 0007-4985

Medical Imaging Research Group, University of Glamorgan. (2004). CTHERM Demo, June 2011, Available from: http://www.comp.glam.ac.uk/pages/staff/pplassma/MedImaging/Resources/CTHERM_Demo/Intro.htm

Mondelli, M.; Reale, F.; Padua, R.; Aprile, I. & Padua, L. (2001). Clinical and neurophysiological outcome of surgery in extreme carpal tunnel syndrome. *Clin Neurophysiol*, Vol.112, No.7, pp. 1237-1242, ISSN 1388-2457

Myers, S.; Vermeire, P.; Sherry, B. & Cross, D. (1988). Liquid crystal thermography: quantitative studies of abnormalities in the carpal tunnel syndrome. *Neurology*, Vol.39, No.11, pp. 1465-1469, ISSN 0028-3878

Ochoa, JL. (2002). Pathophysiology of chronic neuropathic pains, In: *Surgical management of pain*, Burchiel KJ, (Ed.), 25-41, Thieme Medical, ISBN 0865779120, New York, USA

Ochoa, JL. & Verdugo, RJ. (1995). Reflex sympathetic dystrophy. A common clinical avenue for somatoform expression. *Neurol Clin*, Vol.13, No.2, pp. 351-63, ISSN 0733-8619

Ochoa, JL. & Yarnitsky, D. (1994). The triple cold syndrome: Cold hyperalgesia, cold hypoaesthesia and cold skin in peripheral nerve disease. *Brain*, Vol.117, No.1, pp. 185-197, ISSN 0006-8950

O'Gradaigh, D. & Merry, P. (2000). Corticosteroid injection for the treatment of carpal tunnel syndrome. *Ann Rheum Dis*, Vol.59, No.11, pp. 918-919, ISSN 0003-4967

Padua, L.; Padua, R.; Aprile, I.; Pasqualetti, P. & Tonali, P. (2001). Multiperspective follow-up of untreated carpal tunnel syndrome: a multicenter study. *Neurology*, Vol.56, No.11, pp. 1459-1466, ISSN 0028-3878

Podgorelec, V.; Kokol, P.; Stiglic, B. & Rozman, I. (2002). Decision trees: an overview and their use in medicine. *J Med Syst*, Vol.26, No.5, pp. 445-463, ISSN 0148-5598

Ring, EFJ. (1995a). Cold stress testing of the hand, In: *The Thermal Image in Medicine and Biology*, Ammer K., Ring EFJ., (Eds.), 237-240, Uhlen Verlag , ISBN 3-900-4666-572, Vienna, Austria

Ring, EFJ. (1995b). The history of thermal imaging, In: *The Thermal Image in Medicine and Biology*, Ammer, K. & Ring, EFJ. (Eds.), pp. 13-20, Uhlen-Verlag, ISBN 3-900466-57-2, Vienna, Austria

Rojas, R. (1996). *Neural Networks: A systematic introduction*, Springer-Verlag, ISBN 3540605053, Berlin, Germany

Rosenbaum, RB. & Ochoa, JL. (2002). *Carpal tunnel syndrome and other disorders of the median nerve: Anatomy of the Median Nerve* (2nd ed.), Butterworth - Heinemann, ISBN 0-7506-7314-1, Boston, Massachusetts, USA

Schartelmüller, T. & Ammer, K. (1996). Infrared Thermography for the Diagnosis of Thoracic Outlet Syndrome. *Thermologie Österreich*, Vol.6, pp.130-134, ISSN 1021-4356

Seror, P. (1987). Electroclinical correlations in the carpal tunnel syndrome. Apropos of 100 cases. *Rev Rhum Mal Osteoartic*, Vol.54, No.10, pp. 643-648, ISSN 0035-2659

Seror, P. (1993). Sensitivity of various electrophysical studies for the diagnosis of carpal tunnel syndrome. *Muscle & Nerve*, Vol.16, No.12, pp. 1418-1419, ISSN 0148-639X

So, YT.; Olney, RK. & Aminoff, MJ. (1989). Evaluation of thermography in the diagnosis of selected entrapment neuropathies. *Neurology*, Vol.39, No.1, pp. 1-5, ISSN 0028-3878

Tchou, S.; Costich, JF.; Burgess, RC. & Wexler, CE. (1992). Thermographic observation in unilateral carpal tunnel syndrome: report of 61 cases. *J Hand Surg Am*, Vol.17, No.4, pp.631-637, ISSN 0363-5023

Tortora, JG. & Derrickson, BH. (2008). The Integumentary system. In: *Principles of Anatomy and Physiology*, 12th ed., pp. 140-159, John Wiley & Sons, ISBN 0470279877, New York, USA

Uncini, AD.; Muzio, A.; Awad, J.; Kanente, G.; Tafuro, H. & Cambi, D. (1993). Sensitivity of three median-to-ulnar comparative tests in diagnosis of mild carpal tunnel syndrome. *Muscle & Nerve*, Vol.16, No.12, pp. 1366-1373, ISSN 0148-639X

Verdugo, RJ.;, Bell, LA.; Campero, M.; Salvat, F.; Triplett, B.; Sonnad, J. & Ochoa, JL. (2004). Spectrum of cutaneous hyperalgesias/allodynias in neuropathic pain patients. *Acta Neurol Scand*, Vol.110, No.6, pp. 368–376, ISSN 0001-6314

Verghesse, J.; Galanopoulou, AS. & Herskovitz, S. (2000). Autonomic dysfunction in idiopathic carpal tunnel syndrome. *Muscle Nerve* , Vol.23, No.8, pp. 1209-1213, ISSN 0148-639X

Yarnitsky, D. & Ochoa, JL. (1991). Differential effects of compression-ischaemia block on warm sensation and heat-induced pain. *Brain*, Vol.114, No.2, pp. 907-913, ISSN 0006-8950

13

Middle and Long Latency Auditory Evoked Potentials and Their Usage in Fibromyalgia and Schizophrenia

Hande Turker, Ayhan Bilgici[1] and Huseyin Alpaslan Sahin
Ondokuz Mayis University School of Medicine, Department of Neurology, Samsun
[1]Ondokuz Mayis University School of Medicine,
Department of Physical Therapy and Rehabilitation, Samsun
Turkey

1. Introduction

1.1 Middle and long latency auditory evoked potentials and their usage in fibromyalgia

FM is a chronic syndrome that occurs predominantly in women and is marked by generalized pain, multiple defined tender points, fatigue, disturbed sleep, cognitive difficulty, and numerous other somatic complaints. The etiology and pathophysiology of FM remain unclear. Despite extensive research, no structural pathology has been identified in muscles or other tissues. The general and widespread nature of pain in FM strongly suggests the involvement of central mechanisms (Williams et al., 2006). Although psychological factors associated with chronic distress appear to be important for the development of FM in many patients, abundant evidence now indicates that pain in FM reflects abnormal pain processing in the central nervous system (ie. central sensitivity) (Herrero JF et al., 2000, Staud R. et al, 2001). Recent research suggested that FM patients might have deficiencies in central inhibitory mechanisms, such as diffuse noxious inhibitory control or the endogenous pain inhibitory system. Nevertheless, little is yet known about the brain mechanisms involved in the processing of nonpainful somatosensory information in FM (Monyoto P et al., 2006, Julien N. Et al., 2005).

Central mechanisms related to pathophysiology and hypervigilance have long been discussed for fibromyalgia. Nevertheless, research into this issue has been inconclusive so far. Our aim to design this study (Turker et al., 2008) was to determine whether central mechanisms played an important role in fibromyalgia via examining brain activity elicited by auditory evoked potentials in patients with FM and to assess relationship with clinical variables.

Middle latency evoked potentials (Middle Latency Auditory Evoked Potentials) are composed of several components that can be recorded from 10 to 50 msec after stimulus onset. The most stable components are Na and Pa, with latencies between 16-30 msec and 30-45 msec, respectively. Most of the MLAEP complex is thought to originate near the auditory cortex, although No, Po and Na may be generated by subcortical structures.

1.2 Patients and methods

33 female patients with a diagnosis of FM and 37 healthy women participated in the study. All patients met the American College of Rheumatology (ACR) criteria for FM (Wolfe et al., 1990).

Eighteen tender points accepted by the ACR for FM were evaluated. Each tender point was rated from 0 point (no pain) to 3 points (most severe pain). The sum of the 18 tender points was calculated as the total myalgic score (TMS). Other symptoms of FM were evaluated by using the Fibromyalgia Impact Questionaire (FIQ) and Health Assesment Questionary (HAQ) (Küçükdeveci et al.,2004,Bennett et al.,2005). The HAQ functional disability index was used to assess functional status. The instrument asks 24 questions regarding 8 activities of daily living areas.

The FIQ is a 20-item, self report instrument that measures multiple symptoms, functioning, and overall well-being. The first 10 items comprise a physical functioning scale; each item is rated on a 3-point Likert-type scale. On items 11 and 12, subjects indicate the days that they feel well or miss work because of fibromyalgia symptoms. Items 14 through 20 rate the difficulty in performing their job responsibilities, pain, fatigue, morning tiredness, stiffness, anxiety, and depression on a 10-cm visual analog scales (VAS). All subscores with the exception of the two work-related scores and physical function score were summed to yield the total score of fibromyalgia impact, which ranges from 0 (no impact) to 70 (maximum impact). Global disease severity was assessed with visual analogue scale (VAS) (0=very good, 10=very poor). The Hamilton Rating Scale for Depression and Hamilton Rating Scale for Anxiety were used to evaluate the affective condition of patients with FM (Hamilton et al., 1967).

Patients were excluded if they had evidende of traumatic injury, inflammatory rheumatic disease, a history of seizure, head trauma, or cerebrovascular disease; a lifetime history of pyschosis, or dementia; alcohol or substance dependence; if they received psychiatric treatment in the last 3 weeks or if there was a history of auditory impairment.

1.3 Evoked potentials recording procedure

All recordings of MLAEPs were performed at Dantec Keypoint. Electrode montage was adjusted as active electrode placed on ipsilateral mastoid and reference and ground electrodes at Cz and Fz, respectively. Silver surface electrodes were used for reference and ground electrodes. A scalp needle electrode was used as active electrode. Alternating clicks of 100 μsec duration were used and polarity was adjusted as vertex. The frequency of stimulation was 10/sec and the filtering was chosen as 10 Hz–200 Hz. Analysis time (sweep length) and sensitivity were 100msec and 0,2 μv/d, respectively. The intensity of the stimuli was chosen according to the auditory threshold. The ipsilateral ear was stimulated with an intensity of stimulus such as hearing threshold plus 60 DB, while the contralateral ear was masked with white noise. Averaging of 1000 signals was performed twice and overlapped for each ear. No, Po, Na, Pa, Nb, and Pb were sampled and latencies and amplitudes of each potential were determined and compared with age and gender matched controls. MLAEPs recordings were performed bilateraly i.e. 30 recordings were performed for patients and 30 recordings were performed for controls making a total of 60 recordings. No artifact rejection was employed. As hearing impairment can alter the MLAEPs, prior to beginning testing, the external ear canal was checked with an otoscope to assure that the canal was not blocked by cerumen. Patients with hearing problems assessed by otologic tests were excluded. MLAEPs are known to be affected by medications, however all patients were under treatment and there was no other way to investigate them.

Recordings of MLAEPs and LLAEPs (Long latency auditory evoked potentials) were performed for both patients and controls, using an active electrode placed on ipsilateral mastoid and reference and ground electrodes at Cz and Fz, respectively. Binaural stimulation was performed for LLAEPs. No, Po, Na, Pa, Nb, and Pb were sampled for MLAEPs. N1, P1, N2 and P2 were sampled for LLAEPs. Latencies and amplitudes of each potential were compared with those of controls and correlation between clinical and electrophysiological parameters were investigated statistically. Our study was approved by the local committee of ethics.

1.4 Statistical methods

Statistical evaluation of data was performed via using descriptive statistical methods such as mean and standard deviations while student T test was used for quantitative data showing normal statistical distribution. Pearson and Spearman's correlation analysis methods were used to investigate the correlation between latencies of MLAEP and clinical parameters. The results were evaluated at a confidency interval of 95% and a statistical significancy of $p < 0.05$. Comparisons between groups were made using the chi-square test for categorical variables. No statistically significant differences were recognized in the comparison of demographical data (age, disease duration, education, occupation, education level and marital status) between the groups. Clinical measures of patients are shown in table 1.

Clincal parameter	Mean ± SD
HAQ (0-3)	0,87 ± 0,48
Number of tender points(11-18)	14,90 ± 4,14
Total myalgia score	35,09 ± 13,22
Anxiety score	23,06 ± 9,75
Depression score	19,15 ± 8,94
Global disease severity(0-10)	6,72 ± 1,89
	Mean ± SD
FIQ Total (0-70)	51,57 ± 15,08
Physical function score (0 – 30)	11,63 ± 5,49

HAQ: Health Assesment Questionary FIQ: Fibromyalgia Impact Questionaire

Table 1. Clinical measures of patients.

1.5 Results

The latencies of Na, Nb and Pb of MLAEPs in the patient group were statistically longer when compared with those of the healthy controls ($p < 0.05$, $p < 0.01$ and $p < 0.01$ respectively). However No, Po and Pa did not show any statistical significant difference between the groups (Student t test). Latency of Na had statistically significant positive correlations with disease duration, FIQ total score, physical score and number of tender points ($p < 0.05$). Latency of Pa had statistically significant positive correlations with age, disease duration, FIQ total score, physical score and FIQ 2, FIQ 3, FIQ 4 and FIQ 6 ($p < 0.05$, $p < 0.01$, $p < 0.05$, $p < 0.05$, $p < 0.01$, and $p < 0.05$ for the rest respectively) (Figure 1). Latency of Nb had statistically significant positive correlations with disease duration ($p<0.05$) (Figure 2), FIQ total score ($p<0.05$), FIQ 2 ($p<0.01$), FIQ 6 ($p<0.05$), global disease severity ($p<0.05$). Latency of Pb had statistically significant positive correlations with FIQ total score ($p<0.05$), FIQ 2 ($p<0.05$) and global disease severity ($p<0.05$) (Pearson and Spearman's correlation tests). Evaluation of groups regarding parameters of LLAEP showed that latencies of P1, N2 and P2 were statistically longer when compared with those of the healthy controls ($p<0.05$, $p<0.01$ and $p<0.01$ respectively) whereas N1 did not show any statistical significancy between the groups (Student t test).

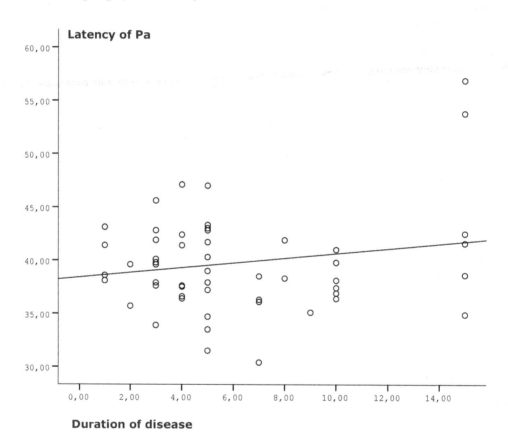

Duration of disease

Fig. 1. Correlation analysis of Pa latency and disease duration.

Correlation studies of latencies of LLAEPs with clinical parameters showed that FIQ total score had a positive and statistically significant correlation with latency of N2 ($p<0.05$), while the same was valid for physical score and FIQ2 with latency of N1 ($p<0.05$). FIQ 5, 7 and 8 were positively correlated with latency of N2 ($p<0.05$, $p<0.01$ and $p<0.01$ respectively), while FIQ 9 and 10 were positively correlated with latency of N1 ($p<0.01$, $p<0.05$ respectively). HAQ and anxiety score had positive correlations with latency of N2 ($p<0.05$).

The amplitudes of Po, Pa and Nb of MLAEPs and P1, N1, P2 and N2 of LLAEPs in the patient group were statistically significantly very low when compared with those of the healthy controls (p<0.01) (Student t test). However, there were not any statistical significant differences of amplitudes of MLAEPs and LLAEPs between patients having different disease durations. Patients suffering from fibromyalgia for five or more than five years did not show statistically higher or lower amplitudes when compared with patients having the disease for less than five years. Patients having myalgia scores equal or more than 40 also did not show any statistical differences of amplitudes of MLAEPs and LLAEPs when compared with patients having myalgia scores less than 40. Patients having anxiety scores equal or more than 25 were also compared with the ones having scores less than 25 and no statistically significant differences of amplitudes were found. Same results were obtained when patients were compared regarding latencies of both MLAEPs and LLAEPs.

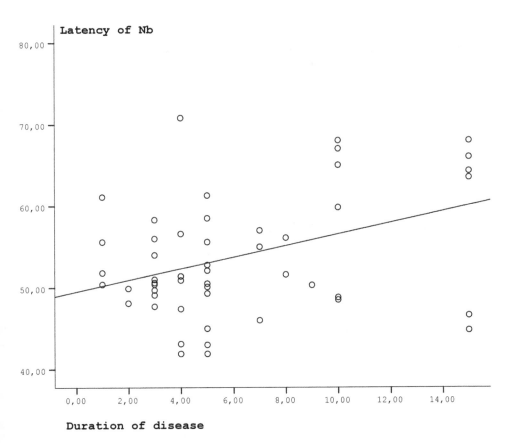

Fig. 2. Correlation analysis of Nb latency and disease duration.

A LLAEP trace of one of the patients with long latencies is shown in Fig. 3.

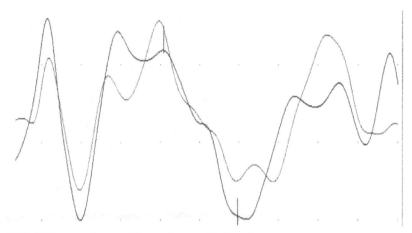

Fig. 3. A LLAEP trace of one of the patients with long latencies.

Correlation studies of amplitudes of LLAEPs with clinical parameters did not point out to any results of statistical significancy, whereas only one electrophysiological parameter in MLAEP amplitudes did. Amplitude of No showed a negative correlation with number of tender points (p<0.05) (Figure 4).

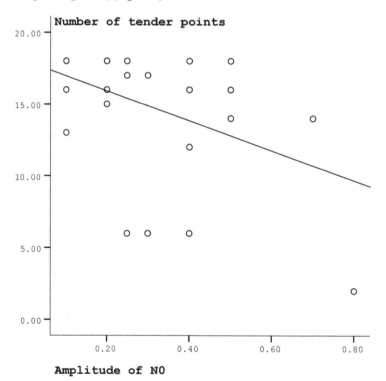

Fig. 4. Correlation analysis of number of tender points and amplitude of No.

Latencies of Na, Nb and Pb were statistically significantly longer in the patient group when compared with controls ($p < 0.05$ and $p < 0.01$ respectively).

The most important results for our study pointed out that Na, Pa and Nb latencies had positive correlations with disease duration which were statistically significant ($p < 0.05$, $p < 0.01$ and $p < 0.05$ respectively) while the correlations between Na and HAQ and myalgia scores were positive although statistically insignificant ($p > 0.05$). On the other hand, the number of tender points had a statistically significant positive correlation with Na ($p < 0.05$). FIQ2 scores had negative and statistically very significant correlations with Pa and Nb ($p < 0.01$ for both) while FIQ3 and FIQ scores had statistically positive correlations with Pa ($p < 0.05$).

1.6 Discussion

Since 1990s, some possible explanations for the involvement of central pathways in fibromyalgia are discussed in various papers, though their number is still limited. To our knowledge, correlation of clinical parameters of fibromyalgia with MLAEPs has not been studied before.

In 1995, Johansson et al., reported significant focal flow decreases in dorsolateral frontal cortical areas of both hemispheres of fibromyalgic patients (Johansson et al., 1995). The AEPs also showed signs of dysfunction at least at the brainstem level. A large group of fibromyalgia patients were studied electrophysiologically by Rosenhall et al. in 1996 and significant differences were found in the study group regarding absolute and interpeak latencies in short latency AEPs, when compared with normals (Rosenhall et al, 1996). However sensorineural hearing loss was reported in 15% of patients. Bayazit et al., also studied short latency AEPs in fibromyalgia patients with and without cochleovestibular symptoms and reported no statistical difference of AEP abnormalities in these subgroups indicating that FM patients might complain of otologic symptoms without having a detectable ear disease and that a neural disintegration or some other events related to neural mediators might be the mechanism involved (Bayazit et al.,2002). Our group of patients did not have otological symptoms, however their MLAEPs showed statistically significant differences when compared with normal controls. This result of our study may be considered as being in agreement with the above study. Fann et al. studied MLAEPs in a similar patient group (chronic low back pain) and found a trend of increased latencies and lower amplitudes of P50 potential in the study group reporting also a decreased habituation of this very potential (Fann et al.,2005). Our study also indicated that Na, Nb and Pb (namely N16, N40 and P50 potentials) had longer latencies in the patient group when compared with normals. The origins of MLAEPs are still controversial. Most authors share the opinion that Pa potential (P30) is generated in the supratemporal auditory center of each hemisphere, but it is not clear that Pa represents the earliest cortical auditory response. Na and Pa are believed to be related with the activation of of the primary auditory cortex. Some authors imply that Pa is generated in the auditory cortex while Na is originated subcortically. No, Po and Na have origins of subcortical structures while most other MLAEP potentials have origins generated from sites near the auditory cortex. In 1991 Erwin RJ et al. reported that P50 (Pb) was generated in thalamus (Erwin RJ et al., 1991). In a review of functional MRI (Magnetic resonance imaging) findings in FM, decreased rCBF (regional cerebral blood flow) in the thalamus and in the caudate nucleus was reported as results of various studies, nevertheless indicating the fact that this finding was not unique to FM.

Latency, on the other hand, has been shown to reflect the efficiency and speed of information processing in cognitive function (Gracely et al., 2002).

Thus results of our study may well be interpreted that FM patients show a slower speed of information processing in areas which are responsible for complex auditory perceptions related highly to cognitive functions. In 2006 Montaya et al. found significant amplitude reductions in FM patients for the auditory but not the somatosensory modality and suggested also that there was abnormal information processing in FM patients characterized by a lack of inhibitory control to repetitive nonpainful somatosensory information during stimulus coding and cognitive evaluation (Montoya et al., 2006). Roth et al. also stated that women with chronic pain were particularly vulnerable to cognitive dysfunction in a study designed as a cross-sectional survey (Roth et al., 2005).

1.7 Conclusion

Our results may be interpreted that central mechanisms may be important in the evolution of fibromyalgia. CNS dysfunction may be both an etiological factor in the fibromyalgia syndrome and a pathophysiological mechanism explaining the clinical symptoms and signs.

2. The relationship between middle latency auditory evoked responses, and the neuropsychological profile in patients with schizophrenia

2.1 Introduction

Although variable time ranges are described for MLAEPs, recent reliable sources report that the middle latency auditory evoked responses (MLAEPs) are far-field potentials that appear between 10-50 ms following an auditory stimulus and are recorded on vertex. The upper range limit is also reported as 80-100 ms in some sources (Buchwald et al., 1989; Buchwald et al., 1991; Erwin et al., 1986; Erwin et al., 1987; Mauguire et al., 2007). Far field potentials are generated by movement of the charge, but the electrode sees the moving front of depolarization and repolarization rather than the direct charge flow between regions of depolarization and repolarization. Most evoked potentials are generated by charge movement in nerve tracts to and from the relay nuclei and are far-field potentials because of the depth of the neural generators. The near-synchronous volley of action potentials in the nerve tracts produces far-field potentials that are recorded at scalp electrodes (Mauguire et al., 2007).

In literature, it has been assumed that MLAEPs are composed of six waves; No, Po, Na, Pa, Nb, Pb. No and Po are the the the earliest responses. Pa and Pb (P1, P50) are defined as positive waves occurring in the 29 msec and 45 msec after a stimulus, while Na and Nb are negative deflections in the 25 msec and 50 msec, respectively. The neural sources of these waves are still controversial (Misulis et al., 2001, Cacace et al., 1990). Most of the MLAEP complex is thought to originate near the auditory cortex, although No, Po and Na may be generated by subcortical structures.

Among components of MLAEPs, the most commonly studied wave is the Pb (synonyms: P1 or P50). The P1 potential is blocked by the muscarinic anticholinergic drugs. It is present during waking and rapid eye movement sleep and does not exist during deep slow wave sleep. It has also been reported that the P1 component may be associated with cognitive processes, especially attention and state. Abnormalities of MLAEPs have been reported in some neurodegenerative and psychiatric diseases such as Alzheimer's disease, Parkinson's disease, schizophrenia, Huntington disease and autism (Buchwald et al.,1989, Woods et al., 1987, Green et al., 1995).

It has been assumed that latency in evoked potential studies reflect the efficiency and speed of information processing. Thus, the prolonged latency may reflect that the information processing speed slowed. Amplitude abnormalites, on the other hand, refer to axonal loss in related areas and show the overall efficiency of neural structures mediating a response.

Over thirty years, various MLAEP studies have been performed in patients with schizophrenia. In most of these studies, the sensory gating paradigm has been investigated and they demonstrated the P1 habituating phenomenon, recovery cycle abnormalities and P1 suppression deficiency (Aminoff et al., 1990; Buchwald et al., 1992; Dickerson et al., 1991). However the relationship between the P1 latencies, amplitudes and neurocognitive status stil remains unclear. In this study (Sahin et al, 2005; Turker et al., 2008) we investigated whether the MLAEPs correlated with the performances of neuropsychological tests in patients with schizophrenia and healthy controls.

2.2 Methods
2.2.1 Subjects
We examined 15 patients (8 female and 7 male) with schizophrenia, who met diagnostic criteria of DSM-IV for schizophrenia and compared them with control subjects (9 females and 6 males). Patients and control subjects were matched for age, gender, education levels and handedness.

Subjects who had other neurological or psychiatric disease, history of substance abuse and head trauma were not included in the study. All patients were psychiatrically stable (there were no psychotic symptoms and medication changes within at least two weeks prior to the assesment). Psychopathological symptoms severity in patiens was assessed by Positive and Negative Syndrome Scale (PANSS) (First, 1997). Informed consent was obtained from patients and control subjects before the study.

2.2.2 Evoked potentials recording procedure
All recordings of MLAEPs were performed at Dantec Keypoint. Electrode montage was adjusted as active electrode placed on ipsilateral mastoid and reference and ground electrodes at Cz and Fz, respectively. Silver surface electrodes were used for reference and ground electrode while a scalp needle electrode was used as active electrode. Alternating clicks of 100 µsec duration were used and polarity was adjusted as vertex. The frequency of stimulation was 10/sec and the filtering was chosen as 10 Hz-200 Hz. Analysis time (sweep length) and sensitivity were 100msec and 0,2 µv/d, respectively. The intensity of the stimuli was chosen according to the auditory threshold. The ipsilateral ear was stimulated with an intensity of stimulus such as hearing threshold plus 60 dB, while the contralateral ear was masked with white noise. Averaging of 1000 signals was performed twice and overlapped for each ear. No, Po, Na, Pa, Nb, and Pb were sampled and latencies and amplitudes of each potential were determined and compared with age and gender matched controls. MLAEPs recordings were performed bilateraly i.e. 30 recordings were performed for patients and 30 recordings were performed for controls making a total of 60 recordings. No artifact rejection was employed.

In MLAEP recording procedure, latency and amplitude measurements are usually done on the display, either manually or by an automatic peak detection algorithm that seeks the maximum value between preset time values. The amplitude can be expressed as a peak to peak value between adjacent positive and negative components or the peak value can be measured against some baseline, usually taken just before the stimulus is presented. Latency for MLAEPs can be described as the time till the peak of the negative or the positive potential has evolved and this may be labelled on the display after the click (Erwin et al., 1987)

As hearing impairment can alter the MLAEPs, the external ear canal was checked with an otoscope to assure that the canal was not blocked by cerumen before the test. Patients with hearing problems assesed by otologic tests were excluded. MLAEPs are known to be affected by medications, however all patients were under treatment and there was no other way to investigate them.

2.2.3 Neuropsychological evaluation

An extensive neuropsychological test battery was used to assess the cognitive functions; attention, language, visuospatial functions, verbal and visual memory, executive functions (Table 3).

2.2.4 Statistical methods

The age, gender, handedness, education, the latencies and amplitudes of MLAEPs the neuropsychological test parameters of the patients and controls groups were compared with student-t test. The pearson correlation coefficient was used to determine the correlation between PANNS scores, the neuropsychological test parameters, and disease duration.

2.3 Results

The demographic features of patient and control groups are presented in Table 2. There were no statistically significant difference between age, gender, handedness, and education levels of patient and control groups.

	Patients (n = 15)		Controls (n = 15)	p
Age	32.9 ± 10.6	29.8±2.3	NS	
Education	12.1 ± 3.7	12.6±2.6	NS	
MMSE	28.1 ± 2.7	29.6±0.8	S	
Gender	8M. 7F	9M. 6F		NS
Duration of disease (month)	135.3± 112.1	(-)		(-)

Table 2. Demographic Features.

2.3.1 Neuropsychological tests

Results are summarized in Table 4. Generally, in all the neuropsychological tests, performance of the patient group was poor when compared to control group. MMSE scores of the patient group were statistically significantly lower than those of the control groups.

There were statistically significant differences regarding the attention and the language tests. The scores of the tests assessing visuospatial functions, except BLO, were significantly different between patient and control groups. Also, patients got statistically significant lower scores on memory tests, and executive functions when compared with controls.

Mini mental state examination (MMSE)
Attention
   WAIS-R Digit Span (DS)
   Verbal Fluency (K-A-S Test)
Language
   Boston Naming Test (30-items)
Visuo-spatial Functions
   Benton's Line Orientation Test (BLO)
   Benton's Facial Recognition Test (BFR)
   WAIS-R BlocK Design (BD)
   Hooper Visual Organization Test (HVOT)
   Clock Drawing
Verbal Memory
   California Verbal Learning Test (CVLT)
Visual Memory
   WAIS-R subtest
Executive Functions
   Wisconsin Card Sorting Test (WCST)
   Stroop Test
   Trail Making Test A and B (TMT A-B)

WAIS = Wechsler Adult Intelligence Scale.

Table 3. Neuropsychological Test Battery.

	Patients (n = 15)		Controls (n = 15)		
	Mean	SD	Mean	SD	p
MMSE	28.1	2.7	29.6	0.8	S
Attention					
WAIS-R DS-fwd	6	1.06	7.2	1.01	S
WAIS-R DS-bwd	3.6	1.29	5.2	1.08	S
Verbal Fluency (K-A-S Test)	35.07	13.96	48.47	12.18	S
K-A-S perseveration	0.67	0.81	0.07	0.25	S
Language					
Boston Naming Test (30-items)	27.60	2.79	29.27	1.28	S
Visuo-spatial Functions					
BLO	23.43	7.94	26.40	2.99	NS
BFR	18.07	3.38	21.93	2.63	S
BD	21.14	11.43	30.20	9.59	S
HVOT	17.79	4.04	21.00	1.89	S
Clock Drawing	9.26	0.79	9.93	0.25	S

	Patients (n = 15)		Controls (n = 15)		
	Mean	SD	Mean	SD	p
Verbal Memory					
CVLT					
Total of 5 trails	38.71	10.57	51.46	6.94	S
Long-delay free recall	7.92	2.97	12.53	2.06	S
Long-delay cued recall	8.21	2.96	13.20	1.65	S
Perseverations	5	4.11	3.40	3.08	NS
Free recall intrusions	2	2.21	1	1.81	NS
Cued recall intrusions	1.21	1.67	0.67	1.11	NS
Recognition	13.21	3.01	15.13	1.06	S
Discriminability (%)	88.09	9	96	3.5	S
False positive	1.5	1.6	0.46	1.06	S
Visual Memory					
WAIS-R subtest	8	3.2	11.67	1.1	S
Executive Functions					
WCST					
Total number of responses	117.50	18.25	95.6	15.37	S
Total categories completed	3.57	2.10	5.93	0.25	S
Number of perseverative responses	43.36	36.23	12.67	4.25	S
Total number of errors	51.64	25.42	22.67	8.30	S
Total number of correct responses	65.86	14.72	72.93	8.40	NS
Stroop 3	14.3	4	11.1	2.7	S
Stroop 5	27.9	9.6	25.1	8.2	NS
TMT A	69.72	25.7	35.35	13.18	S
TMT B	146.44	91.55	75.56	25.13	S

Table 4. Neuropsychological Test Results.

2.3.2 Evoked potentials

The results indicated that most of the MLAEPs data elicited from the patients showed statistically significant differences from controls. The pathological responses from both sides of the brains of patients did not differ significantly from each other as both right and left sides generated MLAEPs which were statistically significantly different from controls (Table 5–6). Apart from NoR and PaL, all latencies of other parameters of MLAEPs were prolonged in the patient group (Table 5). Apart from PbR, amplitudes of parameters of MLAEPs were statistically significantly lower in the patient group when compared with the control group, (Table 6).

We also found no correlations between PANSS scores, the scores of neuropsychological tests, the duration of disease, and the latencies and amplitudes of MLAEPs.

	Patients (n=15)		Control (n=15)		
	Mean	SD	Mean	SD	p
No$_R$	10.67	3.52	8.48	2.64	NS
No$_L$	11.18	3.26	8.04	2.25	S
Po$_R$	18.05	1.55	15.71	2.39	S
Po$_L$	19.14	3.87	15.36	2.38	S
Na$_R$	29.22	2.63	26.26	2.21	S
Na$_L$	29.98	3.55	26.65	2.79	S
Pa$_R$	40.16	3.32	37.70	2.64	S
Pa$_L$	43.01	6.35	39.77	3.31	NS
Nb$_R$	53.44	6.73	48.01	5.37	S
Nb$_L$	55.66	10.09	48.97	3.58	S
Pb$_R$	68.37	7.84	59.19	7.94	S
Pb$_L$	66.54	11.07	59.35	5.76	S

Table 5. Latencies of MLAEPs (Millisecond).

	Patients (n=15)		Control (n=15)		
	Mean	SD	Mean	SD	p
No$_R$	0.17	0.15	0.4	0.2	S
No$_L$	0.22	0.15	0.47	0.27	S
Po$_R$	0.22	0.13	0.49	0.25	S
Po$_L$	0.22	0.15	0.56	0.32	S
Na$_R$	0.39	0.35	0.86	0.50	S
Na$_L$	0.39	0.29	0.76	0.34	S
Pa$_R$	0.26	0.27	0.65	0.51	S
Pa$_L$	0.26	0.25	0.58	0.33	S
Nb$_R$	0.28	0.30	0.55	0.38	S
Nb$_L$	0.25	0.22	0.50	0.33	S
Pb$_R$	0.27	0.29	0.48	0.38	NS
Pb$_L$	0.19	0.10	0.50	0.31	S

Table 6. Amplitudes of MLAEP Potentials (Microvolt).

2.4 Discussion

In this study we found that the many parameters of MLAEPs except NoR and PaL for latency and PbR for amplidute, were significantly abnormal in the patient group. Also, the neuropsychological test performances of the patient group were poor when compared with normals.

According to our data, there were not any correlations between PANSS scores, the scores of neuropsychological test, the duration of disease, and the latencies and amplitudes of MLAEPs.

Although the neural sources of MLAEPs are still controversial, the studies suggest that Pa, Pb and Nb components of MLAEPs have a cortical generator (primary auditory cortex and adjacent areas) while No, Po, and Na have a brainstem-subcortical generator (medial geniculate body, polysensory thalamic nuclei) (Deiber et al., 1988; Diaz et al., 1990) It is well-known that human Pb (P1) potential is blocked by scopalamine, muscarinic cholinergic antagonists, and due to lesions including cholinergic pedunculopontine nucleus (Diaz et al., 1990)

In patients with schizophrenia, the abnormalities in auditory evoked potentials have been reported by other studies. Erwin et al. reported that the recovery cycle of the P1 component of auditory midlatency evoked potential is abnormal (Erwin et al.,1991). Boutros and coworkers suggested that there were morphological abnormalities of the MLAEPs in schizophrenia patients (Boutros et al.,2004). Clementz et al.showed that P50 suppression was deficient in these patients, indicating sensory gating abnormality (Clementz et al., 1997). All these findings were interpreted by authors as a deficiency of generators of MLAEPs, underlying neural structures and neurotransmitter systems in patients with schizophrenia.

We investigated the latency and amplitude features of MLAEPs recorded on dominant and non-dominant hemisphere in patients with schizophrenia but not the recovery cycle and sensory gating features. All patients and control subjects were strongly right-handed according to Edinburgh Inventory (Oldfield et al., 1971).

Our results revealed statistically significant differences both in latency and amplitudes of MLAEP components in the patient group when compared with the normal group.

Lateralization seems to be important in schizophrenic patients since some symptoms of the disease emerge when specific parts of the brain are involved. It was hypothesized that hypermetabolism of the left temporal lobe seemed to occur only if the patient was actively hallucinating for example (Mesulam et al., 1990).

In our study the pathological responses elicited from both sides of the brains of patients did not differ significantly from each other as both right and left sides generated MLAEPs which were statistically significantly different from controls. We believe this is an important finding since all our patients and controls were strongly right-handed. Thoma et al. concluded in one of their studies that converging evidence from EEG, MEG and neuropsychological measures pointed to left hemisphere dysfunction related to the well established sensory gating in schizophrenia (Thoma et al., 2003).

It has been assumed that latency in evoked potential studies reflect the efficiency and speed of information processing. Thus, the prolonged latency may reflect that the information processing speed slowed.

Amplitude abnormalites, on the other hand, refer to axonal loss in related areas and show the overall efficiency of neural structures mediating a response.

Amplitude abnormalities in evoked potentials of patients with schizophrenia have been reported with much more consistency than latency abnormalities. Munkundan and coworkers observed amplitude and recovery abnormalities but normal latencies of MLAEPs in schizophrenia patients (Munkundan et al., 1986). Williams and coworkers similarly found no latency abnormalities in a group of medicated schizophrenia patients (Williams et al, 2000). However, Boutros and coworkers demonstrated that schizophrenia patients had significantly longer latencies for the P50 and N100 components (Boutros et al., 2004). Our findings agree with results of the researchs in literature.

The many previous studies investigated the neuropsychological profile of the patients with schizophrenia. Almost all of these studies demonstrated the neuropsychological impairments in the multiple cognitive areas etc. memory, attention, language, executive functions (Bozikas et al., 2006; Brazo et al., 2005; Mohamed at al., 1999). However, it is still unknown whether there is a relationship between the neuropsychological impairments and neuroanatomical changes. Also, it is unclear whether the negative and positive symptoms are associated with a spesific brain region and/or neuropsychological deficits. Andreasen et al. and Weinberg et al. have reported that the negative symptoms reflected primarily frontal lobe dysfunction (Andreasen, 1986; Weinberger, 1987). Berman et al. observed that negative symptoms associated with poor performances on cognitive tests reflected poor frontal lobe functions while positive symptoms were associated with poor attention representing widespread neural network (Berman et al., 1997). Liu et al. demonstrated that the negative schizophrenic patients had executive function deficits and lower rCBF perfusion in left prefrontal lobes (Liu et al, 2002). On the other hand, Morrison-Stewart et al. found no correlation between frontal lobe assessing neuropsychological tests and negative symptoms (Morrison et al., 2002). Addington et al. reported that there was no relationship between attention and negative and positive symptoms (Addington et al., 1997).

The results of our study showed that the cognitive functions assessing the comprehensive neuropsychological test battery were statistically significantly worse in the patient group when compared with the control group.

Schizophrenia is a heterogeneous mental disease which is characterized with thought disorder, hallucination, delusion and cognitive deficits.[45] Postmortem studies showed low neuron density, cortical volume reduction, pyramidal cell disarray, neurotransmitter disturbances such as glutamate, GABA, dopamine, and acetylcholine (Harrison et al.,1998; Sarter et al.,1998; Simpson at al, 1998). The longitudinal studies support that schizophrenia is largely a static disorder while others suggest a deteriorating course (Harrison et al.,1998; Gur et al., 1998; Vita et al., 1997).

The spectrum of disease duration of our patients was fairly widespread (min: 50 months max: 440 months). In our study there were no correlations between the disease duration, severity of the disease (by PANSS), EP measures, and neuropsychological profiles. This may perhaps support that schizophrenia is a static disorder rather than progressive.

3. Acknowledgements

This second work was partly supported by a research grant from Ondokuz Mayis University. The authors thanks to Prof. Dr. Yuksel Bek for statistical analysis.

4. References

Addington J, Addington D, Gasbarre L. Distractibility and symptoms in schizophrenia. J Psychiatry Neurosci 1997;22(3):180-4.

Andreasen NC, Nasrallan Z, Dunn VD, Olson SC, Grove WM, Ehrhardt JC, Coffman JA. Crossett JH. Structural abnormalities in frontal system in schizophrenia: a magnetic resonance imaging study. Arch Gen Psychiatry 1986;43:136-44.

Aminoff MJ, Goodin A, Goodin DS Electrophysiological features of the dementia of Parkinson's disease. Adv Neurol 1990;53:361-3.

Bayazit YA, Gursoy S, Ozer E, Karakurum G, Madenci E. Neurotologic manifestations of the fibromyalgia syndrome. J Neurol Sci. 2002 Apr 15;196(1-2):77-80.

Bennett R. The Fibromyalgia Impact Questionnaire(FIQ):a review of its development, current version, operating characteristics and uses. Clin Exp Rheumatol 2005;23(Suppl. 39):154-162.

Berman I, Viegner B, Merson A, Allan E, Pappas D, Green AL. Differential relationships between positive and negative symptoms and neuropsychological deficits in schizophrenia. Schizophr Res 1997;25(1):1-10.

Boutros NN, Korzyuko O, Oliwa G, Feingold A, Campbell D, Mcclain-Furmansk D, Struve F, Jansen BH. Morphological and latency abnormalities of the mid-latency auditory evoked responses in schizophrenia: a preliminary report. Schizophrenia Res 2004;70(2-3):303-13.

Bozikas Vp, Kosmidis MH, Kiosseoglou G, Karavatos A. Neuropsychological profile of cognitively impaired patients with schizophrenia. Compr Psychiatry 2006;47(2):136-43.

Brazo P, Delamillieure P, Morello R, Halbecq I, Marié RM, Dollfus S. Impairments of executive/attentional functions in schizophrenia with primary and secondary negative symptoms. Psychiatry Res 2005;133(1):45-55.

Buchwald JS, Erwin RJ, Read S, Lancker Dv, Guthrie D, Schawfel J, Tanhguay P. Midlatency auditory evoked responses: differential abnormality of P1 in Alzheimer disease. Electroencephalogr Clin Neurophysiol 1989;74(5):378-4.

Buchwald Js, Rubinstein EH, Schwafel J, Strandburg RJ. Midlatency auditory evoked responses. Electroencephalogr Clin Neurophysiol 1991;80(4):303-9.

Buchwald JS, Erwin RJ, Read S, Lancker DV, Cummings JL. Midlatency auditory evoked responses: P1 abnormalities in adult autistic subjects. Electroencephalogr Clin Neurophysiol 1992;84(2):164-71.

Cacace AT, Satya-Murti S, Wolpaw JR. Human middle latency auditory evoked potentials: vertex and temporal components. Electroencephalogr Clin Neurophysiol 1990;77(1):6-18.

Clementz BA, Geyer MA, Braff Dl. P50 suppression among schizophrenia and normal comparison subjects: a methodological analysis. Biol Psychiatry 1997;41(10):1035-44.

Deiber MP, Ibañez V, Fischer C, Perrin F, Mauguière F. Sequential mapping favours the hypothesis of distinct generators for Na and Pa middle latency auditory evoked potentials. Electroencephalogr Clin Neurophysiol 1988;71(3):187-97.

Diaz F, Cadaveria F, Grau C. Short- and middle-latency auditory evoked potentials in abstinent chronic alcoholics: preliminary findings. Electroencephalogr Clin Neurophysiol 1990;77(2):145-50.

Dickerson LW, Buchwald JS. Midlatency auditory evoked responses: Effects of scopolamine in cat and implication for brain stem cholinergic mechanisms. Exp Neurol 1991; 112(2):229-39.

Erwin RJ, Buchwald JS. Midlatency auditory evoked responses: differential recovery cycle characteristics. Electroencephalogr Clin Neurophysiol 1986;64(5):417-23.

Erwin RJ, Buchwald JS. Midlatency auditory evoked responses in the human and the cat model. Electroencephalogr Clin Neurophysiol Suppl 1987;40:461-7.

Erwin RJ, Mawhinney-Hee M, Gur RC, Gur RE. Midlatency auditory evoked responses in schizophrenia. Biol Psychiatry 1991;30(5):430-42.

Fann AV, Preston MA, Bray P, Mamiya N, Williams DK, Skinner RD, Garcia-Rill E. The P50 midlatency auditory evoked potential in patients with chronic low back pain (CLBP). Clin Neurophysiol. 2005 Mar;116(3):681-9. Epub 2004 Nov 23.

First MB, Spitzer RL, Gibbon M, Williams JBW. Structured Clinical Interview for DSM-IV Axis I disorders (SCID-I), clinical version. Washington, DC: American Psychiatric Press. 1997.

Gracely RH, Petzke F, Wolf JM, Clauw DJ. Functional magnetic resonance imaging evidence of augmented pain processing infibromyalgia. Arthritis Rheum. 2002 May;46(5):1333-43.

Green JB, Elder WW, Freed DM. The P1 component of tha middle latency auditory evoked potential predicts a practice effect during clinical trials in Alzheimer disease. Neurology 1995;45(5):962-6.

Gur RE, Cowell P, Turetsky BI, Gallacher F, Cannon T, Bilker W, Gur RC. A follow-up magnetic resonance imaging study of schizophrenia. Relationship of neuroanatomical changes to clinical and neurobehavioral measures. Arch Gen Psychiatry 1998;55(2):145-52.

Hamilton M. Development of a rating scale for primary depressive illness. Br J Soc Clin Psychol 1967;6:278-296.

Harrison PJ. The neuropathology of schizophrenia: a critical rewiew of the data and their interpretation. Brain 1999;122(4):593-624.

Herrero JF, Laird JM, Lopez-Garcia JA (2000) Wind-up of spinal cord neurones and pain sensation:much ado about something? Progress in Neurobiology 61(2);169-203.

Johansson G, Risberg J, Rosenhall U, Orndahl G, Svennerholm L, Nystrom S. Cerebral dysfunction in fibromyalgia:evidence from regional cerebral blood flow mesurements, otoneurological tests and cerebrospinal fluid analysis. Acta Psychiat Scand 1995;91:86-94.

Julien N, Goffaux P, Arsenault P, Marchand S. Widespread pain in fibromyalgia is related to a deficit of endogenous pain inhibition. Pain 2005;114:295-302.

Küçükdeveci AA, Sahin H, Ataman S, Griffiths B, Tennant A. Issues in cross-cultural validity: example from the adaptation, reliability, and validity testing of a Turkish version of the Stanford Health Asessment Questionnaire. Arthritis Rheum 2004;51:14-9.

Mauguire F, Butler SR, Ceranic B, Cooper R, Holder GE. Normal Findings by Modality in Clinical Neurophysiology Vol 1, eds. Binnie C, Cooper R, Mauguire F, 2007; 422.

Liu Z, Tam WC, Xie Y, Zhao J. The relationship between regional cerebral blood flow and the Wisconsin Card Sorting Test in negative schizophrenia. Psychiatry Clin Neurosci 2002;56(1):3-7.

Mesulam M. Schizophrenia and the brain. NEJM 1990; 322(12):789-94.

Mesulam M. From sensation to cognition. Brain 1998;121(6):1013-52.

Misulis KE, Fakhouri T. Spehlmann's Evoked Potential Primer, 3rd edition. Oxford Press, Butterworth Heinemann, Boston, 2001;6-7.

Mohamed S, Paulsen JS, O'leary D, Arndt S, Andreasen N. Generalized cognitive deficits in schizophrenia. Arch Gen Psychiatry 1999;56(8):749–54.

Montoya P, Sitges C, Garcia-Herrera M et al (2006) Reduced brain habituation to somatosensory stimulation in patients with fibromyalgia. Arthritis Rheum 2006;54(6);1995-2003.

Morrıson-Stewart Sl, Williamson PC, Cornıng WC, Kutcher SP, Snow WG, Merskey H. Frontal and non-frontal lobe neuropsychological test performance and clinical symptomatology in schizophrenia. Psychol Med 1992;22(2):353-9.

Munkundan CR. Middle latency components of evoked potential responses in schizophrenics. Biol Psychiatry 1986;21(11):1097-100.

Oldfield RC. The assessment and analysis of handedness: the Edinburgh Inventory. Neuropsychologia 1971;9(1):97-113.

Roth SR, Geisser ME, Theisen-Goodvich M, Dixon PJ. Cognitive complaints are associated with depression, fatigue, female sex, and pain catastrophizing in patients with chronic pain. Arch Phys Med Rehabil 2005;86:1147-54.

Rosenhall U, Johannsen G, Orndahi G. Otoneurologic and audiologic findings in fibromyalgia. Scand J Rehabil Med. 1996 Dec;28(4):225-32.

Şahin, HA., M. Sarıca, H. Türker, M. Baydın, Ö. Böke, B. Diren, "Şizofrenide semptom profili, kognitif durum ile beyin atrofisi arasındaki ilişki", 41. Ulusal Nöroloji Kongresi, Cilt 11, 70, İstanbul, 2005.

Sarter M, Bruno JP. Cortical acetylcholine, reality distortion, schizophrenia, and Lewy Body Dementia: too much or too little cortical acetylcholine? Brain Cogn 1998;38(3):297-316.

Simpson MD, Slater P, Deakin JF. Comparison of glutamate and gamma-aminobutyric acid uptake binding sites in frontal and temporal lobes in schizophrenia. Biol Psychiatry 1998;44(6):423-7.

Staud R, Domingo M(2001) Evidence for abnormal pain processing in fibromyalgia syndrome. Pain Med 2(3);208-215.

Turker, H., A. Bilgici, M.K. Onar, " The investigation of the correlation between middle and long latency auditory evoked potentials and clinical parameters in fibromyalgic patients," Proc. 13th European Congress of Clinical Neurophysiology, Istanbul, Clin Neurophysiol, Vol.119,104, Elsevier, Amsterdam, 2008.

Turker, H., H. Şahin, M. Sarica, O. Böke, " Middle latency auditory evoked responses in schizophrenia and correlation with hemishpere dominance," Proc. 13th European Congress of Clinical Neurophysiology, Istanbul, Clin Neurophysiol, Vol.119,103-104, Elsevier, Amsterdam, 2008.

Thoma RJ, Hanlon FM, Moses SN, Edgar JC, Huang M, Weisend, MP, Irwın J, Sherwood A, Paulson K, Bustillo J, Adler LE, Mıller GA, Cañive JM. Lateralization of auditory sensory gating and neuropsychological dysfunction in schizophrenia. Am J Psychiatry 2003;160(9):1595-605.

Vita A, Dieci M, Giobbio GM, Tenconi F, Invernizzi G. Time course of cerebral ventricular enlargement in schizophrenia supports the hypothesis of its neurodevelopmental nature. Schizophr Res 1997;23 (1):25-30.

Weinberger DR. Implications of normal brain development for the pathogenesis of schizophrenia. Arch Gen Psychiatry 1987;44(11):660-9.

Williams DA, Gracely RH. Biology and therapy of fibromyalgia. Functional magnetic resonance imaging findings in fibromyalgia. Arthritis Res Ther 2006;8(6):224

Williams LM, Gordon E, Wright J, Bahramali H. Late component ERPs are associated with three syndromes in schizophrenia. Int J Neurosci 2000;105(1-4):37-52.

Woods Dl, Clayworth CC, Knight RT, Simpson GV, Naeser MA. Generators of middle- and long-latency auditory evoked potentials: implications from studies of patients with bitemporal lesions. Electroenceph Clin Neurophysiol 1987;68(2):132-48.

Wolfe F, Smythe HA, Yunus MB et al. The American College of Rheumatology 1990 Criteria for the Classification of Fibromyalgia. Report of the Multicenter Criteria Committe. Arthritis Rheum 1990;33;160-172.

14

Functional Significance of Facilitation Between the Pronator Teres and Extensor Carpi Radialis in Humans: Studies with Electromyography and Electrical Neuromuscular Stimulation

Akira Naito[1], Hiromi Fujii[2], Toshiaki Sato[2],
Katsuhiko Suzuki[2] and Haruki Nakano[1]
[1]Yamagata University
[2]Yamagata Prefectural University of Health Sciences
Japan

1. Introduction

Excitatory (facilitation) or inhibitory spinal reflex arcs (inhibition) mediated by group I afferent fibers from the muscle spindles (group Ia afferents) and Golgi tendon organs (group Ib afferents) among muscles in the human upper limb have been studied (Fig. 1) (Aymard et al., 1995; Baldissea et al., 1983; Cavallari & Katz, 1989; Cavallari et al., 1992; Creange et al., 1992; Day et al., 1984; Fujii et al., 2001; Katz et al., 1991; Kobayashi et al., 2000; Lourenço et al., 2007; Marchand-Pauvert et al., 2000; Miyasaka et al., 1995, 1996, 1998, 2007; Naito et al., 1996, 1998a, 2001; Naito, 2003, 2004; Nakano et al., 2005, 2006; Ogawa et al., 2005; Pierrot-Deseilligny & Mazevet, 2000; Rossi et al., 1995; Sato et al., 2002; Shinozaki et al., 2001; Suzuki et al., 2005, 2007; Wargon et al., 2006). These reflex arcs modulate motoneuron excitabilities to coordinate smooth muscular movements (Naito, 2003, 2004; Pierrot-Deseilligny et al., 1981; Rothwell, 1994; Tanaka, 1989). The facilitation must function for co-contraction of muscles and the inhibition for alternating or reciprocal contraction among muscles (Naito, 2003, 2004).

Musculus (m.) pronator teres (PT) arises from the medial epicondyle of the humerus (humeral head) and the coronoid process of the ulna (ulnar head) and attaches on the lateral surface of the shaft of the radius (Basmajian, 1982; Jenkins, 2008; Standring et al., 2005). It is innervated by the median nerve. M. extensor carpi radialis longus (ECRL) arises mainly from the distal third of the supracondylar ridge of the humerus and attaches to the radial side of the dorsal aspect of the base of the second metacarpal. M. extensor carpi radialis brevis (ECRB) arises mainly from the lateral epicondyle of the humerus and attaches on the radial side of the base of the third metacarpal. Both muscles (ECR) are innervated by the radial nerve. Most textbooks of anatomy describe that PT acts as a forearm pronator and ECR as a wrist extensor and abductor. Our previous studies have demonstrated facilitation between PT and ECR (ECRL, ECRB) in humans (Fig. 1) (Nakano et al., 2005, 2006). The facilitation seems to be mediated by group Ia afferents through a monosynaptic path. It is known that monosynaptic facilitation mediated by group Ia afferents is usually observed

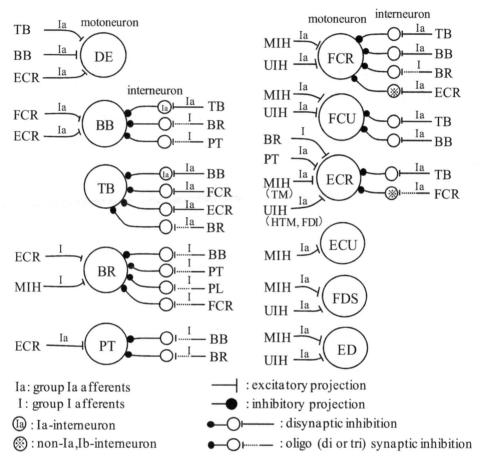

Fig. 1. Excitatory (facilitation) and inhibitory spinal reflex arcs (inhibition) studied among muscles in the human upper limb (homonymous facilitation mediated by group Ia afferents and homonymous inhibition mediated by group Ib afferents are omitted). The facilitation is illustrated on the motoneuron's left, the inhibition on the right. DE: musculus (m.) deltoideus (anterior fibers), BB: m. biceps brachii, TB: m. triceps brachii, BR: m. brachioradialis, PT: m. pronator teres, PL: m. palmaris longus, ECR: m. flexor carpi radialis, FCU: m. flexor carpi ulnaris, ECR: mm. extensor carpi radialis longus and brevis, ECU: m. extensor carpi ulnaris, FDS: m. flexor digitorum superficialis, ED: m. extensor digitorum, MIH: hand muscles innervated by the median nerve, UIH: hand muscles innervated by the ulnar nerve, TM: thenar muscles, HTM: hypothnar muscles, FDI: m. interosseus dorsalis prima, Abbreviations in this as well as Figs. 2-7.

among synergistic muscles (Naito, 2003, 2004; Pierrot-Deseilligny et al., 1981; Tanaka, 1989). However, since PT and ECR are not synergistic, the functional significance of the facilitation is still unclear. This chapter describes the significance elucidated by studies using an electromyography (EMG) and electrical neuromuscular stimulation (ENS).

Functional Significance of Facilitation Between the Pronator Teres and Extensor Carpi Radialis in Humans:
Studies with Electromyography and Electrical Neuromuscular Stimulation

261

2. EMG study

Observations of activities of two muscles during repetitive movements must reveal activation of facilitation or inhibition between them. The facilitation must be active during co-contraction of the muscles and the inhibition must be during alternating or reciprocal contraction between the muscles. Since PT belongs to forearm pronators and ECR (ECRL, ECRB) to wrist extensors, activities of the muscles during repetitive movements of dynamic forearm pronation/supination, and those of static (isometric) wrist extension and dynamic wrist extension/flexion were studied using EMG.

For EMG recording, bipolar intramuscular electrodes made of teflon-coated stainless steel wire (75 μm in diameter, SUS 316, AM system, Carlsborg WA, USA) with distance of about 4 mm were used (Basmajian & Deluca, 1985; Fujii et al., 2007; Naito et al., 1998b; Perotto, 1994). The electrodes were implanted percutaneously into the muscles with 25 gauge-injection needles (Naito et al., 1998b, Riek et al., 2000). A wet bandage was put round the shoulder and used as reference. EMGs were amplified, band pass filtered (10-1,000 Hz), and sampled at 2,048 Hz. Then they were integrated (rectified and averaged) with an EMG integration program (Multi-Computer System, Giga Tex Co., Osaki, Japan).

2.1 The repetitive movements of dynamic forearm pronation/supination

EMGs of m biceps brachii (BB), PT, ECRL, ECRB, m. extensor carpi ulnalis (ECU), and m. flexor carpi ulnaris (FCU) were recorded in five normal subjects (male, age range 23-46 years). Movements tested were repetitive movements of dynamic forearm pronation/supination between the maximum prone (90 degrees of pronatioon) and spine positions (90 degrees of supination) with maintenance of the wrist neutral position (0 degrees of flexion/extension, 0 degrees of adduction/abduction). The subject sat on a chair with the shoulder joint flexed to 0 degrees of flexion and the elbow joint flexed to 90 degrees of flexion (Fig. 2A). In order to obtain adequate EMGs of the muscles (Basmajian and Deluca, 1985; Naito et al., 1998b), a belt weighing 1.0-2.0 kg was wound around the hand (palm) as a load. The movements were pictured with three digital video cameras (NW-GS 100, Panasonic, Tokyo, Japan) (anterior, superior, and medial aspects). Trajectories of the styloid process of the radius during the movements were traced using a 3-D-position sensor (3DPS) system (Liberty, POLHEMUS, USA), which delivered coordinate (x, y, z). A terminal probe of the 3DPS system was put on the skin of the styloid process with adhesive tape. Lissajou's curves (trajectories in the coronary plane) was drawn with the data (x, y) using a 2-D Lissajou presentation program (RO299-4588G, Gigatex, Osaki, Japan). Video pictures and data of the 3DPS system were fed into a simultaneous recording system of digital video pictures and electric signals (The Teraview, Gigatex, Osaki, Japan) with EMGs (Sagae et al., 2010; Sato et al., 2007).

During the movements, BB showed activities increasing and decreasing and PT, ECRL, and ECRB parallel activities decreasing and increasing at the supination and pronation phases, respectively, in all the five subjects (Fig. 2B, C). These fluctuations resulted in peaks and troughs of BB activities, and troughs and peaks of PT, ECRL, and ECRB activities at the maximum supination and pronation, respectively (Table 1). ECU showed parallel activities to PT, ECRL, and ECRB activities in all the subjects and those to BB activities (Fig. 2C) in two subjects. Peaks of the parallel activities of the latter were much lower than those of the former. FCU showed parallel activities to BB activities in three subjects (Fig 2B). In one subject, large and regular activities of which peaks followed the peaks of BB activities and small irregular activities were observed (Fig. 2C). In the remaining one subject, FCU showed no activities during the movements.

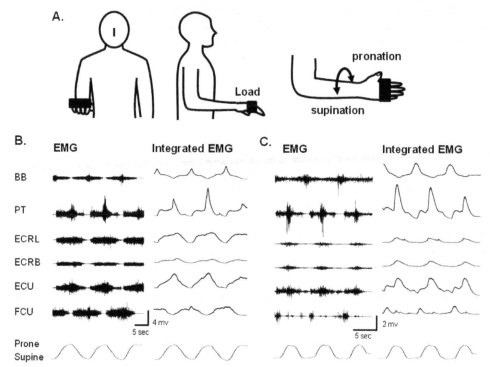

Fig. 2. An electromyographic (EMG) study of repetitive movements of dynamic forearm pronation/supination with maintenance of wrist neutral position in normal human subjects. **A**: The posture of the subject. During the experiment, the subject sits on a chair and keeps the shoulder joint at 0 degrees of flexion/extension, adduction/abduction, and external/internal rotation, the elbow joint at 90 degrees of flexion, and the wrist joint at 0 degrees of flexion/extension and adduction/abduction (neutral position). In order to evoke adequate EMG activities, a belt weighing 1.0-2.0 kg is surrounded around the hand. **B, C**: EMGs of BB, PT, ECRL, ECRB, ECU, and FCU during the movements in two subjects. The bottom solid lines indicate changes in the position of the forearm. Note that parallel activities of ECRL, ECRB, and PT increasing and decreasing at the pronation and supination phases, respectively, are observed in both the subjects.

Among BB, PT, ECR (ECRL, ECRB), ECU, and FCU in humans, facilitation between PT and ECR (Nakano et al., 2005, 2006), and from ECR to BB (Cavallari & Katz, 1989) and inhibition between BB and PT (Miyasaka et al., 1996; Naito et al., 1998a), and from BB to FCU (Cavallari et al., 1992) have been studied (Fig. 1). The EMG study showed that activities of BB increased and decreased and those of PT and ECR decreased and increased at the supination and pronation phases, respectively, in all the five subjects. This observation suggests that reciprocal contraction between BB and PT, and BB and ECR, and co-contraction of PT and ECR occur during the movements. The inhibition between BB and PT

Functional Significance of Facilitation Between the Pronator Teres and Extensor Carpi Radialis in Humans:
Studies with Electromyography and Electrical Neuromuscular Stimulation

263

	Peaks		Troughs	
	MaxS	MaxP	MaxS	MaxP
BB	5	0	0	5
PT	0	5	5	0
ECRL	0	5	5	0
ECRB	0	5	5	0
ECU	0	5	5	0
FCU	3	0	0	4

MaxS: the maximum supination, MaxP: the maximum pronation, BB: musculus (m.) biceps brachii, PT: m. pronator teres, ECRL: m. extensor carpi radialis longus, ECRB: m. extensor carpi radialis brevis, ECU: m. extensor carpi ulnaris, FCU: m. flexor carpi ulnaris, Abbreviations in this as well as Tables 2, 3.

Table 1. Peaks and troughs of activities of muscles during repetitive movements of dynamic forearm pronation/supination with maintenance of the wrist neutral position in five subjects.

(Miyasaka et al., 1996; Naito et al., 1998a) must be active during the reciprocal contraction and the facilitation between PT and ECR (Nakano et al., 2005, 2006) must be during the co-contraction. The facilitation must work effectively for the parallel activities increasing at the pronation phase. The facilitation from ECR to BB (Cavallari & Katz, 1989) seems to be inactive during the movement. In the EMG study, parallel activities of ECU to PT and ECR activities and BB activities were seen in all and two subjects, respectively. The parallel activities of the latter were much smaller than those of the former. These results suggest that co-contraction of PT, ECR, and ECU, and reciprocal contraction between BB and ECU occur during the movement. The EMG study also showed that parallel activities of FCU to BB activities were observed in three subjects and activities of FCU of which peaks followed the peaks of BB activities in one subject. This observation suggests that co-contraction of BB and FCU, and reciprocal contraction between FCU and PT, and FCU and ECR occur during the movements. The inhibition from BB to FCU (Cavallari et al., 1992) seems to be inactive during the movements. Observations of the co-contraction and reciprocal contraction suggest a possibility that facilitation between PT and ECU, and ECR and ECU, and inhibition between PT and FCU, ECR and FCU, and ECU and FCU exist in humans. Further studies are required to elucidate existences of the facilitation and inhibition.

2.2 The repetitive movements of static wrist extension and dynamic wrist extension/flexion

EMGs of PT, ECRL, ECRB, and FCR were recorded in twelve normal human subjects (male 9, female 3, age range 20-40 years) (Fujii et al., 2007). EMGs were fed into a data recorder (RECTI-HORIZ-8K, NEC, Tokyo, Japan) and pen recorder (RCD-928, Shinko, Tokyo, Japan). Movements tested were repetitive movements of static (isometric) wrist extension and dynamic wrist flexion/extension in the prone (about 80 degrees of pronation), semiprone (neutral), and supine positions (about 80 degrees of supination) of the forearm (Fig. 3A). The subject sat on a chair and put the forearm on an experimental table with the shoulder joint flexed to 0-20 degrees of flexion and the elbow joint flexed to 70-90 degrees of flexion (Fig. 3A). In the movements of the static wrist extension, the subject made an effort to extend the wrist in the position of 0-20 degrees of extension against resistance for about 5 sec. The resistance was produced by the experimenter's hand. The hand pressed the dorsum of the subject's hand to prevent the wrist from extending. The effort was performed 3-5 times at interval of about 5 sec. In the movements of the dynamic wrist flexion/extension, the subject performed a to-and-fro motion from the maximum flexion to the maximum extension of the wrist 5 times for about 25 sec. Angular changes of the wrist in flexion/extension direction were measured using an electrogoniometer (PH510, Denkikeisoku Hanbai, Tokyo, Japan). Data of the angular changes were fed into the data recorder and pen recorder with EMGs.

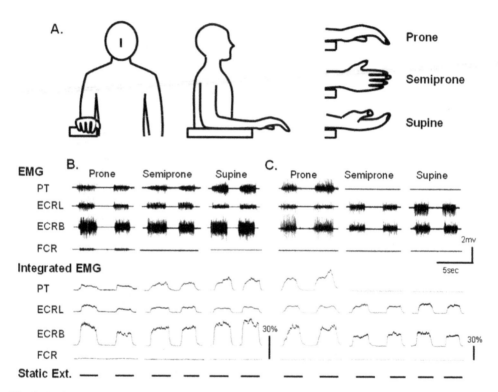

Fig. 3. An EMG study of repetitive movements of static (isometric) wrist extension with maintenance of the forearm in the prone, semiprone (neutral), and supine positions in normal human subjects. **A**: The posture of the subject. During the experiment, the subject sits on a chair and puts the pronated, semipronated, and supinated forearm on an experimental table with the shoulder joint at 0-20 degrees of flexion/extension, 0 degrees of adduction/abduction, and external/internal rotation, the elbow joint at 70-90 degrees of flexion. Static wrist extension is performed against the resistance produced by the experimaner's hand. **B, C**: EMGs of ECRL, ECRB, PT, and FCR during the movements in two subjects. The bottom thick lines indicate the period of the extension. Parallel activities of PT, ECRL, and ECRB are observed in the prone, semiprone, and supine positions in one subject (**B**) and in the prone position in another (**C**). Calibration bars for integrated EMGs: a percentage of the amplitude produced by the maximum contraction. Reproduced with permission from Fujii et al. (2007).

Functional Significance of Facilitation Between the Pronator Teres and Extensor Carpi Radialis in Humans: Studies with Electromyography and Electrical Neuromuscular Stimulation

265

During the movements of the static wrist extension, ECRL and ECRB showed activities in the prone, semiprone, and supine positions of the forearm in all the twelve subjects (Table 2, Fig. 3B, C). Slight or no activities were seen in FCR. PT showed activities in the prone, semiprone, and supine positions in all, eight, and eight subjects, respectively. The activities were parallel with those of ECRL and ECRB. In the remainders, PT showed no activities during the movements.

During the movements of the dynamic wrist flexion/extension, activities of ECRL and ECRB increased at the extension phase and those of FCR at the flexion phase in all the twelve subjects (Fig. 4). Therefore peaks of the activities of ECRL and ECRB appeared at the extension phase and those of FCR at the flexion phase (Table 3). Activities of PT increased at the extension phase in all, eight and five subjects, respectively, and at the flexion phase in zero, four, and five subjects, respectively, in the prone, semiprone, and supine positions. In three subjects (YE, SY, SK in Table 3), the activities increased at both the extension and flexion phases in the semiprone and supine positions. The activities of PT at the extension and flexion phases were parallel with those of ECRL and ECRB, and FCR (Fig. 4A), respectively.

Subject	Prone				Semiprone				Supine			
	ECRL	ECRB	PT	FCR	ECRL	ECRB	PT	FCR	ECRL	ECRB	PT	FCR
K.S.	+	+	+	−	+	+	+	+	+	+	−	−
Y.E.	+	+	+	−	+	+	−	−	+	+	−	−
H.F.	+	+	+	−	+	+	−	−	+	+	−	−
M.S.	+	+	+	−	+	+	−	−	+	+	−	−
K.S.	+	+	+	−	+	+	+	−	+	+	+	−
S.Y.	+	+	+	+	+	+	+	−	+	+	+	−
H.T.	+	+	+	−	+	+	+	+	+	+	+	−
Y.K.	+	+	+	−	+	+	−	+	+	+	+	−
A.M.	+	+	+	−	+	+	+	−	+	+	+	+
Y.U.	+	+	+	−	+	+	+	−	+	+	+	−
S.K.	+	+	+	+	+	+	+	+	+	+	+	−
Y.W.	+	+	+	−	+	+	+	−	+	+	+	−

FCR: m. flexor carpi radialis. Abbreviations in this as well as Table 3.

Table 2. Activities of muscles during repetitive movements of static wrist extension in twelve subjects.

Among PT, ECR, and FCR in humans, inhibition between ECR and FCR (Aymard et al., 1995; Baldissera et al., 1983; Day et al., 1984), and facilitation between PT and ECR (Nakano et al., 2005, 2006) have been studied (Fig. 1). In the EMG study, during the repetitive movements of the dynamic wrist flexion/extension ECR (ECRL and ECRB) and FCR showed increments of activities at the extension and flexion phases, respectively, regardless of the positions of the forearm in all the subjects. Therefore alternating contraction between the muscles occurred during the movements. The inhibition between ECR and FCR (Aymard et al., 1995; Baldissera et al., 1983; Day et al., 1984) must be active during the alternating contraction. In the EMG study, in the prone, semiprone, and supine positions of the forearm, PT and ECR showed parallel activities during the movements of the static wrist extension in all, eight, and eight subjects and at the extension phase of the movements of the dynamic wrist extension/flexion in all, eight and five subjects, respectively. Therefore co-contraction of the muscles occurred during the wrist extension movements at least with the prone forearm. The facilitation between PT and ECR (Nakano et al., 2005, 2006) must be

Subject	Prone				Semiprone				Supine			
	ECRL	ECRB	PT	FCR	ECRL	ECRB	PT	FCR	ECRL	ECRB	PT	FCR
K.S.	E	E	E	F	E	E		F	E	E		F
Y.E.	E	E	E	F	E	E	E F	F	E	E	E F	F
H.F.	E	E	E	F	E	E		F	E	E		F
M.S.	E	E	E	F	E	E	E F	F	E	E	F	F
K.S.	E	E	E	F	E	E	E	F	E	E		F
S.Y.	E	E	E	F	E	E	E F	F	E	E	E F	F
H.T.	E	E	E	F	E	E		F	E	E	F	F
Y.K.	E	E	E	F	E	E	E	F	E	E	E	F
A.M.	E	E	E	F	E	E	E	F	E	E		F
Y.U.	E	E	E	F	E	E		F	E	E		F
S.K.	E	E	E	F	E	E	E F	F	E	E	E F	F
Y.W.	E	E	E	F	E	E	E	F	E	E	E	F

E: extension phase, F: flexion phase

Table 3. Peaks of activities of muscles during repetitive movements of dynamic wrist flexion/extension in twelve subjects.

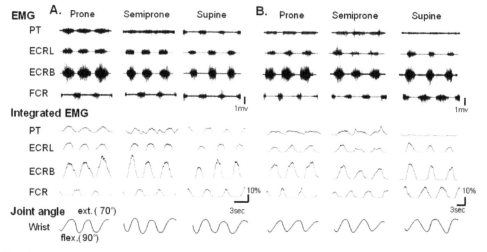

Fig. 4. An EMG study of repetitive movements of dynamic wrist flexion/extension with maintenance of the forearm in the prone, semiprone (neutral), and supine positions in normal human subjects. The subject performed the movements in the posture as well as Fig. 3A. **A, B**: EMGs of ECRL, ECRB, PT, and FCR during the movements in two subjects. The bottom trace represents the position of the wrist in flexion/extension direction. Parallel activities of PT, ECRL, and ECRB are seen at the extension phase in the prone and semiprone positions in both subjects (**A, B**). PT and FCR show parallel activities at the flexion phase in the supine and semiprone positions in one subject (**A**). Calibration bars for integrated EMGs: a percentage of the amplitude produced by the maximum contraction. Reproduced with permission from Fujii et al. (2007).

active during the co-contraction. In the EMG study, during the movements of the dynamic wrist flexion/extension parallel activities of PT and FCR were seen at the flexion phase in the semiprone and supine positions in four and five subjects, respectively. This observation

Functional Significance of Facilitation Between the Pronator Teres and Extensor Carpi Radialis in Humans:
Studies with Electromyography and Electrical Neuromuscular Stimulation

267

of co-contraction seems to indicate existence of facilitation between PT and FCR. It therefore seems likely that the facilitation between PT and ECR is activated with pronating the forearm and that between PT and FCR is with supinating the forearm. Further studies are required to elucidate influence of the forearm position on the facilitation.

3. ENS study

Motions of the forearm and wrist produced by ENS to PT and ECRL were examined in the same twelve subjects of the EMG study in 2.2 (Fujii et al., 2007). The subject sat on a chair the shoulder joint flexed to 0-20 degrees of flexion and the elbow joint flexed to 70-90 degrees of flexion as well as in EMG study in 2.2 (Fig. 3A). The forearm was put on an experimental table in the prone, semiprone, and supine positions. For electrical stimulation, monopolar electrodes made of teflon-coated stainless steel wire (above-mentioned product) were implanted percutaneously into each motor point of ECRL and PT with 27 gauge injection-needles (Fujii et al., 2007; Naito et al., 1994, 2002; Sagae et al., 2010). A guide needle of a 25 gauge spinal-needle (length: 89 mm, Top Co., Tokyo, Japan) was percutaneously inserted into the subcutaneous tissue along to the lateral intermuscular septum of the arm and used as reference. Before the implantation, locations of the motor points were examined by electrical stimulation with surface electrodes. During the implantation, electrical rectangular pulses (duration: 0.2 ms, amplitude: -20-0 V, frequency: 1 or 20 Hz) were occasionally delivered to the muscles through the wire electrodes and contraction of individual muscles was confirmed by inspecting and palpating the tendon or belly of them (Albright & Linburg, 1978; Basmajian, 1982; Standring, 2005; Yoshida, 1994). Also it was carefully checked that no contraction of any other muscles was induced by the stimulation. For the ENS study, electrical rectangular pulses (duration: 0.2 ms, amplitude: -20 - 0 V, frequency: 20 Hz) were delivered using a computer-controlled multi-channel functional electrical stimulation (FES) system which we had developed to restore motor functions of paralyzed extremities with intramuscular wire electrodes (Handa et al., 1989; Hoshimiya et al., 1989). EMGs of ECRL and PT were recorded with two pairs of surface electrodes (Ag/AgCl Paste Applied with PVC Tape, Vitrode, NIHON KODEN, Tokyo, Japan), which were put on the central part of the contracted muscle belly longitudinally with the distance of about 1 cm. EMGs were amplified and band pass filtered (10-350 Hz). A wet bandage put round the shoulder was used as reference. Stimulation intensities (voltage) for the motor threshold (MT) and maximum contraction (MC) in individual muscles were determined by monitoring EMGs (motor wave) of the muscles and palpating the belly and tendon of them. In order to stimulate each of the muscles with the intensity between MT and MC, the voltage data for MT and MC were put into the FES system. Before ENS, the examined forearm was in the prone, semiprone, and supine positions. Then motions of the forearm and wrist induced by ENS were taken video with a digital video system (NV-MX2500, Panasonic, Tokyo). Angular changes of the motions of the wrist in flexion/extension direction and the forearm in pronation/supination direction were measured with the electrogoniometers mentioned above. A motion of the wrist in abduction/adduction direction was checked with video pictures. During ENS, EMGs of PT and ECRL were recorded with the pairs of the surface electrodes mentioned above. Data of the angular changes and EMGs were fed into the data recorder and pen recorder. ENS to ECRL was examined in all the twelve subjects. Since ENS to PT resulted in activation of PT and the other muscles innervated by the median nerve, i.e. FCR, m. palmaris longus, in one subject, it was examined in the remaining eleven subjects. The stimulus intensity was increased linearly from MT to MC for 4-5 sec.

ENS to PT induced a motion of forearm pronation from the prone, semiprone, and supine positions to the maximum pronation (90 degrees of pronation) in all the eleven subjects. ENS to ECRL induced motions of wrist extension to the maximum extention (70 degrees of extension) and abduction (radial flexion) to 5-20 degrees of abduction regardless of the positions of the forearm in all the twelve subjects. When the forearm was pronated before ENS, 30-80 degrees supination of the forearm from the prone position was induced in all the twelve subjects (Fig. 5).

Combined ENS to PT and ECRL was examined in the eleven subjects. An increase of the stimulus intensity of ENS to PT from MT to MC fixed the forearm in the maximum pronation (Fig. 6). Then an increase for ENS to ECRL from MT to MC resulted in motions of wrist extension to the maximum extension and abduction to 5-20 degrees of abduction without a motion of supination in all the eleven subjects. In this situation, a decrease of the intensity of ENS to PT from MC to MT resulted in a motion of 40–90 degrees supination from the maximum pronation while holding the wrist extension and abduction. Then the increase of the intensity of ENS to PT from MT to MC resulted in a motion of pronation to the maximum pronation while holding the extension and abduction (Fig. 6D).

4. Functional significance of the facilitation between PT and ECR

The ENS study showed that ENS to PT produced forearm pronation from the prone, semiprone, and supine positions to the maximum prone position and that to ECRL wrist extension to the maximum extension and abduction to 5-20 degrees of abduction in the forearm prone, semiprone, and supine positions in all subject. These results suggest that PT acts as a forearm pronator and ECRL as a wrist extensor and abductor independent of the forearm position. The EMG study of the repetitive movements of dynamic forearm pronation/supination with maintenance of the wrist neutral position showed parallel activities of PT, ECRL, and ECRB increasing and decreasing at the pronation and supination phases, respectively, in all subject. This result suggests that the facilitation between PT and ECR is active during the co-contraction and works effectively at the pronation phase of the movements. Since at the pronation phase pronating force of PT must be used to pronate the forearm and extending and abducting force of ECR must be to support the weight of the hand, the facilitation seems to be convenient for maintenance of the wrist position.

The ENS study showed that ENS to ECRL produced 30-80 degrees forearm supination from the prone position in all subject. This result suggests that ECRL act as not only a wrist extensor and abductor but also a forearm supinator when the forearm is in the prone position. Hence forearm supination from the prone position should be added to one of the actions of ECRL. The EMG study showed parallel activities of PT, ECRL, and ECRB during the movements of static wrist extension and at the extension phase of the movements of dynamic wrist extension/flexion in the prone position of the forearm in all subject. This result suggests that co-contraction of PT and ECR occurs during both static and dynamic wrist extension movements at least with the prone forearm. The facilitation must be active during the co-contraction. Since during the wrist extension movements extending and abducting force of ECRL must be used to extend the wrist and pronating force of PT must be to counteract supinating force of ECRL, the facilitation seems to be very convenient for maintenance of the forearm position. Actually the ENS study confirmed that combined ENS to PT and ECRL resulted in wrist extension and abduction with maintenance of the forearm prone position. The results of the EMG and ENS studies suggest that the facilitation is between antagonistic muscles. It is of no ordinary type.

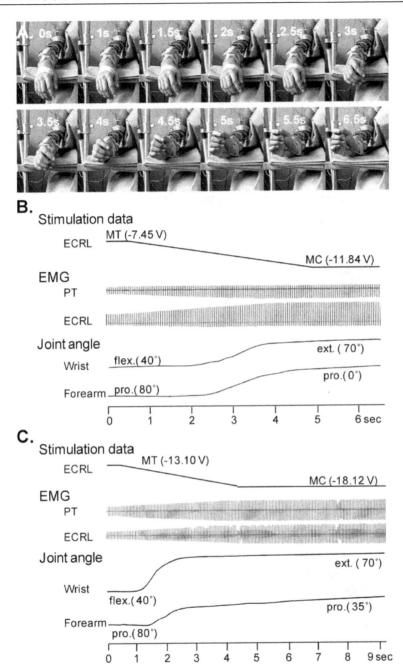

Fig. 5. An electrical neuromuscular stimulation (ENS) study: Motions produced by ENS to ECRL in normal human subjects. **A**: Pictures showing a sequence of the motions in a subject at 0.5-1 s interval. Before ENS (0 s), the forearm is in the prone position. Motions of wrist

extension and abduction (radial flexion), and forearm supination are induced (1-6.5 s). **B, C:**
Results in two subjects, of which one (**B**) is of the subject in **A**. Prior to ENS, the forearm in
the prone position. The stimulation intensities increased linearly from the motor threshold
(MT) to the maximum contraction (MC) for 4.5 s in **B** and 4 s in **C**. Motions of wrist
extension from 40 degrees of flexion to 70 degrees of extension and forearm supination from
80 to 0 degrees of pronation are induced in **B** and those of extension from 50 degrees of
flexion to 70 degrees of extension and supination from 80 to 35 degrees of pronation are in
C. No voluntary contraction of ECRL and PT are observed in EMG in both subjects (**B, C**).
Abbreviations in this as well as Fig. 6. Reproduced with permission from Fujii et al. (2007).

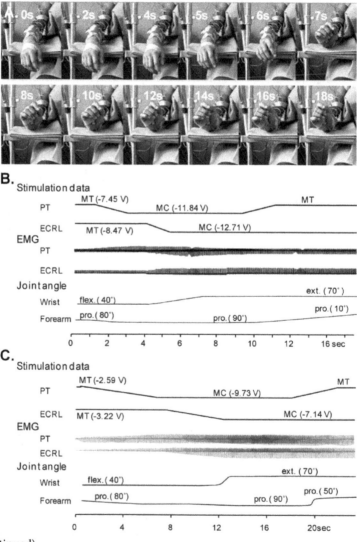

Fig. 6. (Continued)

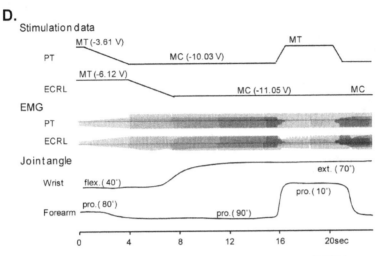

Fig. 6. An ENS study: Motions produced by a combined ENS to PT and ECRL in normal human subjects. **A**: Pictures showing a sequence of the motions in one subject at 1-2 s interval. Before ENS (0 s), the forearm is in the prone position. ENS to PT induces a motion of pronation to the mamimum pronation of the forearm (1-4 s). Then ENS to ECRL produces a motion of wrist extension and abduction with maintenance of the maximum pronation (4-8 s). Then a reduction of ENS to PT results in a motion of supination with maintenance of the extension and abduction (8-18 s). **B-D**: Results in three subjects, of which one (**B**) is of the subject in **A**. In all the three subjects (**B-D**), an increase of the stimulation intensity of ENS to PT from MT to MC induces a motion of pronation from 80 to 90 degrees of pronation (from the prone position to the maximum pronation). Then an increase of the intensity of ENS to ECRL from MT to MC induces a motion of wrist extension from 40 degrees of flexion to 70 degrees of extension (the maximum extension) with maintenance of the maximum pronation. Then a decrease of the intensity of ENS to PT from MC to MT results in a motion of supination from the maximum supination to 10 (**B**), 50 (**C**), and 10 degrees of pronation (**D**) with maintenance of the maximum extension. In one subject (**D**), then an increase of the intensity of ENS to PT induces a motion of pronation to the maximum pronation with maintenance of the maximum extension. No voluntary contraction is observed in EMG in all the subjects (**B-D**). Reproduced with permission from Fujii et al. (2007).

5. Effects of wrist extension and flexion on forearm supinating force

It is known that FCR acts as not only a wrist flexor and abductor but also a forearm pronator (American Society for Surgery of the Hand, 2011; Basmajian, 1982). The ENS study has shown that ECRL acts as a wrist extensor and abductor and a forearm supinator when the forearm is in the prone position (Fujii et al., 2007). It therefore is support an idea that forearm supinating force is increased and decreased by wrist extension and flexion, respectively.

Our previous study showed effects of wrist extension and flexion on forearm supinating force in humans (Otaki et al., 2009). In our study, the forces produced by maximal supination with the wrist relaxed (R-Sup), maximally flexed (F-Sup), and maximally extended (E-Sup) in the forearm 90° (prone), 60°, 30°, and 0° pronated (neutral) positions were measured in eight normal human subjects (male 7, female 1, age range 20-41 years). Also activities of BB, which acts as an elbow flexor and forearm supinator, FCR, and ECR (ECRL and ECRB) were recorded with EMG using surface electrodes. In the EMG study, FCR and ECR respectively showed activities during wrist flexion and extension (Fig. 7A, B). BB showed activities increasing concomitantly with increased the force. Usually, E-Sup produced larger BB activities than R-Sup and F-Sup; and F-Sup decreased FCR activities and increased ECR activities. In the force study, the respective force of R-, F-, and E-Sup decreased with changing position from prone to neutral. Assuming the force of R-Sup in each position as 100%, that of E-Sup was 163±20%(mean ±S.D.), 142±17%, 134±15%, and 118±23%, and those of F-Sup was 81±7%, 90±14%, 78±13%, and 80±10%, respectively, in the prone, P60°, P30°, and neutral positions (Fig. 7C). In every position, the force of E-Sup was larger and that of F-Sup was smaller than that of R-Sup. The increment of the force of E-Sup decreased with changing the position from prone to neutral.

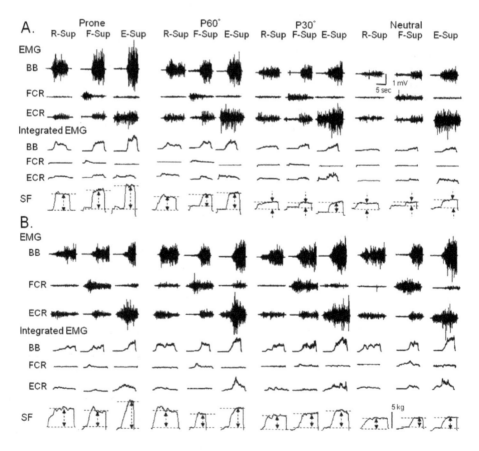

Fig. 7. (Continued)

Functional Significance of Facilitation Between the Pronator Teres and Extensor Carpi Radialis in Humans:
Studies with Electromyography and Electrical Neuromuscular Stimulation

273

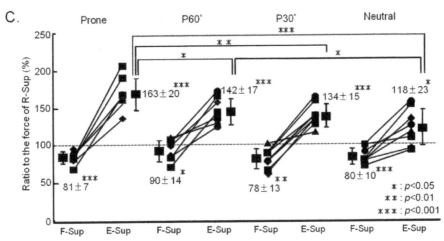

Fig. 7. Effects of wrist extension and flexion on forearm supinating force (SF) in normal human subjects. **A, B**: EMGs of BB, FCR, and ECR, and SF during maximal forearm supination with the wrist relaxed (R-Sup), maximally flexed (F-Sup), and maximally extended (E-Sup) in the forearm 90 degrees (Prone), 60 degrees (P60°), 30 degrees (P30°), and 0 degrees pronated (Neutral) positions in two normal human subjects. SF is indicated by the length of double broken arrow or the distance between two broken arrows. In every forearm position, E-Sup produces larger BB activities than R- and F-Sup. A decrease of FCR activities and an increase of ECR activities are observed during F-Sup. **C**: A graph showing ratio (%) of SF of F- and E-Sup to that of R-Sup in the forearm Prone, P60°, P30°, and Neutral positions in eight subjects. Individual data of the ratio of SF, and average and standard deviation are illustrated in the graph. In every position, SF of E-Sup is larger and that of F-Sup is smaller than that of R-Sup. Note that the increment of SF of E-Sup decreases with the forearm position from Prone to Neutral. Reproduced with permission from Otaki et al. (2009).

The results of the force study suggest that the supinating force is reinforced by the extension and weakened by the flexion and the reinforcement effect decreases with supination of the forearm. Since reflex arcs of facilitation from ECR to BB, inhibition between FCR and ECR, and from BB to FCR exist in humans (Fig. 1) (Aymard et al., 1995; Baldissera et al., 1983; Cavallari & Katz, 1989; Cavallari et al, 1992), the results of the EMG study suggest that the effects result not only from actions of the muscles but also from activations of the reflex arcs. Our recent study further showed an increase and decrease of forearm pronating force by wrist flexion and extension, respectively, in humans (Sato et al., 2011).

6. Summary

The functional significance of facilitatory spinal reflex arcs (facilitation) between musculus (m.) pronator teres (PT) and m. ectensor carpi radialis (ECR; ECR longus: ECRL, ECR brevis: ECRB) in humans was studied using an electromyography (EMG) and electrical neuromuscular stimulation (ENS). The EMG study of dynamic forearm pronation/ supination movements with maintenance of the wrist neutral position (PS-movements) showed parallel activities (co-contraction) of PT and ECR increasing and decreasing at the pronation and supination phases, respectively. The facilitation must be active during the co-contraction and work effectively at the pronation phase. The EMG study of static and dynamic wrist extension movements with the prone forearm (WE-movements) also showed co-contraction of the muscles. The facilitation must be active during the co-contraction. The ENS study showed that ENS to PT produced forearm pronation and that to ECRL wrist extension and abduction independent of the forearm position. Since at the pronation phase of the PS-movements pronating force of PT must be used to pronate the forearm and extending and abducting force of ECR must be to support the weight of the hand, the facilitation seems to be convenient for maintenance of the wrist position. The ENS study also showed that ENS to ECRL produced forearm supination from the prone position. This result suggests that ECRL acts as not only a wrist extensor and abductor but also a forearm supinator when the forearm is in the peone position. Since during the WE-movements extending force of ECR must be used to extend the wrist and pronating force of PT must be to counteract supinating force of ECR, the facilitation seems to be convenient for maintenance of the forearm position. The results of EMG and ENS studies suggest that the facilitation is between antagonistic muscles. Finally, an increase and decrease of forearm supinating force respectively by wrist extension and flexion were briefly described.

7. Acknowledgment

The authors thank Dr. Takuji Miyasaka, Dr. Shinji Kobayashi, Dr. Katuhiro Shinozaki, Dr. Masaaki Sagae, Dr. Aya Narita, Mr. Makoto Nagamuma, Mr. Hiroto Kobayashi, Mr. Wataru Hashizume, Ms. Saori Yoshida, Mr. Katsuhiko Kato, and Mr. Inazo Eguchi for their excellent assistance. Thanks are also tendered to students of Yamagata University School of Medicine and Yamagata Prefectural University of Health Sciences for their helpful cooperation. This study was supported, in part, by a Grant-in-Aid from Japanese Ministry of Education, Science, Sport and Culture (17590146) and by grants from the Yamagata Health Support Society Foundation.

8. References

Albright, J.A. & Linburg, R.M. (1978) Common variations of the radial extensors. *J Hand Surg*, Vol. 3, pp.134-138, ISSN 1531-6564

American Society for Surgery of the Hand (2011) *The electric textbook of hand surgery. Anatomy of the hand. Muscles*. E-HAND. COM,
        http://www.eatonhand.cpm/hom/hom033.htm

Aymard, C.; Chia, L.; Katz R.; Lafitte, C. & Penicaud, A. (1995) Reciprocal inhibition between wrist flexors and extensors in man: a new set of interneurones? *J Physiol (Lond)*, Vol. 487, pp.221-235, ISSN 0022-3751

Baldissera, F.; Campadelli, P. & Cavallari, P. (1983) Inhibition of H-reflex in wrist flexors by group I afferents in the radial nerve. *Electromyogr Clin Neurophysiol*, Vol.23, pp.187-193, ISSN 0301-150X

Basmajian, J.V. (1982) *Primary Anatomy* (8th Ed.), Williams and Wilkins, ISBN 0-683-00550-2, Baltimore, pp 150-164

Basmajian, J.V. & Deluca, C.J. (1985) *Muscle Alive: Their Functions Revealed by Electromyography* (5th Ed.), Williams and Wilkins, ISBN 0-683-00414-X, Baltimore, pp 265-289

Functional Significance of Facilitation Between the Pronator Teres and Extensor Carpi Radialis in Humans:
Studies with Electromyography and Electrical Neuromuscular Stimulation

275

Cavallari, P. & Katz, R. (1989) Pattern of projections of group I afferents from forearm muscles to motoneurones supplying biceps and triceps muscles in man. *Exp Brain Res*, Vol. 78, pp.465-478, ISSN 0014-4819

Cavallari, P.; Katz, R. & Penicaud, A. (1992) Patterns of projections of group I afferrents from elbow muscles to motoneurones supplying wrist muscles in man. *Exp Brain Res*, Vol. 91, pp. 311-319, ISSN 0014-4819

Creange, A.; Faist, M.; Katz, R. & Panicaud, A. (1992) Distributions of heteronymous Ia facilitation and recurrent inhibition in the human deltoid motor nucleus. *Exp. Brain Res*, Vol. 90, pp. 620-624, ISSN 0014-4819

Day, B.L.; Marsden, C.D.; Obeso, J.A. & Rorhwell, J.C. (1984) Reciprocal inhibition between the muscles of the human forearm. *J Physiol (Lond)*, Vol. 349, pp.519-534, ISSN 0022-3751

Fujii, H.; Kobayashi, S.; Shinozaki, K.; Naito, A.; Sato, T.; Miyasaka, T. & Shindo, M. (2001) Inhibitory projections of muscle afferents between the brachioradialis and flexor carpi radialis in humans. *Neurosci Res*, Suppl 25, S87, ISSN 0168-0102

Fujii, H.; Kobayashi, S.; Sato, T.; Shinozaki, K. & Naito, A. (2007) Co-contraction of the pronator teres and extensor carpi radialis during wrist extension movements in humans. *J Electromyogr Kinesiol*, Vol. 17, pp.80-89, ISSN 1050-6411

Handa, Y.; Hoshimiya, N.; Iguchi, Y. & Oda, T. (1989) Developments of percutaneous intramuscular electrode for multi-channel FES system. *IEEE Trans Biomed Eng*, Vol. 36; pp.705-710, ISSN0018-9294

Hoshimiya, N.; Naito, A.; Yajima, M. & Handa, Y. (1989) A multichannel FES system for the restoration of motor functions in high spinal cord injury patients: A respiration-controlled system for multijoint upper extremity, *IEEE Trans Biomed Eng*, Vol. 36; pp.754-760, ISSN0018-9294

Jenkins, D.B. (2008) *Hollinshead's Functional Anatomy of the Limbs and Back* (9th ed.), WB Saunders, ISBN 978-1-4160-4980-7, Philadelphia

Katz, R.; Penicaud, A. & Rossi, A. (1991) Reciprocal Ia inhibition between elbow flexors and extensors in the human. *J Physiol (Lond)*, Vol. 437; pp.269-286, ISSN 0022-3751

Kobayashi, S.; Naito, A.; Hayashi, M.; Ogino, T.; Fujii, H. & Tonosaki, A. (2000) Inhibitroy projections of muscle afferents from the brachioradialis to the flexor carpi radialis motoneurones in humans. *Acta Anat Nippon*, Vol. 76, p.130 (in Japanese), ISSN 0022-7722

Lourenço, G.; Iglesias, C. & Marchand-Pauvert, V. (2007) Effects produced in human arm and forearm motoneurones after electrical stimulation of ulnar and median nerves at wrist level. *Exp Brain Res*, Vol. 178, pp.267-284, ISSN 0014-4819

Marchand-Pauvert, V.; Nicolas, G. & Pierrot-Desilligny, E. (2000) Monosynaptic Ia projections from intrinsic hand muscles to forearm motoneurones in humans. *J Physiol (Lond)*, Vol. 525, pp.241-252, ISSN 0022-3751

Miyasaka, T.; Sun, Y.-J.; Naito, A.; Morita, H.; Shindo, M.; Shimizu, Y. & Yanagisawa, N. (1995) Reciprocal inhibition between biceps brachii and brachioradialis in the human. In abstract, *4th IBRO World Congress of Neuroscience*; Rapid Communications, Oxford New York, p.334

Miyasaka, T.; Sun, Y.-J.; Naito, A. & Shindo, M. (1996) Inhibition projections from the biceps brachii to the pronator teres motoneurones in the human. *Neurosci Res*, Suppl 20, S183, ISSN 0168-0102

Miyasaka, T.; Naito, A.; Morita, H.; Sun, Y.-J.; Chishima, M. & Shindo, M. (1998) Inhibitory neural connection from the brachioradialis to the pronator teres in human. *Neurosci Res*, Suppl 22, S159, ISSN 0168-0102

Miyasaka, T.; Naito, A.; Shindo, M.; Kobayashi, S.; Hayashi, M.; Shinozaki, K. & Chishima, M. (2007) Modulation of bracioradialis motoneuron excitabilities by group I fibers of the median nerve in humans. *Tohoku J Exp Med*, Vol. 212, pp.115-131, ISSN 0040-8727

Naito, A.; Handa, Y.; Handa, T.; Ichie, M.; Hoshimiya, N. & Shimizu, Y. (1994) Study on the elbow movement produced by functional electrical stimulation (FES). *Tohoku J Exp Med*, Vol. 174, pp.343-349, ISSN 0040-8727

Naito, A.; Shindo, M.; Miyasaka, T.; Sun, Y.-J. & Morita, H. (1996) Inhibitory projections from brachioradialis to biceps brachii in human. *Exp Brain Res*, Vol. 111, pp.483-486, ISSN 0014-4819

Naito, A.; Shindo, M.; Miyasaka, T.; Sun, Y.-J.; Momoi, H. & Chishima, M. (1998a) Inhibitory projections from pronator teres to biceps brachii motoneurones in human. *Exp Brain Res*, Vol. 121, pp.99-102, ISSN 0014-4819

Naito, A.; Sun, Y.-J.; Yajima, M.; Fukamachi, H. & Ushikoshi, K. (1998b) Electromyographic study of the elbow flexors and extensors in a motion of forearm pronation/supination while maintaining elbow flexion in humans. *Tohoku J Exp Med*, Vol. 186, pp.267-277, ISSN 0040-8727

Naito, A.; Shinozaki, K.; Kobayashi, S.; Fujii, H.; Sato, T.; Miyasaka, T. & Shindo, M. (2001) Excitatory projections of muscle afferents between the bracchioradialis and extensor carpi radialis in humans. *Neurosci Res*, Suppl 25, S87, ISSN 0168-0102

Naito, A.; Yajima, M.; Chishima, M. & Sun, Y.-J. (2002) A motion of forearm supination with maintenance of elbow flexion produced by electrical stimulation to two elbow flexors in humans. *J Electromyogr Kinesiol*, Vol. 12, pp.259-265, ISSN 1050-6411

Naito, A. (2003) Spinal mechanism for motor control: neural connections among muscles in the human upper limb. *Yamagata Med J*, Vol. 21, pp.155-169 (in Japanese) , ISSN 0288-030X

Naito, A. (2004) Electrophysiologircal studies of muscles in the human upper limb: the biceps brachii. *Anat Sci Int*, Vol. 79, pp.11-20, ISSN 1447-6959

Nakano, H.; Miyasaka, T.; Sagae, M.; Fujii, H.; Sato, T.; Suzuki, K.; Ogawa, K.; Shindo, M. & Naito, A. (2005) Facilitation from the pronator teres to extensor carpi radialis motoneurons in humans: Studies using a post-stimulus time-histogram technique. Acta Anat Nippon, 80 suppl, p.5, ISSN 0022-7722

Nakano, H.; Miyasaka, T.; Sagae, M.; Fujii, H.; Sato, T.; Suzuki, K.; Shindo, M.; Ogino, T. & Naito, A. (2006) Facilitation between pronator teres and extensor carpi radialis: Studies with a PSTH method. *Clin Neurophysiol*, Vol. 117, S160, ISSN 1388-2457

Ogawa, K.; Suzuk,i K.; Fujii, H.; Sato, T.; Nakano, H.; Sagae, M.; Miyasaka, T.; Naito, A. & Watanabe, H. (2005) Facilitation from thernar muscles to extensor carpi radialis in humans: A study using an electromyogram-averaging method with mechanical conditioning stimulation. *Yamagata Med J*, Vol. 23, pp.107-105 (in Japanese with English abstract and figure legends), ISSN 0288-030X

Otaki, R.; Sato, T.; Naganuma, M.; Suzuki, K.; Narita, A.; Sato, A.; Miyasaka, T.; Fujii, H. & Naito, A. (2009) Effects of wrist flexion and extension on forearm supination force.

Functional Significance of Facilitation Between the Pronator Teres and Extensor Carpi Radialis in Humans:
Studies with Electromyography and Electrical Neuromuscular Stimulation

277

Structure Function, Vol. 8, pp.13-18 (in Japanese with English abstract and figure legends), ISSN 1347-7145

Perotto, A.O. (1994) *Anatomical Guide for the Electromyographer: The Limb and Trunk* (3rd ed.), Charles C. Thomas, ISBN 0-398-05900-4, Springfield IL

Pierrot-Deseilligny, E.; Morin, C.; Bergego, C. & Tankov, N. (1981) Pattern of group I fiber projections from ankle flexor and extensor muscles in man. *Exp Brain Res*, Vol. 42:, pp.337-350, ISSN 0014-4819

Pierrot-Deseilligny, E. & Mazevet, D. (2000) The monosynaptic reflex: a tool to investigate motor control in humans. Interest and limits. *Neurophysiol Clin*, Vol. 30, pp.67-80, ISSN 0987-7053

Riek, S.; Carson, R.C. & Wright, A. (2000) A new technique for the selective recording of extensor carpi radialis longus and brevis EMG. *J Electromyogr Kinesiol*, Vol. 10, pp.249-253, ISSN 1050-6411

Rossi, A.; Decchi, B.; Zalaffi, A. & Mazzocchio, R. (1995) Group Ia non-reciprocal inhibition from wrist extensor to flexor motoneurones in humans. *Neurosci Lett*, Vol. 191, pp.205-207, ISSN 0304-3940

Rothwell, J. (1994) *Control of Human Voluntary Movement* (2nd ed.) Chapman & Hall, ISBN 0-412-47700-9, London, pp149–181

Sagae, M.; Suzuki, K.; Fujita, T.; Sotokawa, T.; Nakano, H.; Naganuma, M.; Narita, A.; Sato, T.; Fujii, H.; Ogino, T. & Naito, A. (2010) Strict actions of the human wrist extensors: A study with an electrical neuromuscular stimulation method. *J Electromyogr Kinesiol*, Vol. 20, pp.1178-1185, ISSN 1050-6411

Sato, T.; Fujii, H.; Naito, A.; Tonosaki, A.; Kobayashi, S.; Shinozaki, K.; Miyasaka, T. & Shindo, M. (2002) Inhibition of muscle afferents from the brachioradialis to triceps brachii motoneurones in humans: Central pathway. *Acta Anat Nippon*, Vol. 77 Suppl, H511, ISSN 0022-7722

Sato T, Suzuki K, Sotokawa T, Fujita T, Sagae M, Nakano H, Naganuma M, Fujii H, Kato K & Naito A (2007) Simultaneous recording system for digital video pictures and electric signals. *Structure Function*, Vol. 6, pp.3-8 (in Japanese with English abstract and figure legends), ISSN 1347-7145

Sato, T.; Sato, T.; Konishi, Y.; Naganuma, M.; Suzuki, K.; Narita, A.; Fujii, H.; Hashizume, W. & Naito, A. (2011) Effects of wrist flexion and extension on forearm pronation force. *Structure Function*, Vol. 9, pp.59-63 (in Japanese with English abstract and figure legends), ISSN 1347-7145

Shinozaki, K.; Naito, A.; Kobayashi, S.; Miyasaka, T.; Shindo, M. & Tonosaki, A. (2001) Pathways of facilitatory projections between the bracioradialis and extensor carpi radialis in humans. *Acta Anat Nippon*, Vol. 76, p.130 (in Japanese) , ISSN 0022-7722

Standring, S.; Ellis, H.; Healy, C.; Johnson, D. & Williams, A. (2005) *Gray's Anatomy* (39th ed.) Elsevier, Churchill Livingstone, ISBN 0-443-07168-3, Edinburgh, pp.879–880

Suzuki, K.; Nakano, H.; Sato, T.; Fujii, H.; Ogawa, K.; Watanabe, H. & Naito, A. (2005) Facilitation from the median nerve innervating hand muscles to extensor carpi radialis in humans: A study using an electromyogram-averaging method. *Yamagata Med J*, Vol. 23, pp.59-68 (in Japanese with English abstract and figure legends), ISSN 0288-030X

Suzuki, K.; Fujita, T.; Sotokawa, T.; Naganuma, M.; Sato, T.; Fujii, H.; Nakano, H.; Narita, A.; Miyasaka, T.; Shindo, M. & Naito, A. (2007) Facilitation from hand muscles innervated by the ulnar nerve to extensor carpi radialis in humans: A study using an electromyogram-averaging method. *Jpn J Clin Neurophysiol*, Vol. 35, p.449-450 (in Japanere), ISSN 1345-7101

Tanaka, R. (1989) Spinal mechanisms for human motor control. In: *Annual Review of Neuroscience*, edited by M. Ito & H. Narabayashi, Igaku-Shoin, IBSN4-260-17303-0, Tokyo, pp. 61-91 (in Japanese)

Wargon. I.; Lamy, J.C.; Baret, M.; Ghanim, Z.; Aymard, C.; Penicaud, A. & Katz, R. (2006) The disynaptic group I inhibition between wrist flexor and extensor muscle revisited in humans. *Exp Brain Res*, Vol. 168, pp.203-217, ISSN 0014-4819

Yoshida, Y. (1994) Anatomical studies on the extensor carpi radialis longus and brevis muscles in Japanese. *Okajima's Folia Anat Jpn*, Vol. 71, pp.123-136, ISSN 0030-154X

Permissions

The contributors of this book come from diverse backgrounds, making this book a truly international effort. This book will bring forth new frontiers with its revolutionizing research information and detailed analysis of the nascent developments around the world.

We would like to thank Mark Schwartz, for lending his expertise to make the book truly unique. He has played a crucial role in the development of this book. Without his invaluable contribution this book wouldn't have been possible. He has made vital efforts to compile up to date information on the varied aspects of this subject to make this book a valuable addition to the collection of many professionals and students.

This book was conceptualized with the vision of imparting up-to-date information and advanced data in this field. To ensure the same, a matchless editorial board was set up. Every individual on the board went through rigorous rounds of assessment to prove their worth. After which they invested a large part of their time researching and compiling the most relevant data for our readers. Conferences and sessions were held from time to time between the editorial board and the contributing authors to present the data in the most comprehensible form. The editorial team has worked tirelessly to provide valuable and valid information to help people across the globe.

Every chapter published in this book has been scrutinized by our experts. Their significance has been extensively debated. The topics covered herein carry significant findings which will fuel the growth of the discipline. They may even be implemented as practical applications or may be referred to as a beginning point for another development. Chapters in this book were first published by InTech; hereby published with permission under the Creative Commons Attribution License or equivalent.

The editorial board has been involved in producing this book since its inception. They have spent rigorous hours researching and exploring the diverse topics which have resulted in the successful publishing of this book. They have passed on their knowledge of decades through this book. To expedite this challenging task, the publisher supported the team at every step. A small team of assistant editors was also appointed to further simplify the editing procedure and attain best results for the readers.

Our editorial team has been hand-picked from every corner of the world. Their multi-ethnicity adds dynamic inputs to the discussions which result in innovative outcomes. These outcomes are then further discussed with the researchers and contributors who give their valuable feedback and opinion regarding the same. The feedback is then collaborated with the researches and they are edited in a comprehensive manner to aid the understanding of the subject.

Apart from the editorial board, the designing team has also invested a significant amount of their time in understanding the subject and creating the most relevant covers. They scrutinized every image to scout for the most suitable representation of the subject and create an appropriate cover for the book.

The publishing team has been involved in this book since its early stages. They were actively engaged in every process, be it collecting the data, connecting with the contributors or procuring relevant information. The team has been an ardent support to the editorial, designing and production team. Their endless efforts to recruit the best for this project, has resulted in the accomplishment of this book. They are a veteran in the field of academics and their pool of knowledge is as vast as their experience in printing. Their expertise and guidance has proved useful at every step. Their uncompromising quality standards have made this book an exceptional effort. Their encouragement from time to time has been an inspiration for everyone.

The publisher and the editorial board hope that this book will prove to be a valuable piece of knowledge for researchers, students, practitioners and scholars across the globe.

List of Contributors

James W. Fee, Jr. and Freeman Miller
Alfred I. DuPont Hospital for Children, USA

Juhani Partanen
University Hospital of Helsinki, Department of Clinical Neurophysiology, Finland

Ken Nishihara
Department of Physical Therapy, School of Health and Social Services, Saitama Prefectural University, Japan

Takuya Isho
Department of Rehabilitation, National Hospital Organization Takasaki General Medical Center, Japan

Heloyse Uliam Kuriki, Fábio Mícolis de Azevedo, Luciana Sanae Ota Takahashi, Emanuelle Moraes Mello, Rúben de Faria Negrão Filho and Neri Alves
Univ. Estadual Paulista, Univ. de São Paulo, Brazil

Adrian P. Harrison and Stig Molsted
IBHV, Faculty of Life Sciences, Copenhagen University, Denmark

Jessica Pingel and Henning Langberg
Institute for Sports Medicine, Bispebjerg Hospital, Copenhagen NV, Denmark

Else Marie Bartels
The Parker Institute, Frederiksberg Hospital, Frederiksberg, Denmark

Paul S. Sung
Korea University, Seoul, Republic of Korea

Hiroki Takada and Yasuyuki Matsuura
University of Fukui, Fukui, Japan

Tomoki Shiozawa
Aoyama Gakuin University, Shibuya, Tokyo, Japan

Masaru Miyao
Graduate School of Information Science, Nagoya University, Nagoya, Japan

Angkoon Phinyomark, Pornchai Phukpattaranont and Chusak Limsakul
Department of Electrical Engineering, Prince of Songkla University, Songkhla, Thailand

M. R. Al-Mulla
Kuwait University, Kuwait

F. Sepulveda and M. Colley
Essex University, UK

Shinichi Daikuya and Atsuko Ono
Kishiwada Eishinkai Hospital, Japan

Toshiaki Suzuki
Kansai University of Health Sciences, Japan

Tetsuji Fujiwara
Kyoto University, Japan

Kyonosuke Yabe
Nagoya University, Japan

Catherine Disselhorst-Klug
Department of Rehabilitation & Prevention Engineering, Institute of Applied Medical Engineering, RWTH Aachen University, Germany

Breda Jesenšek Papež and Miroslav Palfy
University Clinical Centre Maribor, Slovenia

Huseyin Alpaslan Sahin
Ondokuz Mayis University School of Medicine, Department of Neurology, Samsun, Turkey

Hande Turker, Ayhan Bilgici
Ondokuz Mayis University School of Medicine, Department of Physical Therapy and Rehabilitation, Samsun, Turkey

Akira Naito and Haruki Nakano
Yamagata University, Japan

Hiromi Fujii, Toshiaki Sato and Katsuhiko Suzuki
Yamagata Prefectural University of Health Sciences, Japan

Printed in the USA
CPSIA information can be obtained
at www.ICGtesting.com
JSHW011456221024
72173JS00005B/1096